Military Health System Review – Final Report

August 29, 2014

Appendices

APPENDIX 1. INTRODUCTION 1
    Appendix 1.1 Secretary of Defense Memorandum and Signed Project Plan 1
    Appendix 1.2 Terms of Reference - Military Health System Review 7
    Appendix 1.3 Policies and Reports Reviewed by the MHS Review Group 11
    Appendix 1.4 Site Visit Methodology 23
    Appendix 1.5 Site Visit Town Hall Comment Summary 32
    Appendix 1.6 Web-based Comments 142
    Appendix 1.7 The MHS Comparisons to Three Health Systems and Benchmarks 144
    Appendix 1.8 Data Analytics Summary 147

APPENDIX 2. OVERVIEW 153
    Appendix 2.1 Performance Improvement: Defense Health Agency and the Services 153

APPENDIX 3. ACCESS TO CARE 173
    Appendix 3.1 Code of Federal Regulations 32 CFR 199.17 (p)(5) 173
    Appendix 3.2 Access Improvement Working Group Charter 174
    Appendix 3.3 Summary of Access to Care Policies and Orders 176
    Appendix 3.4 Summary of External Reviews Related to Access to Care 184
    Appendix 3.5 Access to Care Education Courses 187
    Appendix 3.6 Access to Care Standards 190
    Appendix 3.7 MTF-Level Access Data 191
    Appendix 3.8 Percent of Appointments Met Analysis – Direct Component 210
    Appendix 3.9 Overseas and United States Access Measures – Direct Care Component ... 218
    Appendix 3.10 Outlier Analysis 223
    Appendix 3.11 Correlation Analyses 231
    Appendix 3.12 TROSS and HCSDB Questions and Benchmarks 236

APPENDIX 4. QUALITY OF CARE 239
    Appendix 4.1 Summaries of Statute, Regulation, Instructions, and Other Guidance 239
    Appendix 4.2 Internal and External Reports 246
    Appendix 4.3 Quality of Care Education and Training 253
    Appendix 4.4 Data Review: Supporting Data and Figures 257

APPENDIX 5. PATIENT SAFETY 305
    Appendix 5.1 Patient Safety Goals 305
    Appendix 5.2 MHS Governance Related to Patient Safety 306
    Appendix 5.3 Patient Safety Policies 313
    Appendix 5.4 Global Trigger Tool 316
    Appendix 5.5 Education and Training 318
    Appendix 5.6 Hospital Survey on Patient Safety Culture 328

Appendix 5.7 PSI #90 Composite 330
Appendix 5.8 National Health Safety Network 331
Appendix 5.9 Reviewable Sentinel Events 337
Appendix 5.10 Site Visit Patient Safety Questions Analyzed 338
Appendix 5.11 Site Visit Data 339
Appendix 5.12 Performance Improvement Initiatives 349

APPENDIX 6. RECOMMENDATIONS AND COMMENTS 353

Appendix 6.1 Compiled Recommendations and Proposed Action Items and Associated
    Timelines 353
Appendix 6.2 Comments of External Reviewers 376

APPENDIX 7. ACRONYMS 437

Appendix 7.1 List of Acronyms 437

APPENDIX 8. ACKNOWLEDGEMENTS 447

Appendix 8.1 MHS Review Senior Oversight and Working Group Members 447

List of Tables

Table 1.7-1 Access to Care: Direct Care Comparison to Three Health Systems and Benchmarks 144
Table 1.7-2 Quality of Care: Direct Care Comparison to Three Health Systems and Benchmarks 145
Table 1.7-3 Patient Safety: Direct Care Comparison to Three Health Systems and Benchmarks 146
Table 2.1-1 Army Performance Management 157
Table 2.1-2 Alignment of Cells to AFMS Strategic Objectives 168
Table 3.2-1 The Military Health Systems (MHS) Access Improvement Working Group (AIWG) 174
Table 3.6-1 Comparison of MHS Access Standards with those of Other Health Care Providers 190
Table 3.7-1 All Measure Results, by Facility 191
Table 3.10-1 Average Number of Days to an Acute Appointment Summary, FY 2014 to Date 223
Table 3.10-2 Average Number of Days to Third Next Acute Appointment – Summary FY 2014 to Date 224
Table 3.10-3 Average Number of Days to Third Next Routine Appointment – Summary FY 2014 to Date 225
Table 3.10-4 Average Number of Days to Specialty Appointment – Summary FY 2014 to Date 226
Table 3.10-5 Average Number of Days to Third Next Specialty Appointment – Summary FY 2014 to Date 227
Table 3.10-6 Percent of Web-Enabled Appointment for TOL Booking – Summary FY14 to Date 228
Table 3.10-7 Percent Satisfied with Access to Care – By Parent Facility, November 2013 – May 2014 229
Table 3.10-8 TROSS – Percent Satisfied with Access to Care – Summary, FY 2013 230
Table 3.12-1 TROSS and HCSDB Questions and Benchmarks – Access When Needed 236
Table 3.12-2 TROSS and HCSDB Questions and Benchmarks – Getting Care Quickly and Getting Care When Needed 237
Table 3.12-3 CAHPS Percentiles (Benchmark Highlighted), TROSS and HCSDB 237
Table 4.4-1 Number of Accreditations and Certifications by Type and Service 257
Table 4.4-2 HEDIS® rating based on NCQA benchmark 257
Table 4.4-3 Percent of Eligible Patients Receiving Select Care Measures, External Comparison: MHS vs. HEDIS® (2010 - 2013) 258
Table 4.4-4 Service Level & Purchased Care HEDIS® Performance (2013) 259
Table 4.4-5 HEDIS® Measures: CONUS – OCONUS 260
Table 4.4-6 Percent of Eligible Purchased Care Patients Receiving Select Care Measures, External Comparison: MHS vs. HEDIS® (2010 – 2013) 261
Table 4.4-7 Star Ratings for OCONUS from 2010 to 2013 261
Table 4.4-8 Star Ratings for CONUS from 2010 to 2013 262
Table 4.4-9a ORYX® TJC Definitions 271

Table 4.4-9b ORYX® Index Score Criteria 272
Table 4.4-9c Direct Care Average Index Score 272
Table 4.4-10 TJC Oryx® Measures 274
Table 4.4-11 MTF ORYX® Core Measure Status for 4Q 2012 – 3Q2013 278
Table 4.4-12 Military Treatment Facility Joint Commission Top Performers (2010 – 2012) ... 279
Table 4.4-13 TJC Oryx® MTF to External Health System Comparison 280
Tables 4.4-14a-c Descriptive Measures 282
Table 4.4-14a Total Deliveries 282
Table 4.4-14b Percent Deliveries (MHS) 283
Table 4.4-14c Percent C-Section 283
Table 4.4-15 Facility Level Data 289
Table 5.4-1 Adverse Events Reported Across Patient Safety Measures 317
Table 5.6-1 Direct Care Comparison to the National Average – Safety 328
Table 5.6-2 Direct Care Comparison to a National System – Safety 329
Table 5.7-1 National PSI and IQI Results for the Medicare Population – Supplementary
    Information (2010 – 2013) 330
Table 5.11-1 Number of Respondent Types 339
Table 5.11-2 Associated Comments from Site Visits 340

List of Figures

Figure 1.6-1 Breakdown of Comment Types 143
Figure 2.1-1 Strategic Initiatives Process 154
Figure 2.1-2 Standard BCA and BPR Process 155
Figure 2.1-3 MEDCOM LSS Program Process 159
Figure 2.1-4 MEDCOM Initiatives Vetting, Approval, and Transfer Process 160
Figure 2.1-5 MEDCOM FY 2103 LSS Capability Self-Assessment and FY 2014
    Projections 161
Figure 2.1-6 Navy Medicine Strategy Map 162
Figure 2.1-7 Air Force Medical Service Strategy Map 167
Figure 2.1-8 Operational Management of Strategy Execution 168
Figure 3.8-1 Acute Appointments Meeting Access Standard - Direct Care Component
    Overall: MHS Goal >90% 210
Figure 3.8-2 Acute Appointments Meeting Access Standard, by Service – MHS Goal:
    >90% 211
Figure 3.8-3 Acute Appointments Meeting Access Standard, by Facility Type – MHS Goal:
    >90% 212
Figure 3.8-4 Acute Appointments Meeting Access Standard, by Location – MHS Goal:
    >90% 213
Figure 3.8-5 Specialty Appointments Meeting Access Standard – Overall: MHS Goal
    >90% 214
Figure 3.8-6 Specialty Appointments Meeting Access Standard, by Service – MHS Goal:
    >90% 215
Figure 3.8-7 Specialty Appointments Meeting Access Standard, by Facility Type – Goal:
    >90% 216
Figure 3.8-8 Specialty Appointments Meeting Access Standard, by Location – Goal: >90% ... 217
Figure 3.9-1 Average Number of Days to an Acute Appointment, by Location – Direct
    Care Component: MHS Access Standard ≤ 1 day 218
Figure 3.9-2 Average Number of Days to Third Next Acute Appointment, by Location –
    Direct Care Component: MHS Access Standard ≤ 1 day 219
Figure 3.9-3 Average Number of Days Third Next Routine Appointment, by Location –
    Direct Care Component: MHS Access Standard ≤ 1 day 220
Figure 3.9-4 Average Number of Days to Specialty Appointment, by Location – MHS
    Access Standard 221
Figure 3.9-5 Average Number of Days to Third Next Specialty Appointment, by Location –
    MHS Access Standard 222
Figure 3.10-1 Average Number of Days to an Acute Appointment – by Facility, FY 2014 to
    Date 223
Figure 3.10-2 Average Number of Days to Third Next Acute Appointment – by Facility,
    FY 2014 to Date 224
Figure 3.10-3 Average Days to Third Next Routine Appointment – by Facility, FY2014 to
    Date 225
Figure 3.10-4 Average Number of Days to Specialty Appointment – by Facility, FY 2014
    to Date 226

Figure 3.10-5 Average Days to Third Next Specialty Appointment – by Facility, FY 2014 to date 227
Figure 3.10-6 Percent of Web-Enabled Appointments for TOL Booking – by Parent Facility, FY 2014 to date 228
Figure 3.10-7 Percent Satisfied with Access to Care – By Parent Facility, November 2013 – May 2014 229
Figure 3.10-8 TROSS – Percent Satisfied with Access to Care – by Facility, FY2013 230
Figure 3.11-1 Correlation between PCM Continuity and Average Number of Days to Third Next Available Acute Appointment 231
Figure 3.11-2 Correlation between PCM Continuity and Average Number of Days to Third Next Routine Appointment 232
Figure 3.11-3 Correlation between Average Number of Days to Acute Appointment and Satisfaction with Getting Care When Needed (Service Surveys) 233
Figure 3.11-4 Correlation between Average Number of Days to Third Next Available Appointment and Satisfaction with Getting Care When Needed 234
Figure 3.11-5 Correlation between Average of Days to Third Next Available Routine Appointment and Satisfaction with Access to Care 235
Figure 4.4-1 Hospital Compare Measures in Purchased Care Component 263
Figure 4.4-1a Purchased Care Acute Myocardial Infarction (AMI) Rate, FY09 – FY12 263
Figure 4.4-1b Purchased Care Heart Failure (HF) Rate, FY09 – FY12 264
Figure 4.4-1c Purchased Care Surgical Care (SCIP) Rate, FY09 – FY12 264
Figure 4.4-1d Purchased Care Children's Asthma Care (CAC) Rate, FY09 – FY12 265
Figure 4.4-1e Purchased Care Pneumonia Rate, FY09 – FY12 265
Figure 4.4-1f Purchased Overall Rate, FY09 – FY12 266
Figure 4.4-2 TJC Oryx Core Measures 267
Figure 4.4-2a Primary Percutaneous Coronary Intervention (AMI-8a), FY10 – FY13 267
Figure 4.4-2b Home Management Plan of Care Given to Patient/Caregiver (CAC-3), FY10 – FY13 268
Figure 4.4-2c Discharge Instructions (HF-1), FY10 – FY13 268
Figure 4.4-2d Blood Cultures Performed in the ED prior to Initial Antibiotic in Hospital (PN-3b), FY10 – FY13 269
Figure 4.4-2e Surgery Patients on Beta-Blocker Therapy prior to Arrival Who Received a Beta-Blocker During the Perioperative Period (SCIP-Card2), FY10 – FY13 269
Figure 4.4-2f Prophylactic Antibiotic Selection for Surgical Patients (SCIP-2a), FY10 – FY13 270
Figure 4.4-2g Pneumococcal Immunization (IMM-1a), FY12 – FY13 270
Figure 4.4-2h Influenza Immunization (IMM-2) 271
Figure 4.4-3 Thirty-Day Risk-Adjusted Readmission Rate Ratio (Observed/Expected) 281
Figure 4.4-4a MHS Level-Induction of Labor at Less Than 37 Weeks Gestation with Medical Indication, CY10 – CY13 284
Figure 4.4-4b MHS Level C-Section at Less Than 37 Weeks Gestation with Medical Indication, CY10 – CY13 284
Figure 4.4-5 MHS Level Patient Safety Indicator (PSI) 18, CY10 – CY13 285
Figure 4.4-6 Annual Rate of PSI 19 Obstetric Trauma-Vaginal Delivery without Instruments, CY10 – CY13 285

Figure 4.4-7 Annual Rate of Postpartum Readmissions to Delivery Site, CY10 – CY13 286
Figure 4.4-8 Annual Percent of Inborn Readmissions to Birth Site, CY10 – CY13 286
Figure 4.4-9 Annual Rate of Vaginal Deliveries Coded with Shoulder Dystocia by Branch of Service, CY10 – CY13 287
Figure 4.4-10 Annual Rate of Postpartum Hemorrhage by Branch of Service, CY10 – CY13 287
Figure 4.4-11 Annual Rate of PSI 17 Injury to Neonate by Branch of Service, CY10 – CY13 288
Figure 4.4-12 Inborn Mortality Rate (per 1,000 live births) ≥ 500 Grams by Branch of Service, CY10 – CY13 288
Figure 4.4-13 Overall Rating of Health Care, FY10 – FY13 291
Figure 4.4-14 Overall Rating of Health Plan, FY10 – FY13 292
Figure 4.4-15 Overall Rating of Hospital 293
Figure 4.4-15a Rating of Hospital in Medical Care, FY11 – FY13 293
Figure 4.4-15b Rating of Hospital in Surgical Care, FY11 – FY13 293
Figure 4.4-15c Rating of Hospital in Obstetric Care, FY11 – FY13 294
Figure 4.4-16 Willingness to Recommend Hospital 295
Figure 4.4-16a Willingness to Recommend Hospital for Medical Care, FY11 – FY13 295
Figure 4.4-16b Willingness to Recommend Hospital for Surgical Care, FY11 – FY13 295
Figure 4.4-16c Willingness to Recommend Hospital for Obstetric Care, FY11 – FY13 296
Figure 4.4-17 Reported Experience and Satisfaction with Key Aspects of TRICARE 297
Figure 4.4-17a Health Plan, FY11 – FY13 297
Figure 4.4-17b Primary Care Physician, FY11 – FY13 297
Figure 4.4-17c Specialty Physician, FY11 – FY13 298
Figure 4.4-17d Health Care, FY11 – FY13 298
Figure 4.4-18 Trends in Satisfaction with Health Plan Based on Enrollment Status, FY11 – FY13 299
Figure 4.4-19 Trends in Satisfaction with Health Plan Based on Beneficiary Status, FY11 – FY13 300
Figure 4.4-20a Trends in Satisfaction with TRICARE Health Care Based on Beneficiary Category, FY11 – FY13 301
Figure 4.4-20b Trends in Satisfaction with TRICARE Health Care Based on Enrollment Status, FY11 – FY13 301
Figure 4.4-21 Trends in Satisfaction with One's Personal Provider Based on Enrollment Status, FY 11 – FY13 302
Figure 4.4-22 Trends in Satisfaction with One's Personal Provider Based on Beneficiary Status, FY11 – FY13 303
Figure 5.2-1 Central Defense Health Agency Structure 306
Figure 5.2-2 AFMOA/SGHQ Organizational Chart 309
Figure 5.2-3 Army Governance of Patient Safety 311
Figure 5.8-1 CAUTI Med/Surg: Major Teaching CY10 – CY13 331
Figure 5.8-2 CAUTI Med/Surg: Other Hospitals Less Than 15 ICU Beds CY10 – CY13 332
Figure 5.8-3 CLABSI Med/Surg: Major Teaching CY10 – CY13 333
Figure 5.8-4 CLABSI Med/Surg: Other Hospitals with Less Than 15 ICU Beds CY10 – CY13 334

Figure 5.8-5 VAP Med/Surg: Major Teaching Hospitals CY10 – CY13 335
Figure 5.8-6 VAP Med/Surg: Other Hospitals with Less Than 15 ICU Beds CY10 – CY13 336
Figure 5.11-1 Number of Themed Concepts from Patient Safety Site Visit Rollup, CY14 341
Figure 5.11-2 Number of Themed Concepts by Site: Site 1, CY14 342
Figure 5.11-3 Number of Themed Concepts by Site: Site 2, CY14 343
Figure 5.11-4 Number of Themed Concepts by Site: Site 3, CY14 344
Figure 5.11-5 Number of Themed Concepts by Site: Site 4, CY14 345
Figure 5.11-6 Number of Themed Concepts by Site: Site 5, CY14 346
Figure 5.11-7 Number of Themed Concepts by Site: Site 6, CY14 347
Figure 5.11-8 Number of Themed Concepts by Site: Site 7, CY14 348
Figure 5.12-1 PES Nursing Work Index, CY13 351

APPENDIX 1. INTRODUCTION

Appendix 1.1
Secretary of Defense Memorandum and Signed Project Plan

Secretary of Defense Memorandum

MEMORANDUM FOR DEPUTY SECRETARY OF DEFENSE
                            SECRETARIES OF THE MILITARY DEPARTMENTS
                            ACTING UNDER SECRETARY OF DEFENSE FOR PERSONNEL
                            AND READINESS

SUBJECT: Military Health System Review

      Our Service members and their families deserve the highest quality health care possible wherever they are stationed or deployed. In recent years, the Department has made great improvements in our health care delivery system – nowhere more important than in improving trauma care, which has resulted in the highest ever survival rate from battlefield injuries.

      It is our continuing obligation to those who serve, and all beneficiaries of the Military Health System (MHS), to continually review and improve our standards of care and the system that delivers that care. To ensure that we are meeting these standards, I am directing a 90-day comprehensive review ("Review") of the MHS, effective immediately.

      The Review will be led by Deputy Secretary of Defense Bob Work, with the assistance of the Acting Under Secretary of Defense for Personnel and Readiness and the Assistant Secretary of Defense for Health Affairs, and the direct participation of the Secretaries of the Military Departments and the Service Chiefs. In addition, I have asked Deputy Secretary Work to solicit the perspectives of outside experts in the areas of patient safety and quality care, and perform the Review in a fully transparent manner.

      The Review will focus on the following core areas:

- *Access to Health Care*: The Department has issued clear guidance and standards for access to health care, based on the urgency of the care a patient requires. In addition, the Department has issued standards to ensure that patients will not have to travel excessive distances to receive required care. The Review will assess whether or not the MHS is meeting these standards on a facility-by-facility basis. If a particular standard is not being met, the Review will provide a recommendation on how to meet or exceed that standard along with an associated timeline.

- *Safety of Care*: The Review will recommend ways to improve patient safety across the MHS by: (1) examining existing patient safety data; and (2) identifying best practices for patient safety from across the health care provider spectrum.

- *Quality of Care*: The Review will assess whether the quality of care provided by MHS meets DoD and nationally accepted standards. If MHS is found to be falling short of these standards in any particular area of care, the Review will provide specific recommendations for improvement.

A Plan of Action and Milestones for conducting the Review shall be delivered to me by June 6, 2014. I want regular updates on the progress of this review. A final report, complete with specific recommendations to address standards of care and implementation timelines, will be delivered to me no later than August 29, 2014.

The Department must continue to provide the best available health care to our Service men and women, and their families, who have sacrificed so much on behalf of this Nation. They deserve nothing short of our highest level of effort. Accordingly, I fully expect the Review to lead to Departmental standards that exceed the national averages in access to, safety, and quality of health care.

Thank you.

Chuck Hagel

cc:
Chairman of the Joint Chiefs of Staff
Chiefs of the Military Services
Chief of the National Guard Bureau
General Counsel of the Department of Defense
Assistant to the Secretary of Defense for Public Affairs
Assistant Secretary of Defense for Legislative Affairs
Assistant Secretary of Defense for Health Affairs

PERSONNEL AND
READINESS

MEMORANDUM FOR SENIOR ACTION COUNCIL

SUBJECT: Military Health System Review Scope Limitation

I have reviewed your recommendation and the endorsement of the Assistant Secretary of Defense (Health Affairs) to limit the project scope of the Secretary of Defense directed Military Health System (MHS) Review to exclude targeted review of specific Diagnosis-Related Groups (DRGs) and the singling out of specific demographic groups as out of scope.

Given the limited time and resources available to execute the review, I approve your recommendation that DRGs and the singling out of specific demographic groups be considered out of scope for the MHS review.

Jessica L. Wright

Attachment:
As stated

PROJECT TIMELINES AND MILESTONES

PROJECT TIMELINE

Date	Action
23 May – 7 Jul	Policy review and gap analysis
30 May – 9 Jul	Review and analysis of past findings
5 Jun – 3 Jul	Data pulls for working groups
23 Jun – 17 Jul	Working Groups analyze data
20 Jun – 11 Jul	Site visits
2 Jul – 17 Jul	Review of other health systems
10 Jul – 23 Jul	Consultants' review
25 Jul – 31 Jul	Final edits
28 Jul – 29 Jul	Preliminary Legal sufficiency review
31 Jul – 2 Aug	Internal Military Health System (MHS) Staffing
14 Aug – 28 Aug	Formal staffing

MILESTONES

The following represent key project milestones, with estimated completion dates:

Milestone	Estimated Completion Date
Plan of Action and Milestone (POA&M) and Time of Release (TOR) to Senior Executive Review Committee (SERC)	5 Jun, 2014
POA&M and TOR to Secretary of Defense (SECDEF)	6 Jun, 2014
Final report out to Military Health System Executive Review (MHSER)	31 Jul, 2014
MHS overview brief to the SERC	4 Aug, 2014
Final report out to Deputy's Management Action Group/DEXCOM/TANK	13 Aug, 2014
Final report to SECDEF	29 Aug, 2014

PERSONNEL AND
READINESS

MEMORANDUM FOR SENIOR ACTION COUNCIL

SUBJECT: Military Health System Review Scope Modification

I have reviewed your recommendations and the endorsement of the Assistant Secretary of Defense (Health Affairs) regarding the exclusion of Wounded Warrior Units and dental care reviews from the current Military Health System (MHS) review.

Given the limited time and resources available to execute the review, I approve your recommendation that Wounded Warrior Units and dental care be considered out of scope for the MHS Review.

Jessica L. Wright

PERSONNEL AND
READINESS

MEMORANDUM FOR SENIOR ACTION COUNCIL

SUBJECT: Military Health System Review Metric Modification

I have reviewed your recommendations and the endorsement of the Assistant Secretary of Defense (Health Affairs) regarding the recommendation to modify the proposed metrics to be utilized for the Secretary of Defense directed Military Health System Review

I approve your recommendation to measure routine appointment access standard compliance by using the "3rd available" metric and combining the routine and established appointment types.

Jessica L. Wright

Appendix 1.2
Terms of Reference - Military Health System Review

Purpose

These Terms of Reference establish the objectives and process for the Military Health System (MHS) Review. This review will assess health care access, patient safety, and health care quality across the MHS, as directed by the Secretary of Defense. Health care provided in support of the Combatant Commands and operational forces is excluded from this review.

Background

On May 28, 2014, the Secretary of Defense (SECDEF) ordered a review of the MHS. The review will focus on health care access, patient safety and quality of care, and be performed in a fully transparent manner consistent with law. Further, the review will include both the direct care component composed of Department of Defense (DoD) operated and staffed health care facilities, as well as the purchased care system operated through our TRICARE managed care support contracts. The review will incorporate the perspectives of outside experts in patient safety and health care quality. The report will include recommendations for Departmental standards that exceed national averages in access to, safety, and quality of health care. The final report will be delivered to the SECDEF not later than August 29, 2014.

The MHS is a comprehensive, global and integrated system of health support that includes combat medical services, peacetime health care delivery, public health, medical education and training, and medical research and development. The MHS is comprised of Army, Navy, Air Force and Defense Health Agency medical facilities, supported by a private sector network of civilian providers and hospitals. With an annual budget of approximately $50 billion, the MHS is staffed with over 150,000 military and civilian personnel -- working in 56 hospitals, over 300 clinics, a fully accredited university, and a broad array of other research and educational institutions.

Goals and Objectives

This review has three goals:
1) To determine if the MHS provides ready access to medical care as defined by the access standards in OSD and Military Department policies and guidance, and TRICARE contract specifications.
2) To determine if the MHS has created a culture of safety with effective processes for safe and reliable care.
3) To determine if the MHS meets or exceeds the benchmarks for health care quality as defined in OSD and Military Department policies and guidance, and TRICARE contract specifications, with a particular focus on how the MHS performs relative to known national benchmarks.

To accomplish these three goals, we have defined eight objectives:

- Assess prior recommendations and findings from relevant internal and external reports, including the last ten years of Government Accountability Office (GAO) and DoD Inspector General (IG) reports. The assessment will include what problems were identified, what actions were taken to remedy the problems, and whether the remedy has been sustained.

- Review all relevant OSD, Service and TRICARE policy standards and assess the degree to which the policies have been implemented.

- Evaluate data to assess compliance with existing policy or national standards. Determine how the MHS can consistently exceed these standards. Determine if any variance from the standards is due to data inaccuracy or inconsistency.

- Review education and training documentation of health care professionals and staff regarding the execution of policies and assess knowledge of existing standards.

- Compare MHS performance to at least three civilian health systems, where standards are relevant and comparable.

- Assess the experiences and perceptions of the MHS patients' regarding access, quality and safety standards.

- Determine the effectiveness of governance in policy and system performance.

- Identify current resources for access, safety and quality efforts to the extent possible.

The final report will also include a senior level review of the current federated MHS governance structure and its effectiveness in supporting enterprise management. Governance will be reviewed within the context of existing roles and responsibilities. Recommendations to improve or enhance the decision making process with respect to the goals of this review will be provided to the Secretary of Defense.

Deliverables

Not later than August 29, 2014, the Deputy Secretary of Defense will deliver a full report on this review to include recommendations for improving access, safety, and quality to the Secretary of Defense. Where the MHS is falling short of meeting standards as defined in OSD or Military Department policies, or as defined in TRICARE contracts, specific recommendations will be provided to improve performance. The report will also include identified, proven practices from the MHS and from other health care systems that demonstrate higher levels of performance in access, patient safety, and quality.

To the extent that the MHS Review report's recommendations identify areas requiring additional study, the Secretary may direct follow-on action through the MHS Review processes and structures.

Periodic updates will be provided to the Secretary of Defense through the Deputy Secretary of Defense.

Process

This review will begin immediately and will be led by the Deputy Secretary of Defense, assisted by the Acting Under Secretary of Defense for Personnel and Readiness and the Assistant Secretary of Defense for Health Affairs (ASD(HA)), with the direct participation of the Secretaries of the Military Departments, the Service Chiefs, and the Joint Staff. The review will also include the individual perspectives of outside experts in the areas of patient safety and quality of care, along with their individual assessment of the MHS's performance in safety and quality.

The Deputy Secretary of Defense has established a Senior Executive Review Committee (SERC) to guide the review process, remove any barriers to successful completion of the review, and achieve concurrence regarding the plan, milestones, timeline and final report. Chaired by the Deputy Secretary of Defense, membership on the SERC includes the Acting Under Secretary of Defense for Personnel and Readiness, the Under Secretaries of the Military Departments, the Assistant Secretary of Defense for Health Affairs, the Director of the Joint Staff, the Military Departments' Surgeons General, and the Director of the Defense Health Agency.

The SERC will also review the existing MHS governance process and make recommendations to the Secretary of Defense to improve or enhance its performance. In addition to the SERC, the Deputy Secretary of Defense will call upon the Deputy's Executive Committee (DEXCOM), the TANK, or the Deputy's Management Action Group (DMAG) as appropriate over the period of the review. The DEXCOM membership includes the Secretaries of the Military Departments, the Under Secretaries of Defense, and General Counsel. The TANK consists of the Chairman and Vice Chairman of the Joint Chiefs of Staff, along with the Service Chiefs and Chief of the National Guard Bureau. The DMAG includes the Secretaries of the Military Departments, Under Secretaries of Defense, Deputy Chief Management Officer, Chiefs of the Military Services, Chief of the National Guard Bureau, Commander of United States Special Operations Command, and Director of Cost Assessment and Program Evaluation.

Prior to the SERC review, the Military Health System Executive Review group (MHSER) will review deliverables to ensure alignment with other ongoing MHS initiatives. The MHSER membership includes the Under Secretary of Defense for Personnel and Readiness, Under Secretary of Defense (Comptroller), Assistant Secretary of Defense for Health Affairs, Director of the Cost Assessment and Program Evaluation Office, Service Vice Chiefs, Assistant Commandant of the Marine Corps, the Surgeons General, and the Military Department Assistant Secretaries for Manpower and Reserve Affairs.

The review will be supported by an Action Group composed of action officers from each of the Military Departments' medical programs, the Defense Health Agency, and the Joint Staff, Service Senior Enlisted personnel, and a representative from the National Guard Bureau, chaired by an OSD Health Affairs action officer. This group will be responsible for reviewing the identified internal and external studies and reports regarding access, safety and quality. They will identify recommendations and findings from those studies and reports, determine the extent to which they have been acted upon by the MHS and assess whether the remedy has been sustained. They will also be responsible for the coordination and structure of selected military treatment facilities site reviews, to include town hall meetings, as well as collecting and analyzing all data relevant to this review. During the site visits, they will conduct in-person interviews with staff and patients. The Action Group will conduct a review and analysis of relevant health care professional and staff educational and training programs regarding access, quality and safety. It will assess the MHS performance in all three areas compared to stated OSD and Military Department and Service policy standards and benchmarks, along with national standards and benchmarks.

The Action Group will be supported by a Senior Action Council (SAC), chaired by the Principal Deputy Assistant Secretary of Defense for Health Affairs, composed of the Deputy Assistant Secretaries of Defense in the Office of the Assistant Secretary of Defense for Health Affairs, the Deputy Director of the Defense Health Agency, the Deputy Surgeons General, and the Joint Staff Surgeon. The SAC will provide support to and supervision of the Action Group. The SAC will ensure that resources are available to the effort and that action and activities are coordinated to ensure success. The SAC will provide progress reports to the Acting Under Secretary of Defense for Personnel and Readiness through the Assistant Secretary of Defense for Health Affairs. The SAC will review all deliverables to ensure that goals and objectives are met.

The MHS Review directed by the Secretary of Defense does not encumber the authority of the Secretaries of the Military Departments with respect to any necessary administrative actions or investigations required for their respective Departments. The Secretaries of the Military Departments shall coordinate with the Under Secretary of Defense for Personnel and Readiness with regard to any implementing actions as a result of investigation findings or recommendations during the period of the MHS Review.

Strategic Communication

This review is intended to be transparent for all stakeholders. All strategic communications will be coordinated through the Deputy Secretary of Defense and supported by the Office of the Assistant to the Secretary of Defense for Public Affairs and Office of the Assistant Secretary of Defense for Legislative Affairs. In addition to our stakeholders, it is important to communicate the intent, scope and results of the review to our MHS workforce.

Appendix 1.3
Policies and Reports Reviewed by the MHS Review Group

Reviewed Policies: Access

Legislation Level

10 U.S. Code, Chapter 55, Sections 1073, 1079, 10 USC Chapter 55 - Medical and Dental Care
32 CFR 199.17, Code of Federal Regulations, TRICARE Program

DoD/MHS Level

DoDD 1241.01, Reserve Component Medical Care and Incapacitation Pay for Line of Duty Conditions
MHS Guide to Access Success, 15 Dec 2008
DoDI 6000.14, Patient Bill of Rights and Responsibilities in the Military Health System (MHS)
DODD 6010.4, Healthcare for Uniformed Services Members and Beneficiaries
HA 09-015, Policy Memorandum Implementation of the Patient Centered Medical Home, Model of Priority Care in MTFs
HA 11-005, Health Affairs Policy 11-005, TRICARE Policy for Access to Care
HA 01-015, Health Affairs Policy 01-015, Policy Memorandum to Refine Policy for Access to Care in MTFs and Establish the TRICARE Plus Program
RTC FY2010 S721(e)(1), Report to Congress, Health Care Needs of Active Duty Families
RTC FY2010 S721(e)(1) Initial, Report to Congress, Study and Plan to Improve Military Health Care
RTC FY2010 S721(e)(1) follow-up, Report to Congress, Study and Plan to Improve Military Health Care (follow-up)
TRICARE Policy Manual 6010.57M, Chapter 1, Section 1.1, General Policy and Responsibilities
TRICARE Policy Manual 6010.57M, Chapter 12, Section 1.3, Outside the 50 US and the District of Columbia Locality-based Reimbursement Rate Waiver
TRICARE Operations Manual 6010.56-M, Chapter 1, Section 3, TRICARE Processing Standards
TRICARE Operations Manual 6010.56-M, Chapter 5, Section 1, Network Development
TRICARE Operations Manual 6010.56-M, Chapter 6, Section 1, Enrollment Processing
TRICARE Operations Manual 6010.56-M, Chapter 6, Section 4, TRICARE Plus
TRICARE Operations Manual 6010.56-M, Chapter 8, Section 5, Referrals/Preauthorizations/Authorizations
TRICARE Operations Manual 6010.56-M, Chapter 11, Section 3, BCAC, DCAO & HBA Relations
TRICARE Operations Manual 6010.56-M, Chapter 16, TRICARE Prime Remote Program
TRICARE Operations Manual 6010.56-M, Chapter 18, Demonstrations
TRICARE Operations Manual 6010.56-M, Chapter 21, TRICARE Alaska
TRICARE Operations Manual 6010.56-M, Chapter 22, Reserve Component Health Coverage Plans

DoD/MHS Level

TRICARE Operations Manual 6010.56-M, Chapter 24, TRICARE Overseas Program (TOP)
TRICARE Operations Manual 6010.56-M, Chapter 25, TRICARE Young Adult
TRICARE Operations Manual 6010.56-M, Chapter 26, Continued Health Care Benefit Program (CHCBP)

Service Level

NAVMED Policy 08-001, Implementation of TRICARE Prime Access Standards for Mental Health
NAVMED Policy 09-004, Access to Care Management Policy for Navy MTFs
BUMED Instruction 6300.19, Primary Care Services in Navy Medicine
BUMED Instruction 6500.15, Navy Medicine Referral Management Program
OTSG/MEDCOM Policy 12-006 MEDCOM MTF, Enrollment, Access and Appointment Standards for all Uniformed Service Members, with Special Emphasis on Enhanced Access to Care for Specified populations
OTSG/MEDCOM Policy 12-085 NTF, Appointing Policy to Support Patient Appointing and PCMH Access
OTSG/MEDCOM Policy 13-061 MEDCOM MTF, Referral Management Office - Overarching Core Business
OTSG/MEDCOM Policy 11-089, Improving MTF Practices for Provider Template and Schedule Management
OTSG/MEDCOM Policy 14-007, No-Show Policy
OTSG/MEDCOM Policy 13-065, AMEDD Enrollment Policy
MEDCOM OPORD 09-36 with FRAGOs Access to Care Campaign
MEDCOM OPORD 11-05 with FRAGOs Community Based Primary Care Clinics
MEDCOM OPORD 11-20 with FRAGOs Army Patient Centered Medical Home
MEDCOM OPORD 12-50 with FRAGOS Soldier Centered Medical Home
Army PCMH Operations Manual Leaders Guide to Army PCMH
AFI 44-176, Access to Care Continuum, 12 Sept 2011
AFI 44-171, Patient Centered Medical Home and Family Health Operations, 18 Jan 2011
AFMS Referral Management Guide v9, 1 May 2014
NCR 6015.01 Joint Task Force National Capital Region Medical Instruction: Appointing, Template, Demand and Referral Management

Reviewed Studies and Reports: Access

GAO Studies

GAO-14-384 GAO #291141, DEFENSE HEALTH CARE: More-Specific Guidance Needed for Assessing Nonenrolled TRICARE Beneficiaries' Access to Care

GAO-07-941R GAO #290602 TRICARE: Changes to Access Policies and Payment Rates for Services Provided by Civilian Obstetricians

GAO-13-205 GAO #291029, DOD HEALTH CARE: Domestic Health Care for Female Service members

GAO Studies

GAO-10-402 GAO #290762, DEFENSE HEALTH CARE 2008 Access to Care Surveys Indicate Some Problems, but Beneficiary Satisfaction Is Similar to Other Health Plans

GAO-11-500 #290858, DEFENSE HEALTH Access to Civilian Providers under TRICARE Standard and Extra

GAO-13-364, TRICARE Multilayer Surveys Indicate Problems with Access to Care for Nonenrolled Beneficiaries

GAO-07-48, Access to Care for Beneficiaries who have not enrolled in TRICARE's Managed Care Option

GAO-12-453SP (no code), Follow-up on 2011 Report: Status of Actions Taken to Reduce Duplication, Overlap, and Fragmentation, Save Tax Dollars, and Enhance Revenue

GAO-08-1137 GAO #130663, MILITARY DISABILITY SYSTEM Increased Supports for Service Members and Better Pilot Planning Could Improve the Disability Evaluation Process

GAO-11-318SP, Opportunities to Reduce Potential Duplication in Government Programs, Save Tax Dollars, and Enhance Revenue

GAO-11-570 GAO #290866, VA AND DOD: HEALTH CARE: First Federal Health Care Center Established, but Implementation Concerns Need to Be Addressed

GAO-11-551 GAO #290870, DEFENSE HEALTH CARE: DOD Lacks Assurance That Selected Reserve Members Are Informed about TRICARE Reserve Select

GAO-12-571R 14 GAO #291017, Military Personnel: Prior GAO Work on DOD's Actions to Prevent and Respond to Sexual Assault in the Military

GAO-12-992 GAO #290974, VA AND DOD HEALTH CARE: Department-Level Actions Needed to Assess Collaboration Performance, Address Barriers, and Identify Opportunities

GAO-09-178 GAO #360855, VETERINARIAN WORKFORCE: Actions Are Needed to Ensure Sufficient Capacity for Protecting Public and Animal Health

GAO-10-850 GAO #460599, BIOLOGICAL LABORATORIES: Design and Implementation Considerations for Safety Reporting Systems

GAO-11-69 GAP #130971, MILITARY AND VETERANS DISABILITY SYSTEM: Pilot Has Achieved Some Goals, but Further Planning and Monitoring

GAO-11-114 GAO #130967, HEARING LOSS PREVENTION Improvements to DOD Hearing Conservation Programs Could Lead to Better Outcomes

GAO-07-195 GAO #290492, MILITARY HEALTH: Increased TRICARE Eligibility for Reservists Presents Educational Challenges

GAO-07-647 GAO #290559, MILITARY HEALTH CARE: TRICARE Cost-Sharing Proposals Would Help Offset Increasing Health Care Spending, but Projected Savings Are Likely Overestimated

GAO Studies

GAO-06-105 GAO #350604, MILITARY PERSONNEL: Top Management Attention Is Needed to Address Long-standing Problems with Determining Medical and Physical Fitness of the Reserve Force

GAO-12-27R GAO #290921, Department of Defense: Use of Neurocognitive Assessment Tools in Post-Deployment Identification of Mild Traumatic Brain Injury

GAO-08-495R GAO #290646, VA and DOD Health Care: Progress Made on Implementation of 2003 President's Task Force Recommendations on Collaboration and Coordination, but More Remains to Be Done

GAO-11-837R GAO #290935, DOD Health Care: Cost Impact of Health Care Reform and the Extension of Dependent Coverage

GAO-11-445 GAO #290756, Value in Health Care: Key Information for Policymakers to Assess Efforts to Improve Quality While Reducing Costs

GAO-07-317R GAO #290465, Military Personnel: Medical, Family Support, and Educational Services Are Available for Exceptional Family Members

GAO-12-224, Applying Key Management Practices Should Help Achieve Efficiencies within the Military Health System

DoD IG Review

Report No. DODIG-2014-040 (Project No. D2010-D00SPO-0209.007, Assessment of DoD Wounded Warrior Matters: Managing Risks of Multiple Medications

Report No. DODIG-2012-106 (Project No. D2011-D000LF-0041.000), DoD Needs to Improve the Billing System for Health Care Provided to Contractors at Medical Treatment Facilities in Southwest Asia

Department of Defense Report No.1E-2008-005 (Project No. D2006-DIPOE2-137.000), DoD/VA Care Transition Process for Service Members Injured in OIF/OEF

Report No. DODIG-2012-088 (Project No. D2011-D000LF-0093.000) Guam Medical Staffing Plan Needs Improvement to Ensure Eligible Beneficiaries Will Have Adequate Access to Health Care

DODIG-2013-135 (Project No. D2012-D000DA-0190.000) The Department of Defense and Veteran Affairs Health Care Joint Venture at Tripler Army Medical Center Needs More Management Oversight

Report No. D-2007-054 Quality Assurance in the DoD Healthcare System

Report No. D-2008-045 (Project No. D2005-D000LF-0267.000), Controls Over the TRICARE Overseas Healthcare Program

Reviewed Policies: Quality of Care

Legislation Level

10 U.S. Code § 1102, Confidentiality of medical quality assurance records: qualified immunity for participants

10 U.S .Code 1079, Inpatient mental health benefit limitations

32 CFR 199.15, Quality and utilization review peer review organization program.

Public Law 101-629, Safe Medical Devices Act of 1990

Title 32, Code of Federal Regulations, National Defense

Title 42, Code of Federal Regulations, Public Health

Title 48, Code of Federal Regulations, Federal Acquisition Regulations System

DoD/MHS Level

DoDI 6000.14, DoD Patient Bill of Rights and Responsibilities in the MHS

PR006342-11_Memofinal_Signed, Amplifying Guidance Relating to Preparing of Sentinel Events and Personally Identifiable Information Breaches

6010.51-M, TRICARE Operations Manual Chapter 7, Section 4

6010.51-M, TRICARE Operations Manual Chapter 17, Section 3

DoDM 6025.13, Medical Quality Assurance (MQA) and Clinical Quality Management in the Military Health System (MHS)

DoDD 5010.42, DoD-Wide Continuous Process Improvement (CPI)/Lean Six Sigma (LSS) Program

DoDI 5010.43, Implementation and Management of the DoD-Wide Continuous Process Improvement/Lean Six Sigma (CPI/LSS) Program

HA Policy 98-010, Policy for Improving Access and Quality in Military Health system

DoDI 6025.20, Medical Management (MM) Programs in the Direct Care System (DCS) and Remote Areas

HA Policy 12-010, Waiver of Restrictive Licensure and Privileging Procedures to Facilitate the Expansion of Telemedicine Services in the Military Health System

HA Policy 10-008, Policy Memorandum for Military Health System Health Care Quality Assurance Data Transparency

HA Policy 09-019, Policy Memorandum - Military Health System Data Quality Management Control Program, Revised Reporting Documents

HA Policy 03-027, Codification of Business Rules for Mandatory Inclusion of Certain Providers/Practitioners in the Centralized Credentials Quality Assurance System (CCQAS)

HA Policy 02-016, Military Health System Definition of Quality in Health Care

DoDM 6440.02, Lab Accreditation

DoD/MHS Level

HA Memo, "Comprehensive Pain Management (March 2011)"

Executive Order 13410, Promoting Quality and Efficient Health Care in Federal Government Administered or Sponsored Health Care Programs

Service Level

Air Force Policy Directive 41-2, Medical Support

Air Force Instruction 44-171, Patient-Centered Medical Home and Family Health Operations

Air Force Instruction 44-176, Access to the Care Continuum

Air Force Policy Directive 44-1, Medical Operations

Air Force Instruction 46-101, Nursing Services and Operations

Air Force Instruction 44-108, Infection Prevention and Control Program

Air Force Instruction 44-102, Medical Care Management

Air Force Instruction 44-119, Medical Quality Operations

Implementation guidance in response to 44-119, E6: Reduce Variation to Create Reliability Initiative Implementation

Air Force Instruction 90-201, Special Management - The Air Force Inspection System

Air Force Medical Service, Wart Treatment Support Staff Protocol (SSP)

Air Force Medical Service, Pregnancy Test Support Staff Protocol (SSP)

Air Force Medical Service, Implementation of AFMS Support Staff Protocol (SSP)

Air Force Medical Service, AFMS Strategic Plan Objective E6 Reduce Variation to Create Reliability

Air Force Medical Service, AFMS Surgical Safety Performance Improvement Program (Memo and 4 attachments)

USAF/SG3 Continued Implementation of 6000.14

Air Force Medical Operations Agency, Standardized Use of Medical Readiness Decision Support System to document TeamSTEPPS®

SG Doc 08-027, Report to Congress DoD MTF Satisfaction Surveys

SG Doc 11-002, Partnership for Patients

SG DOC 10-0014, Requirement to Attend the Lean for Healthcare Course

MEDCOM Regulation Nos. 40-41, Medical Services: The Patient Safety Program

OTSG/MEDCOM Policy Memo 13-048, Memorandum for Commanders, MEDCOM Regional Medical Commands (RMC) and Regional Dental Commands (RDC)

MEDCOM Regulation No. 40-XX, EMERGENCY DEPARTMENT AND OBSTETRIC COMANAGEMENT OF THE PREGNANT TRAUMA PATIENT-EVIDENCE-BASED GUIDELINES

OTSG/MEDCOM Policy Memo 12-014, Fluoroscopy Training and Credentialing for Non-radiologist Physicians (NRP)

Service Level

OTSG/MEDCOM Policy Memo 12-061, Medical and Dental Provider Credentialing and Privileging Requirements

MEDCOM Regulation 40-48, Fires Associated with the Performance of Surgical Procedures

MEDCOM Regulation 40-54, UNIVERSAL PROTOCOL: PROCEDURE VERIFICATION POLICY

OTSG/MEDCOM Policy Memo 13-050, Root Cause Analysis (RCA) Reporting Requirements for Sentinel Events

Operation Order 11-38, AMEDD-Wide Implementation of TeamSTEPPS®

MEDCOM Regulation 40-57, TRIAL OF LABOR FOR PATIENTS ATTEMPTING VAGINALBIRTH AFTER PREVIOUS CESAREAN DELIVERY

OTSG/MEDCOM Policy Memo 13-052, Color-Coded Wristband Standardization for Patient Alerts

OTSG/MEDCOM Policy Memo 11-051, Prevention of Ventilator-Associated Pneumonia

Army Regulation 40-68, Clinical Quality Management

Army Medicine 2020 Campaign Plan

AR 40-3, Medical Dental and Veterinary Care

MEDCOM Regulation 40-49, Surgical Counts

MEDCOM Regulation 40-59, Standardization of Inpatient Falls Risk Assessment and Documentation Falls Prevention Program

WRMC OPORD 14-55, (Healthcare Effectiveness Data and Information Set (HEDIS®) Campaign Plan)

SMRC Policy 13-045, Designations Duties and Functions for the Director of Health Services

SMRC Policy 13-047, External Privileged Provider Peer Review

ERMC Policy 004, Primary Care Manager Continuity Standard

MEDCOM Cir 40-15, Pain Assessment Documentation

MEDCOM Cir 40-13, Depression Out-Patient forms

MEDCOM Cir 40-12, Tobacco Cessation outpatient forms

MEDCOM Cir 40-8, Diabetes Outpatient forms

MEDCOM Cir 40-7, Asthma outpatient forms

MEDCOM Cir 40-6, Low Back Pain Documentation

AR 40-3, Army CAP Policy, Medical Dental and Vet Care

OTSG/MEDCOM Policy Memo 14-046, Transition of Care Process for Preventing Readmissions

BUMED INSTRUCTION 6010.13, Quality Assurance (QA) Program

BUMED INSTRUCTION 6000.2E, Accreditation of Fixed Medical Treatment Facilities

BUMED INSTRUCTIONS 6320.66E, Change Transmittal 2- Credentials Review and Privileging Program

Service Level

BUMED INSTRUCTION 6320.66E, Credentials Review and Privileging Program

BUMED INSTRUCTION 5830.1A, Health Care Investigation-Procedures for Specialty Reviews

BUMED INSTRUCTION 6010.17B, Naval Medical Staff Bylaws

BUMED INSTRUCTION 6220.9B, Health Care Associated Infection Prevention and Control Program

BUMED INSTRUCTION 6010.18A, Participation in the National Practitioner Data Bank

BUMED INSTRUCTION 6010.21, Risk Management Program

BUMED INSTRUCTION 6010.28, Healthcare Resolutions Program

BUMED INSTRUCTION 6320.67A, Change Transmittal 1-Adverse Privileging Actions, Peer Review Panel Procedures, and Health Care Provider Reporting

BUMED INSTRUCTION 5220.5, Navy Medicine Continuous Process Improvement/ Lean Six Sigma

NavMed West Instructions 6010.1C, Policy and Procedures for Reporting Regional Quality Assurance and Accreditation to Navy Medicine West

NavMed East Instructions 6010.1A, Policy and Procedures for Reporting Regional Quality Assurance and Accreditation Initiatives to Navy Medicine East

NavMed P-117 Manual of the Medical Department

6025.01, JTF Clinical Quality Manual

Reviewed Studies and Reports: Quality of Care

Direct Review

Lumetra External Review

Evaluation of Tobacco Use Cessation Programs (2008)

Evaluation of Hypertension among Beneficiaries with Diabetes Mellitus – Study Arm #1: Blood Pressure Control in the TRICARE Direct Care System (2008)

Evaluation of Hypertension among Beneficiaries with Diabetes Mellitus – Study Arm #2: MHS Angiotensin-Converting Enzyme Inhibitor Formulary Change (2008)

Evaluation of Influenza Immunization Rates among Enrolled Beneficiaries with Diagnosed Asthma, Heart Failure, and/or Acute Myocardial Infarction In the Military Health System (2008)

Case Management Services for TRICARE Beneficiaries with Serious Mental Health Conditions - Part 1 (2010) and Part 2 (2011)

Case Management Services for TRICARE Beneficiaries with Serious Mental Health Conditions - Part 2 (2011)

TRICARE Three-Tier COPAYMENT STRUCTURE & MEDICATION SWITCHING Among Department of Defense (DoD) Beneficiaries (2010)

Direct Review

Prenatal Care Among Women with Uncomplicated Deliveries (2011)

TRICARE Three-Tier Copayment Structure & Medication Compliance among DoD Beneficiaries (2011)

Cervical Cancer Screening Within DoD (2011)

Evaluation of the RESPECT-MIL PROGRAM: PHASE II Study #1: Evaluating RESPECT-Mil Initial Screening & Assessment Procedures (2009)

Evaluation of the RESPECT-MIL PROGRAM: PHASE II Study #2: Mental Health Services Following Initial RESPECT-Mil Assessment

Evaluation of the RESPECT-MIL PROGRAM: PHASE II Study #3: Pre- vs. Post-RESPECT-Mil Program Implementation Comparisons on Antidepressant Medication Management

Evaluation of the RESPECT-MIL PROGRAM: PHASE II Study #4: Post-Deployment Health Assessment & RESPECT-Mil Assessment

Clinical Outcomes of a Step Therapy Program for Proton Pump Inhibitors (2009)

Emergency Department Utilization in the Military Health System

Low Back Pain Evaluation and Treatment in the Military Health System

Evaluating Improvement in Patients Seen in Military Treatment Facility PAIN MANAGEMENT CLINICS (2010)

SLEEP APNEA & Military Health System Beneficiaries: DEMOGRAPHICS, DIAGNOSIS, TREATMENT & FOLLOW-UP (2010)

Department of Defense INTENSIVE CARE UNITS: Influence of Organizational Structure on Patient Outcomes (2010)

Childhood and Adolescent Overweight / Obesity Evaluation, Recognition, and Counseling in Direct Care System Outpatient Care (2012)

Prenatal Care Among Women with Uncomplicated Deliveries (2012)

Chronic Opioid Therapy Report (2012)

Evaluation of Chlamydia Trachomatis Screening for Active Duty Women (2007)

Evaluation of the RESPECT – MIL Program (2007)

Congestive Heart Failure Care Performance Measures In the Military Health System (2007)

A Study of Organizational Structure and Function on Clinic Performance

Postpartum depression in the military health system

Clinical Practice Guidelines in MHS (2006)

Process of care for high blood pressure treatment (2005)

Association of prehypertension with the development of subsequent hypertension (2005)

Post-deployment Post-traumatic stress disorder screening (2005)

MHS Clinical Practice Guideline Implementation Evaluation Phase 1 Quest dev.

Discharge instructions following hospitalization for heart failure (2005)

Pregnancy Among Active Duty Women In the Military Health System (2008)

Direct Review

Obstetric Utilization and Quality of Care (KePRO, Purchased Care only)

30-Day Readmissions (KePRO, Purchased Care only) (2013)

Epidemiological Review of Military Health System Data Repository: Inpatient Claims (KePRO, Purchased Care only)

Chest Pain (KePRO, Purchased Care only) (2014)

Global Trigger Tool (KePRO, Purchased Care only)

Hysterectomy Focused Study (KePRO, Purchased Care only) (2014)

TRICARE Low Back Pain Final Report (KePRO, Purchased Care only) (2012)

A Report to Congress: Study Incidence of Breast Cancer among Members of Armed Services

Views of Quality of Care in MTF and Civilian Systems Among TRICARE Prime Beneficiaries

Volume of Complex Procedures and Conditions at MTFs

GAO-08-901GAO #130663, VETERANS' DISABILITY BENEFITS Better Accountability and Access Would Improve the Benefits Delivery at Discharge Program

GAO-12-703 GAO #131100, VETERANS PARALYMPICS PROGRAM: Improved Reporting Needed to Ensure Grant Accountability

GAO-12-483 GAO 290927, VA ADMINISTRATIVE INVESTIGATIONS Improvements Needed in Collecting and Sharing Information

GAO-08-399 GAO #541033, VA HEALTH CARE: Additional Efforts to Better Assess Joint Ventures Needed

GAO-04-767 GAO #290324, DEPARTMENT OF VETERANS AFFAIRS: Federal Gulf War Illnesses Research Strategy Needs Reassessment

Reviewed Policies: Patient Safety

Legislation Level

32 CFR 199.17, Code of Federal Regulations Title 32 (Civilian Health and Medical Program of the Uniformed Services, Part 199.17 (32 CFR 199.17); TMA Version, April 2005

Public Law 106-398, "Floyd D. Spence National Defense Authorization Act for Fiscal Year 2001", Appendix H.R. 5408, (114Stat.1654A-1); Oct 30, 2000

DoD/MHS Level

DoDI 6000.14, DoD Patient Bill of Rights and Responsibilities in the Military Health System (MHS)

DoD Patient Safety Improvement Guide

HA-POLICY 12-005, Reporting Infection Prevention and Control Data to the Centers for Disease Control and Prevention Using the National Healthcare Safety Network

Service Level

Policy memo from Deputy Chief for Dental Operations Support. Related to Dental Safety Program

SER 00/08UM00147 Navy Medicine's health care mediation program - signed by Chief BUMED, 13 Jun 08

BUMED 6010.28, Healthcare Resolutions Program

SER M3/5HCS 08UM3374 22 Jan 09 Memo from Chief BUMED - application of TJC UP

SER M3B2/13UM3B20994, Policy Memo from Chief BUMED - Culture of Safety in Navy Medicine to Commander, Navy Medicine East/West, 3 Jan 2014

Policy memo to Commander, Navy Medicine East/West, Commander Naval Medicine National Capital Area and Commander, Navy Medicine Support Command - reporting Infection Prevention and Control Data to CDC, 8 Jan 2009

BUMED 6220.9B, Healthcare-Associated infection prevention and control program

BUMED 6010.23, Participation in the military health system patient safety program

BUMED 3100.1 9 Oct 13, Commander's Critical Information Requirements

MEDCOM Memo 10-005, Prevention of Central Line Associated Bloodstream Infections (CLABSI)

MEDCOM Memo 10-015, Implementation of Rapid Response Systems (RSS)

MEDCOM Memo 10-017, Common Emergency Codes

MEDCOM Memo 11-096, Mandatory After Action Reviews (AAR) for Suicides Completed within 90 days of Behavioral Health (BH) Visit

MEDCOM Memo 11-051, Prevention of Ventilator-Associated Pneumonia (VAP)

MEDCOM Memo 13-052, Color-Coded Wristband Standardization for Patient Alerts

MEDCOM Memo 13-050, Root Cause Analysis (RCA) Reporting Requirements for Sentinel Events

MEDCOM Memo 13-068, Privacy Act (PA) and Health Insurance Portability and Accountability Act (HIPAA) Privacy and Security Training

MEDCOM Reg 40-48, Fires Associated with the Performance of Surgical Procedures

MEDCOM Reg 40-57, Trial of Labor for Patients Attempting Vaginal Birth after Previous Cesarean Delivery

MEDCOM Reg 40-59, Standardization of Inpatient Falls Risk Assessment and Documentation Falls Prevention Program

MEDCOM Reg 40-54, Universal Protocol: Procedure Verification Policy

MEDCOM Reg 40-41, The Patient Safety Program

MEDCOM Reg 40-49, Surgical Counts

DoDI 6000.14, DoD Patient Bill of Rights and Responsibilities in the Military Health System (MHS)

Army Reg 40-68, Clinical Quality Management

AR 40-68, MEDCOM Regulation 40-41

Reviewed Studies and Reports: Patient Safety

Direct Review

PO GS 10FO183S Task Order W81XWH-07-F-0511, External Review of the DoD Medical Quality Improvement Program (Lumetra) October 2007 - July 2008

Chest Pain (KePRO, Purchased Care only)

30-Day Readmissions (KePRO, Purchased Care only)

CHRONIC OPIOID THERAPY

Obstetric Utilization and Quality of Care (KePRO, Purchased Care only)

Volume of Complex Procedures and Conditions at MTFs

Epidemiological Review of Military Health System Data Repository: Inpatient Claims (KePRO, Purchased Care only)

Global Trigger Tool For Measuring Adverse Events (KePRO, Purchased Care only)

Focus Study Ventilator-Associated Pneumonia

Pregnancy Among Active Duty Women In the Military Health System

OTSG/MEDCOM Policy Memo 11-051, A Study of Organizational Structure and Function on Clinic Performance

KePRO Focused Study on 30 day Readmissions, 03 Mar 13

Volume of Complex Procedures and Conditions at MTFs

DoD Medical Treatment Facilities Patient Safety Indicator 17, Birth trauma, 05 Aug

GAO Studies

GAO-08-399 GAO #541033, VA HEALTH CARE: Additional Efforts to Better Assess Joint Ventures Needed

DoD IG Review

Department of Defense 2011 Tri-Service Survey on Patient Safety

Patient Safety Culture Survey Report

DoD MHS Study

Multidrug-Resistant Organism (MDRO) Control In the Military Health System

TMA MHS Clinical Quality Management Study

A Comparison of Administrative and Medical Records Data in the Identification of Hospital-Acquired Infections

Appendix 1.4
Site Visit Methodology

Standard Questions Used at Site Visits

The site visit review team asked consistent questions at each visit for leadership, MTF functional subject matter experts, health care staff, and patients.

Access Questions for Health Care Staff

1. Is there a designated Access Manager? (yes or no)
2. Who comprises the Access to Care multidisciplinary team? (list)
3. What is the role of the Access to care team in your facility?
4. What information/metrics do you review and what actions do you take? (open ended follow on question)
5. How effectively are you meeting patient access demands? (Score between 1-5, 1= Not at all; 2= Marginally; 3= Neutral; 4= Effective; 5= Very effective; 0 = not applicable)
6. Given the TRICARE standard of 24 hours for urgent care, 7 days for routine care, and 28 days for wellness visits and specialty care, how well are these standards being met? (Score between 1-5, 1= Never; 2= Rarely; 3= Half the time; 4= More than half the time; 5= Always; 0 = not applicable)
7. If you're unable to offer the patient's desired appointment timeline, what do you do? (open ended)
8. Are you using waitlists (CHCS or other processes) if appointments are not available?
9. If a waitlist is being used for unavailable appointment dates, how is the waitlist being managed? (open ended)
10. If a waitlist is being used, patients are seen within appropriate/designated timeframe (Score between 1-5, 1= Never; 2= Rarely; 3= Sometimes; 4= Often; 5= Always; 0 = not applicable)
11. How often do the Command's PCMH clinics utilize $ appointment types and PBO detail codes within their CHCS schedules or templates? (Score between 1-5, 1= Always; 2= Often; 3= Sometimes; 4= Seldom; 5= Never; 0 = not applicable)
12. Schedules are created and released within timeline required by policy. (Score between 1-5, 1= Never; 2= Rarely; 3= Sometimes; 4= Often; 5= Always; 0 = not applicable)
13. How often are appointing agents (contract, active duty, and civilian) trained? Who does the training and is it documented? (open ended)
14. Follow up visits are booked prior to the patient leaving the clinic. (Score between 1-5, 1= Never; 2= Rarely; 3= Half the time; 4= More than half the time; 5= Always; 0 = not applicable)
15. For referral to a specialty clinic, initial visits are booked prior to the patient leaving the MTF. (Score between 1-5, 1= Never; 2= Rarely; 3= Half the time; 4= More than half the time; 5= Always; 0 = not applicable)
16. How effectively is the MTF utilizing TRICARE Online for appointing? (Score between 1-5, 1= Not at all; 2= Marginally; 3= Neutral; 4= Effective; 5= Very effective; 0 = not applicable)

17. How effectively is the MTF utilizing Secure Messaging to support the patient's experience of health care? (Score between 1-5, 1= Not at all; 2= Marginally; 3= Neutral; 4= Effective; 5= Very effective; 0 = not applicable)
18. How often are patients asked to call back to get an appointment? (Score between 1-5, 1= Never; 2= Rarely; 3= Half the time; 4= More than half the time; 5= Always; 0 = not applicable)
19. How often are appointing agents monitored for quality of service? (open ended)
20. What problems have you encountered in your appointing practices? (open ended)

Access Questions for Beneficiaries

1. Scheduling an appointment at the military clinic when I would like to be seen is: (Score between 1-5, 1= Very Difficult; 2= Difficult; 3= Neutral; 4= Easy; 5= Very easy; 0 = not applicable)
2. Scheduling an appointment at a network clinic when I would like to be seen is: (Score between 1-5, 1= Very Difficult; 2= Difficult; 3= Neutral; 4= Easy; 5= Very easy; 0 = not applicable)
3. I am asked by the scheduling clerk/clinic to call back to get an appointment: (Score between 1-5, 1= Always; 2= More than half the time; 3= Half the time; 4= Rarely; 5= Never; 0 = not applicable)
4. I am satisfied with getting a same-day appointment: (Score between 1-5, 1= Always; 2= More than half the time; 3= Half the time; 4= Rarely; 5= Never; 0 = not applicable)
5. Given the TRICARE standard of 24 hours for urgent care, 7 days for routine care, and 28 days for wellness visits and specialty care, how well are these standards being met? (Score between 1-5, 1= Never; 2= Rarely; 3= Half the time; 4= More than half the time; 5= Always; 0 = not applicable)

Access Questions for MTF Leadership

1. Is there a command policy in place governing Access to Care (ATC)? (open ended)
2. How often does your executive committee the access to care metrics? (Score between 1-5; 1=Not at all; 2= Semi-annually; 3= Quarterly; 4= monthly; 5= weekly)
3. What actions do you take with the information you receive? (open ended follow on question)
4. How often do you review patient satisfaction results? (Score between 1-5; 1=Not at all; 2= Semi-annually; 3= Quarterly; 4= monthly; 5= weekly)
5. What actions do you take to respond to patient satisfaction survey results? (open ended)
6. How effectively are you meeting patient access demands? (Score between 1-5, 1= Not at all; 2= Rarely; 3= Neutral; 4= Effective; 5= Very effective; 0 = not applicable)
7. Given the TRICARE standard of 24 hours for urgent care, 7 days for routine care, and 28 days for wellness visits and specialty care, how well are these standards being met? (Score between 1-5, 1= Never; 2= Rarely; 3= Half the time; 4= More than half the time; 5= Always; 0 = not applicable)

Safety Questions for Health Care Staff

1. Describe your role in the Patient Safety program in this organization?
2. What is your level of responsibility in the organization Patient Safety Program?

1=Not at all responsible
2=Somewhat responsible but no active participation
3=Responsible; have a role; and participate
4=Responsible; complete my role, and report to patient safety
5=Responsible; complete my role, report, and disseminate patient safety findings/updates

3. Describe your safety measures currently in place and being monitored.
   1=Not able to answer the question; 2=Unsure of safety measures currently in place; 3=Able to describe at least one safety measure; 4=Described more than one safety measure and monitoring process; 5= Described several safety measures and monitoring process
4. What are you doing to improve patient safety? (Descriptive)
5. How do you ensure effective communication across teams and with patients?
6. Has TeamSTEPPS® been implemented across the MTF?
7. How are you tracking the impact of TeamSTEPPS®?
8. How extensively are safety metrics tracked, reported, and used for improvement at all levels?
9. How effective are these metrics in driving improvement efforts at the MTF?
10. What are the metrics used?
11. Who is responsible for tracking these metrics at the unit/MTF/Service level?
12. What barriers did you overcome to prevent harm (HACs)?
    a. What are they?
    b. What is the process for eliminating them?
    c. Who is responsible for addressing barriers on the unit/MTF/Service levels?
13. What programs are in place to support/ensure sustained improvements over time?
    a. How often are they reviewed/ updated and by whom?
14. How does the MTF apply safe practices to prevent harm?
    a. How have these practices been monitored through PfP Hospital Acquired Conditions/ Infections and Readmissions activities?
    b. Did your MTF improve with your PfP initiatives?
15. How OFTEN are safety event/unsafe condition findings SHARED WITH YOU? 1=NEVER; 2 ALMOST NEVER; 3=OCCASIONALLY/SOMETIMES; 4= ALMOST EVERYTIME; 5= EVERY TIME
16. Describe how your organization creates an environment where staff feels safe reporting errors and failures? GIVE AN EXAMPLE.
a. HOW LIKELY ARE YOU TO REPORT ERRORS AND RELATED CONCERNS?
17. 1-EXTREMEMLY UNLIKELY; 2-UNLIKLEY; 3-NEUTRAL; 4-LIKELY; 5-EXTREMELY LIKELY
18. DESCRIBE YOUR PROCESS FOR MANAGING DISRUPTIVE PROBLEMATIC BEHAVIORS AND/OR SITUATIONS. (Descriptive)
19. Does management use information to encourage behavior changes?
    1= Negative response, have not ever witnessed; 2= Problematic behaviors are ignored here; 3=Problematic behaviors are addressed, but no transparency; 4=Problematic behaviors are addressed and appropriate action taken; 5= Problematic behaviors are addressed, appropriate action, and leadership commitment to zero tolerance

20. How do you reinforce improved behaviors? 1=Not sure; 2=Slightly important; 3=Empower staff to self-monitor / set expectation; 4=Routine feedback to member / teams; 5=Extremely important / routinely addressed
21. WERE THE RESULTS OF THE 2011 CULTURE SURVEY a priority/COMMUNICATED TO YOU? 1=Not a priority; 2=Low priority; 3=Moderate priority; 4=High priority; 5=Essential to our organization
22. 1. Is Patient Safety part of the strategic goals/Core Values? (yes/no)
23. PROVIDE TWO EXAMPLES OF HOW PATIENT SAFETY IS PART OF your core value? 1 = Cannot speak to compliance or give specific example; 2 = Able to speak to compliance but not give an example; 3 = Speaks to compliance and gives one example; 4 = Strong answer for compliance with two examples; 5 = Complete answer with more than two examples
24. WHAT IS YOUR PROCESS FOR DISCLOSING UNEXPECTED EVENTS TO THE PATIENT/FAMILY? (descriptive)

Patient Safety Questions for MTF Leadership

1. Do you make leadership rounds? How frequently do you conduct leadership rounds?
1 – Annually; 2 – Quarterly; 3- monthly; 4- weekly; 5- daily
2. Describe the process and results. (Descriptive)
3. How effectively has leadership fostered a culture of safety?
1 – Totally ineffective; 2 – Slightly ineffective; 3– Neutral; 4 – Effective; 5– Perfectly Effective
4. Describe how the vision and goals focus your organization on improvement in patient safety? (Subjective)
5. What is the role of the Patient Safety Manager (PSM) at your facility? (Describe)
6. How visible/engaged is the PSM in daily activities at your MTF?
1 – Not at all visible/engaged; 2 – slightly visible/engaged; 3 – somewhat visible/engaged; 4 – very visible/engaged; 5 – extremely visible/engaged
7. How do you become aware of patient safety events? What actions are taken?
Level of Awareness
1 – not at all aware/safety events not communicated; 2 – Slightly aware/notified of events eventually; 3 – Somewhat aware/notified but too late to take action; 4 – Moderately aware/notified in time to take action; 5 – Extremely aware/notified immediately
8. How frequently are safety events and unsafe conditions reported, reviewed, and used for improvement at all levels?
1 – Never; 2 – Almost never; 3 – Occasionally/Sometimes; 4 – Almost every time; 5 – Every time
9. How do you communicate and share lessons learned?
1 – Never; 2 – Rarely/informal process; 3 – Sometimes/policy but not routinely followed; 4 – Often/policy and routine dissemination; 5 – Always/policy and documentation at unit level (minutes capture)
10. Are you aware of any patient Safety concerns in the network? (Yes/No)
a. If a patient safety concern from the network were brought to your attention, what would you do with that information?

1 – Would not consider; 2 – Might or might not consider; 3 – Definitely consider but no action; 4 – Consider and assign responsibility; 5- Take action; assign responsibility; and ensure resolution

11. How are patient safety concerns from the network addressed (descriptive)

12. How do you involve patients in their care?

1 = not able to answer/articulate patient involvement; 2 = speaks around question with no specifics 3 = speaks to patient involvement with 1 specific example; 4 = speaks to patient involvement with 2 specific examples; 5= addresses question confidently with examples

13. When a patient expresses concerns about their care, how often are the patient concerns resolved?

1 – Never; 2 – Rarely; 3 – Occasionally; 4 – A moderate amount; 5 – A great deal

14. Explain process and/or if the concerns are not resolved, what steps do you take? (Descriptive)

15. Describe efforts initiated to assist patients to be active participants in their care.
Level of Participation
1 – No, and not considered; 3 – No, but considered (talks but no examples); 5 – Yes (provides examples)

16. What resources/tools are available for engaging patients in their care?
Level of Influence
1 – not at all influential (no resources/tools); 2 – slightly influential (talks subject but no specifics); 3 – somewhat influential (answers question with 1 example); 4 – very influential (answers question with 2 examples); 5 – extremely influential (addresses question confidently with examples)

Patient Safety Questions for Beneficiaries

1. Do you feel you receive safe care here? (yes/no)
2. Do you feel comfortable asking questions to your care providers and MTF staff?
Graded response if asking a beneficiary:
1= no I am not comfortable; 2 = comfortable addressing by survey; 3 = comfortable addressing questions to patient advocate; 4= comfortable addressing questions with nursing staff 5= comfortable addressing questions directly with provider

3. How do you report a safety issue or concern? (descriptive)
a. If you don't know how to report a problem, what steps do you take? (Subjective Response)

4. Do you receive easy to follow instructions/information (I/I) around your care plans?
Graded response if asking a beneficiary:
1 = no I/I received; 2 = received minimal I/I (verbal instructions); 3= received basic I/I (printed and verbal instructions); 4= received detailed I/I (printed/verbal/and required brief back); 5= received detailed I/I and follow-up at home phone call/relay health (after inpatient/outpatient visit)

5. Have you been referred for care in the civilian sector? (yes/no)
a. Did you have any problems in making an appointment? (yes/no)
b. How were you treated?
1-Strongly disagree with treatment; 2-Disagree with treatment; 3-Neither agree nor disagree with treatment; 4-Agree with treatment; 5-Strongly agree with treatment

6. Did you encounter any problems that you had to tell someone about? (yes/no)

i. Who did you contact? (list name/position/title)
7. Did you get a reply? (Yes/No)
8. Was your issue resolved? (Subjective)
9. How responsive is/was your facility (clinic and Managed Care Support Contract) in processing referrals?
1 = no response/complicated/no appointment in 60 days; 2 = referral completed with intervention w/appoint in >30 days; 3 = referral completed no problems w/appoint in >30 days; 4 = referral completed with intervention and appointment in <30 days; 5 = referral process no problems w/appoint in <30 days

Quality of Care Questions for MTF Leadership and Health Care Staff

1. Does the MTF have performance improvement techniques to improve the quality of care?
   (Score between 1-5, 1= Not correlated; 2= Marginally correlates; 3= Partially correlates; 4= Correlates; 5= Exceeds; 0 = not applicable)
2. Is leadership committed to quality?
   (Score between 1-5, 1= Not correlated; 2= Marginally correlates; 3= Partially correlates; 4= Correlates; 5= Exceeds; 0 = not applicable)
3. Does leadership communicate quality initiatives throughout the facility?
   (Score between 1-5, 1= Not correlated; 2= Marginally correlates; 3= Partially correlates; 4= Correlates; 5= Exceeds; 0 = not applicable)
4. Have local policies on orientation requirements for new staff have been developed and are being followed?
   (Score between 1-5, 1= Not correlated; 2= Marginally correlates; 3= Partially correlates; 4= Correlates; 5= Exceeds; 0 = not applicable)
5. Is the facility using data to improve performance?
   (Score between 1-5, 1= Not correlated; 2= Marginally correlates; 3= Partially correlates; 4= Correlates; 5= Exceeds; 0 = not applicable)
6. Is patient survey information incorporated in performance improvement activities
   (Score between 1-5, 1= Not correlated; 2= Marginally correlates; 3= Partially correlates; 4= Correlates; 5= Exceeds; 0 = not applicable)
7. Is quality data communicated across the facility?
   (Score between 1-5, 1= Not correlated; 2= Marginally correlates; 3= Partially correlates; 4= Correlates; 5= Exceeds; 0 = not applicable)
8. Does the MTF conduct regular, systematic, and comprehensive reviews of the quality of health care provided in their facilities, using accreditation standards, national consensus measures, evidence-based practice standards, and medical management guidelines
   (Score between 1-5, 1= Not correlated; 2= Marginally correlates; 3= Partially correlates; 4= Correlates; 5= Exceeds; 0 = not applicable)
9. Is a performance measurement system for clinical quality implemented as a dedicated program to confirm quality-of-care outcomes and identify areas for improvement: (1)(a) must maintain accreditation by TJC under the applicable accreditation manual or through an accreditation source approved by the ASD/HA)?
   (Score between 1-5, 1= Not correlated; 2= Marginally correlates; 3= Partially correlates; 4= Correlates; 5= Exceeds; 0 = not applicable)

10. If the MTF participates in National Quality Programs (based on mission priorities and current health care environment), are appropriate BAA and DSA completed?
    (Score between 1-5, 1= Not correlated; 2= Marginally correlates; 3= Partially correlates; 4= Correlates; 5= Exceeds; 0 = not applicable)
11. Is evidence-based data used in the development of all clinical performance measures, if local clinical performance measures and guidelines are developed by MTF?
    (Score between 1-5, 1= Not correlated; 2= Marginally correlates; 3= Partially correlates; 4= Correlates; 5= Exceeds; 0 = not applicable)

Quality of Care Questions for Beneficiaries

1. Does the MTF have performance improvement techniques to improve the quality of care?
   (Score between 1-5, 1= Not correlated; 2= Marginally correlates; 3= Partially correlates; 4= Correlates; 5= Exceeds; 0 = not applicable)
2. Is leadership committed to quality?
   (Score between 1-5, 1= Not correlated; 2= Marginally correlates; 3= Partially correlates; 4= Correlates; 5= Exceeds; 0 = not applicable)
3. Is the facility using data to improve performance?
   (Score between 1-5, 1= Not correlated; 2= Marginally correlates; 3= Partially correlates; 4= Correlates; 5= Exceeds; 0 = not applicable)
4. Is quality data communicated across the facility?
   (Score between 1-5, 1= Not correlated; 2= Marginally correlates; 3= Partially correlates; 4= Correlates; 5= Exceeds; 0 = not applicable)

A questionnaire was sent to regional commanders when a facility in their region was visited. The purpose of the questionnaire was to measure alignment of what the site review team found at the MTF and regional commander's assessment. See questionnaire below.

Questions for Regional Commanders

1. How often does their executive committee review the access to care metrics?

1	2	3	4	5	0
Not at all	Semi-annually	Quarterly	Monthly	Weekly	N/A

2. How often do they review patient satisfaction results?

1	2	3	4	5	0
Not at all	Semi-annually	Quarterly	Monthly	Weekly	N/A

3. How effectively are they meeting patient access demands?

1	2	3	4	5	0
Not at all	Partially	Neutral	Effective	Very effective	N/A

4. Given the TRICARE standard of 24 hours for urgent care, 7 days for routine care, and 28 days for wellness visits and specialty care, how well are these standards being met?

1	2	3	4	5	0
Never	Rarely	Half the time	More than half the time	Most of the time	N/A

5. How effectively are they promoting Virtual Care (Secure Messaging, TOL)?

1	2	3	4	5	0
Not at all	Partially	Neutral	Effective	Very effective	N/A

6. Rate the MTFs commitment to quality.

1	2	3	4	5	0
Not at all committed		Neutral		Extremely committed	N/A

7. How clear is guidance on quality goals and expectations by the MTF senior leadership?

1	2	3	4	5	0
Not at all clear		Neutral		Extremely clear	N/A

8. Are you familiar with the performance of this MTF's participation in NSQIP, NPIC, NHSN, HEDIS, ORYX, etc.?

1	2	3	4	5	0
Not at all familiar		Familiar		Familiar with all data	N/A

9. How familiar are you with this MTF's quality improvement activities and are you aware of their outcomes?

1	2	3	4	5	0
Not at all familiar		Familiar		Familiar with all data	N/A

10. How do you think the MTF staff would rate the MTF's senior leadership on communication of quality goals and initiatives?

1	2	3	4	5	0
Poor communication		Neutral		Excellent communication	N/A

11. How many examples of patient safety practices or measures to reduce patient harm are in place that the MTF Leadership would identify?

1	2	3	4	5	0
None	One example	Two examples	Three examples	Four or more examples	N/A

12. How many examples of patient safety monitoring activities in place to reduce patient harm would the MTF Leadership identify?

1	2	3	4	5	0
None	One example	Two examples	Three examples	Four or more examples	N/A

13. How many examples would they list where the staff members feel comfortable reporting safety errors would the MTF Leadership identify?

1	2	3	4	5	0
None	One example	Two examples	Three examples	Four or more examples	N/A

14. How many examples of areas where they have made improvements based upon the results of the 2011 cultural survey would the MTF Leadership identify?

1	2	3	4	5	0
None	One example	Two examples	Three examples	Four or more examples	N/A

15. Tell us where the MTF is doing well related to Access, Quality and Patient Safety.

16. Tell us where the MTF needs improvement related to Access, Quality and Patient Safety.

17. For those areas where the MTF needs improvement, have you identified them with the MTF and are you working on an action plan with the MTF to improve these areas?

Appendix 1.5
Site Visit Town Hall Comment Summary

Background

As part of the 90-day Review of the Military Health System (MHS), seven military treatment facilities were visited. At each facility a contract facilitator conducted two town hall meetings: one for staff and one for beneficiaries. The comments and remarks made at the town halls were captured as notes, and reviewed for personal or health identifying information (which was removed) (see below sections for summaries). As noted in the feedback from one of the external subject matter experts, Dr. Brent James, input received from both the town hall meetings may be biased toward individuals dissatisfied with their access or service, and do not represent a valid sample population. Nonetheless, this information is informative, and it has been shared with the MTF Commanders of each site for follow-up or corrective action as necessary.

Discussion

There were 395 comments made that expressed either a positive or negative opinion concerning the performance of the MHS: 218 of these comments (55 percent) came from beneficiaries and the remaining 177 (45 percent) came from staff. Of those, 240 (61 percent) were negative, with 128 negative comments from beneficiaries and 112 from staff.

There were clear and distinct themes identified by each audience that remained consistent across the site visits. These themes included difficulty in getting access to care for beneficiaries and challenges for staff posed by an emphasis on efficiency. Also, while some comments concerning access for beneficiaries focus on being asked to call back to book an appointment, it is important to note that a number of those comments come from individuals who are not enrolled to the MTF (e.g., TRICARE Standard or TRICARE for Life beneficiaries). Access standards apply to TRICARE Prime beneficiaries. For other beneficiary categories, access is provided as space is available so asking them to call back if there are no other appointments available is appropriate.

More detailed discussion of the feedback, including summary tables, is below. The data are segregated between beneficiaries and staff and organized by major area of focus, with an additional "general comments" section for staff.

Beneficiaries

Beneficiaries made 218 comments that expressed either a positive or negative opinion concerning the performance of MHS access to care.

Comments concerning access made up 100 (46 percent) of all feedback and 56 percent (71 of 128) of the negative feedback provided. Difficulty in getting an appointment made up 64 percent of all negative access to care comments.

Beneficiaries felt that they received quality care, with 39 percent of all positive comments discussing the high quality of care experienced. In particular, there was positive feedback concerning tools such as secure messaging via RelayHealth, which made up 18 percent of all positive comments.

Issue	# of Mentions
General / Multi-Category (Negative)	
Difficulty getting appointments as a non TRICARE Prime beneficiary	4
No face-to-face TRICARE representative at MTF to assist beneficiary	4
Poor customer service – *(General: includes negative interactions with providers and/or admin staff)*	4
Long pharmacy wait times	4
Difficult to see the same PCM/Provider	5
Total	**21**

Issue	# of Mentions
Access (Positive)	
Positive feedback on RelayHealth	16
Quick/effective follow-up scheduling	5
No trouble getting general appointment	4
No trouble getting specialty care	2
Faster access than TRICARE network	2
Total	**29**

Issue	# of Mentions
Access (Negative)	
Difficulty in getting an appointment - *(All appointments: none available, too long until first availability, difficult to secure an appointment)*	24
Difficulty in getting specialty appointment	14
Beneficiary forced to resort to visiting ER to receive care	14
Beneficiary told to call back another time due to lack of availability	11
Long time between appointments / difficult to book follow-up appointments	6
Variability in ease of access on clinic by clinic level	2
Total	**71**

Appendix 1. Introduction

Issue	# of Mentions
Quality (Positive)	
I receive good/quality care	35
Care is as good/better than network	5
I receive good/quality specialty care	5
Good continuity of care	4
Good communication with provider	3
Total	**52**

Issue	# of Mentions
Quality (Negative)	
Poor communication – *(Between patient/provider and provider/provider)*	6
Concern about inexperienced providers – *(interns / young providers)*	3
Provider Error	2
Lack of transparency	1
Total	**12**

Issue	# of Mentions
Patient Safety (Positive)	
I receive safe care	6
I feel safe	3
Total	**9**

Issue	# of Mentions
Patient Safety (Negative)	
Beneficiary felt rushed or did not have sufficient time with provider	8
Beneficiary felt the MTF was understaffed	6
Medical record issues – *(lack of standardization, failure to maintain records)*	4
Issues with TRICARE network / managed care support contractors	3
Little or no accountability for complaints of poor performance	3
Total	**24**

Staff

Comments concerning quality comprised the largest number of comments (37 percent). The overarching theme was that, while staff felt they delivered quality care, they expressed concern that a focus on efficiency and quantity of visits, coupled with understaffing, was putting quality at risk (27 percent of all negative comments). Staff turnover (9 percent) and IT/equipment challenges (8 percent) were the remaining leading negative comments.

There was positive feedback concerning the use of patient safety reporting tools (20 percent) and RelayHealth and secure messaging (15 percent). There were several troubling, though small in number, references to fear of retaliation or a toxic leadership climate.

Issue	# of Mentions
General / Multi-Category (Negative)	
Staff felt MTF was understaffed or had insufficient personnel for mission	15
Challenges/problems with EHR/Health IT/Technology	6
Burdensome training requirements	5
Challenges with hiring or firing civilians	4
Poor internal communication	4
Lack of leadership accountability	3
Burdensome policy requirements	2
Challenges with the regional contractors	1
Total	40

Issue	# of Mentions
Access (Positive)	
Use/like RelayHealth	10
Clinics effectively providing access	2
Actively recapturing care	1
Total	13

Issue	# of Mentions
Access (Negative)	
Unable to see patients within required access standards	5
Inability to punish/disincentivize no-shows	5
Staff ask patients to call back to schedule appointment due to no availability	4
Large variance between clinics for appointment availability	4
Poor coordination between TRICARE and MTF	3
Need standardized appointing process/centralized appointing center	2
Existing system difficult to work with	1
Total	24

Appendix 1. Introduction

Issue	# of Mentions
Quality (Positive)	
Confident we deliver quality care	10
TeamSTEPPS referenced	6
Good/quality staff	6
Quality is a priority	5
Focused on process improvement	4
Total	31

Issue	# of Mentions
Quality (Negative)	
Leadership focus is on efficiency and quantity, not quality	15
Challenges presented by turnover, both leadership and provider	10
Lack of medical supplies	3
Lack of proper training for new staff – *(providers and admin staff)*	4
Lack of clear standard operation procedure or quality policy guidance	2
Total	34

Issue	# of Mentions
Safety (Positive)	
Staff utilize patient safety reporting tools	13
Patient safety reporting tools and resources are available	4
Open communication on safety issues with leadership	4
Total	21

Issue	# of Mentions
Safety (Negative)	
Lack of follow-up on reported safety issues	6
Fear of retaliation / retaliated against for reporting	5
Lack of training on appropriate use of patient safety reporting system	2
Patient record inconsistency/failure to maintain	1
Total	14

Military Health System Review – Final Report August 29, 2014

Site 1 Beneficiary Town Hall Questions and Answers

The following text reproduces the Town Hall facilitator questions and audience responses, transcribed as close to verbatim as possible during the session. Information that could potentially identify individual participants has been omitted for privacy purposes.

Approximately 13 people attended this Town Hall meeting.

Questions Related to Quality of Care

Question to Audience: Do you think that you get good care here at [this MTF]?

Responses from Audience:
- I think I get good care here. I have no problems seeing my primary care doctor but seeing specialists is difficult. When you actually get to see the specialist it does not appear to me that they do thorough checks in terms of what you are there to be seen for. It should not be that complicated. [Personal information omitted]

- [Personal information omitted] … have not been able to schedule routine appointments. I think that is a problem.

- The care that I am getting here is okay. I think it is about the same as the care that I am getting in town. I don't have a problem with the care that I receive but I do have a problem with getting to the care. [Personal information omitted]… I had to search for a hospital number to call, then when I called them, I explained the situation and they told me to come in. That was the biggest mistake they could have made. What they should have told me to do is pick up the phone and dial 9-1-1. Once I got to the hospital the care that I did get was the best that I could have received anywhere. [Personal information omitted] … I would have bled to death. I don't have any issues with the quality of care that I get.

Question to Audience: How does the quality of care that you get out in the network compare with the quality of care that you received in this hospital?

Responses from Audience:
- I don't get care in this hospital. It seems to me that the hospital caters to active duty and dependents. Retirees have a hard time getting care in this hospital that is why I choose to use civilian care out in the network.

- I had to go on the outside because [personal information omitted] … I went to two different hospitals to get a [personal information omitted] … So something is going on with the specialist care.

- [Personal information omitted] … I don't know how to access TRICARE overseas. If there is an emergency I cannot get help and I pay for the TRICARE – for-life option.

- ... [Personal information omitted] ... Care has improved immensely ... [Personal information omitted] ... I feel like the care was better here. I like my doctors more here. They are more accessible and they are more personable. I also think that pediatrics care is also supreme here. For example the pediatricians now are primarily civilian pediatricians so you have the same pediatrician every time. It is much easier to get appointments and you have a more established relationship with the doctor because [you] have seen your doctor every time. So I think it has gotten a lot better in a decade.

Question to Audience: If you have a concern about the quality of care that you get what do you do? Who do you talk to?

Responses from Audience:
- That is a very important topic. I cannot speak to quality of care. I just found out that enrollment is no longer done here anymore. I now have to enroll online. The TRICARE office has been closed here.

- They do have comment boxes in all of the clinics where you can make comments. In Pediatrics they have signs that say, "If you haven't been seen in 15 minutes to please talk to the people at the front desk." I also speak to the nurses or the person who is treating me if I encounter any issues.

- They used to have a patient advocate that you could speak with. I have not seen them push it lately. I have used them a few times and they were effective.

Question to Audience: What would you do to improve quality health care at this hospital?

Responses from Audience:
- I would ensure that they have qualified doctors.

- In general I feel that the quality of care is good but there are pockets where it is not so good. I find that the civilian people who man the front desks to not be as helpful as some of the military people. That has been my experience. I think that the phone system is pretty good. I just don't think that you have enough staffing. I have been in situations before where they have said we only have one doctor available but really there is two and it is just that one has been deployed. So you have one person to handle the workload of two. I think that is where you run into serious issues because you have one person doing the work of two. Most of the people here do a very good job but you will always have a few bad apples. I also think that military folk have to be willing to take responsibility for their own health care. I think sometimes we have an expectation that is unrealistic. Sometimes we have to be more proactive in our own care.

Questions Related to Access to Care

Question to Audience: How easy or difficult is it for you to get an appointment here?

Responses from Audience:
- I don't have a problem getting an appointment. [Personal information omitted] ... whose husband died in the military cannot get an appointment. So there is a problem there. [They are] ... TRICARE Standard and cannot get an appointment. I don't understand. [They] ... should have the same access as I do ...

- Sometimes it takes 45 minutes for someone to help you book an appointment. You can be on hold for up to an hour waiting to make an appointment

- The lack of urgent care is terrible. There is no urgent care service except for the Emergency Room. If you go to the ER you have to wait 4-5 hours. There need to be urgent care. Regular appointments are good generally.

Question to Audience: How does getting an appointment out in the network compare with getting an appointment in this institution?

Responses from Audience:
- [Out] in the network they call and ask me, when do I want to come in. I am unable to get an appointment here. In the network I can get an appointment whenever I need one. They don't even have me in the system here.

Question to Audience: When you have an appointment, how often are you asked, before you leave, to book your next follow up appointment?

Responses from Audience:
- They never ask me. I just went to my doctor and they said that she is leaving to another clinic so you will have a new provider. They said to expect a call or a letter.

- In some places the appointment is made and in others they say to call back. So it is not "one size fits all" throughout all of the clinics. [Personal information omitted] ... When I call to make an appointment I am able to get scheduled.

- Same day appointments for pediatrics are terrific. The times I have called for myself for back pain, they could not see me for 3 days. So then you have to determine if it is worth going to the ER. I wish there was an urgent care clinic.

- Internal Medicine, you cannot get same day appointments. They will tell you to go to emergency. I agree that they should have urgent care. Otherwise you will have to go to the ER.

Question to Audience: The TRICARE standard is: 24 hours for urgent care, 7 days for routine care, and 28 days for wellness visits and specialty care. Are these standards being met?

Responses from Audience:
- If you have something that is urgent, that means that you have to be seen. You cannot wait 24 hours.

Questions Related to Patient Safety

Question to Audience: Do you feel that the care that you receive here is safe?

Responses from Audience:
- Two comments. I think it is generally very good. The staff is well trained and when you ask them where they are trained it is always very surprising to hear. The military doctors come from great programs and they get excellent training. I generally feel like my care has been good. I also think that our population does not appreciate that we get free health care. I have friend outside that pays $1800 dollars a month for a family of four and I pay nothing form my family of five. I think we get a little spoiled and we expect perfection. I believe the military does a good job on a limited budget for all of its people.

- I feel safe when I come here, otherwise I would not come. We pay for TRICARE Prime. It is not free for retirees. We also have to make other insurance payments so we are not getting a free ride ... [Personal information omitted]...

Question to Audience: When you are with your provider, do you feel comfortable asking questions about your care?

Responses from Audience:
- No comment

Question to Audience: If you have a safety concern, would you know how and to whom to report it?

Responses from Audience:
- No comment

Question to Audience: Is there anything that you would like to share that we have not asked about yet?

Responses from Audience:
- Yes, a couple of things. My neighbor received a letter that he was no longer eligible for care here. He no longer had a PCM here. He had to find his own out in town. When you get to 65, that is what happens. They cut you off from your PCM. You are still eligible for specialty care here. [Personal information omitted] ... Why didn't TRICARE notify him 60 days prior to his 65th birthday that he was going to be cut off from his PCM and he would have to go find another in town. The whole philosophy for [headquarters] is that if we need you, we will keep you in the huddle, if not we will kick you to the curb. That is why you will continue to see problems with regards to health care for retirees. It

is all a smoke screen. The smoke screen is that by the time I come in to get care that was promised to me, [they] have already changed the rules and [I] cannot get access. That is what veterans like myself are angry about.

- I am concerned about military men who have passed on and left their widows. How are they getting care. It appears like they are getting kicked to the curb? They are not getting appointments.

- I have been listening and some of the comments are legitimate, especially in regards to urgent care. I was kicked out on three different occasions. It was very difficult to find a new physician that took Medicare out in the network. I had [personal information omitted] ... and the doctor on the outside wrote me a prescription ... when that was not what I needed. He didn't even see me. I came here and the doctor took care of me right away. The care that I got here has been wonderful compared to what I have had in the network. I think that the staff here always tries to help patients ...

- ... Ophthalmology, they have a walk in clinic. They triage the patents. They give follow up appointments. They have a system where they call people back. They are great.

- You can actually only walk-in one to two times a week.

- [Patient information omitted] ... they [ophthalmology] have walk-ins every day. I don't know where the hang up is but they have a doctor assigned to that clinic every day.

Site 1 Staff Town Hall Questions and Answers

The following text reproduces the Town Hall facilitator questions and audience responses, transcribed as close to verbatim as possible during the session. Information that could potentially identify individual participants has been omitted for privacy purposes.

Approximately 220 people attended this Town Hall meeting.

Questions Related to Quality of Care

Question to Audience: Is quality a priority here? And if it is, what do you see and experience? If not, what is it that you're seeing that it is not?

Responses from Audience:
- Quality is definitely a priority here. ... It is a great place to work here. Quality shines through. We did an outstanding last year on our joint commission. We got many citations for that. In the cancer department, we had the commission on cancer and received our 4th in a row outstanding achievement award for cancer commission in August. 4th achievement award for cancer. I understand that there are only two hospitals that share this distinction. I'm so proud here of this place...

- ... even though many of the primary clinics will tell [HEDIS matrix staff that they are] the bane of their existence because [staff] continually produce reports that show how their clinics are doing, how providers are doing. We also have a top performing clinic award quarterly and annually that we give out and it's basically now like a few years ago, it was like oh this HEDIS stuff, this quality stuff, this is driving me crazy and it's too much work, and now I hear them saying from clinics how our clinic is doing, when is the data coming out. We want to see how our clinic is doing, we know we are improving and if we are the top performing. We know we are getting to green. So, I know in the primary clinics, they get it. They know the importance of the HEDIS matrix and the values, the values for the command not only for the patient care, but also a cost saving measure. It is really neat to work here and feeling a part of the team in every clinic and working with them, and helping them understand what the methods are and what the methodologies are and I think everyone from the front desk through to the providers know about HEDIS.

- ... almost everything we do is going to be focused on process improvement, quality assurance and patient safety. And in terms of the interests of the hospital, command...every single month, they provide detailed documentation and notes to a very eager group, an interested group of individuals which includes directors. The benefit of having worked for several years now and continuing to work in communities as intense as doing moonlighting ... at an executive leadership standpoint, our leadership is very interested in our metrics in the [inpatient departments] and all the different benchmarks that we are meeting.

Question to Audience: What are you seeing in terms of patient outcomes?

Responses from Audience:
- As far as directly related to quality with patients, I believe that it can be reflected on how we're doing. And I was just informed that one patient received a 6 month coin of sobriety and ... she was so excited about it that she wanted to take it back to the clinic. And I think that says quite a bit that someone can go through a program like ours and six months later you receive a coin for success on their own that enabled them to do through their own experiences. So, it says quite a bit about the quality here.
- ... we had a patient [who required immediate assistance] .... We had a team ... made up of surgical, pain management, OB, labor and delivery teammates that all came together so we could to make sure we had a successful outcome. ... To me that shows how our quality is doing every day.
- I just want to say that one of the things I have seen is that there is really a good group of people that work on our staff. One of the things that really helps a patient outcome that we look at is that we help support other departments and the work that folks in the medical boards office with the black belt project two three years ago that transformed the HEDIS and electronic HEDIS process. Second in a row six sigma. We realized [Service members] that weren't functioning well in society, are doing well and shows how our quality. I also want to give a shout out to the customer service folks, [leadership], and

- ... One of the indirect measures that I'll mention that reflects the quality of the care that we give here is that throughout my career and most frequently now, I have consistently received feedback about providers, nurses, ancillary staff, and administrative staff who have since left the facility or retired or transferred elsewhere. People in other health care systems love our people. They always do. I always hear this over and over again. I get feedback from other facilities, you name it, I've heard from Kaiser, I've heard from various facilities around the country. They really take the initiative to tell us we really love the product that you have and that you're sending us. I would be inclined to say that there is no quality of care measurement that occurs here measures that. I would also be inclined to say that probably is one index that is very vital. It's not just us. We don't just get up and look in the mirror every day and say we love me. Other people love us too.

Question to Audience: What kinds of challenges do you face? Or what kinds of things do you face that can make a day rough when you are attempting to implement quality efforts?

Responses from Audience:
- ... We have an issue with supplies. I understand the hospital is trying to save money and centralize ordering but in the last year it has been the absolute worst in the [time] that I have been here. We can't get ear tips to test some kids. There was a day ... we didn't have baby blankets. How as a parent would you feel if you came to a hospital and your baby is wrapped in a towel because there is no baby blanket. We can't even though we've moved on to electronic medical records, there isn't any copy paper. You know our department ran out of copy paper and we had to borrow from another department and then we get the one box, we have to return it to that department because they lent us theirs. Those are just some examples of issues we have ... and it is the worst [in my time here]. I think we need to trust the department supply people to know what that department needs. When we put it up to the [leadership] level, they do not understand what we are doing.

- Supply process [calls for] too many fingers in the approval process

- ... I think our biggest struggle ... is the amount of turnover that we have among our staff. We have very junior nurses that come and they stay for a year or less and that is one of the most critical points of step one. We have [Service members] who are made to go to different departments after a year or less. And we need people that need to learn more than the basics. We need people to stay long enough to get beyond the novice nurses that become you know they will never become experts, we need than to be more than novice especially you know with service lines that are you know like really intense like the cardiothoracic line, you know we have a lot of issues with training, and the volume and high turnover staff.

Question to Audience: What are some other challenges?

Responses from Audience:
- ... working with the HEDIS matrix and wanting to keep the records and enrollment correct. You know patient files are a real problem. We don't know how to make any of it match up with what is in DEERS, what is in AHLTA and ... DEERS handshake annually, you know there are patients still on our provider panels that we know are deceased, network patients that flip flop back and forth that we know enrolled here and going into town. So data management, accurate data, keeping up to date data.

- One of the things that I have noticed with difficulty in providing quality is moving people that provide the quality. People that provide mind body meditation, yoga.

Question to Audience: When you see an issue, when you face a challenge regarding implementing quality, do you know how to address it? Do you know how to solve the problem? Do you know who to talk to?

Responses from Audience:
- ... [on a major survey for the home health model] they have an 1800 number. Out of 1100 emergency room surveys done and 75% had not heard of the number. ... why do I have three domino pizza numbers and no number for TRICARE? You have a problem because that information is not available, no one knows the number. I still have not seen that number so you have more people winding up in the emergency room that may be necessary because they have no one to call.

- ... when I got home from work, I stopped by my mailbox and talked to my neighbor. He was a retired [Service member] who informed me that he had gotten a letter from TRICARE this week that he could no longer be seen here at [this MTF]. And he could call the number on that letter; for two days [he called] and all he could do was leave a message. So if you have a contact number for you, we need it here today. So every time you send the letter out telling a retiree that he can no longer be seen here, that's wrong. People feel like that they have been kicked to the curb and they don't know whether they can come back here.

Questions Related to Access to Care

Question to Audience: Do your appointment templates and schedules meet demand?

Responses from Audience:
- No.

- Our clinic, I would say the answer is yes. I can't speak for all the clinics .... From our perspective system is working. On the other hand if we get routine consultations for low level concerns or something standard, it could be a couple of weeks. But from our perspective it is working.

- ... We have a couple clinics that do really good ... where a patient can come in next week but we have a couple of clinics that are booking beyond the 28 day access. We just don't have an appointment schedule for them. We have a couple of clinics where we literally just don't have anything within the 28 days, there is no appointment times for these patients. We do see where a lot of times we will have to push these patients out for like gynecological issue with abnormal vaginal bleeding, we are scheduling 25 to 30 days out which is which is just not good. Some of the clinics like he was saying oncology there is something available like next week but a lot of them don't. I think it is clinic dependent; some of them work and some of them don't.

- I'm speaking as a consumer of the health care system and I work in inpatient, I used to work in a clinic, you call for an appointment, they say they do not have an opening at the certain time you are asking, we [say] ... okay when can I schedule one, but their answer is from many different clinics that our schedule is just not open yet so you have to put it on your calendar to call back.

Question to Audience: When do you release schedule for booking?

Responses from Audience:
- I don't think there is a hard and fast rule. It is clinically dependent. But I also want to say that there are examples of when it does work. That's what I want to say. They do a good job ... it is amazing. They are very understanding, they do a good job.

- I'm speaking as internal customer, it is very clinic dependent. As an internal customer, trying to get a PHA appointment, it's a dream, you are wishing upon a star. It is clinic dependent. As a female, those female appointments are extremely difficult to obtain. And you have a PHA deadline so I just want to put it out there.

- I think it is dependent on central appointment. Although ped clinic has always been great about giving appointments same day, next day, at the central clinic there were people ahead of me on the phone. When there are 29 people ahead of you on the line, that's at least 30 minutes.

- I just checked on board and I don't even have my name tag yet. And I came on board and I need my PHA appointment. The military health clinic was able to refer me to the OB clinic who checked every single clinic in the area to try and get me an appointment to fit my deadline and in fact they were able to take me in that afternoon. So, I think it is clinic dependent but access to care, they know and they are trying. I was very impressed with that.

Appendix 1. Introduction

Question to Audience: What needs to happen? How can we get this more consistent?

Responses from Audience:

- ... I have to say that we need to standardize the system and I think that is where the problem lies. We need to, I know there are different clinics and it is dependent on the specialty. I have worked in many different areas. And I know that the patient load changes and we probably need to do detailed study to see how many providers we have per you know the amount of patients they see. And try to standardize it. I know it's hard I know its military and it is very different than working in the outside world so we need to maybe copy system that works in other areas.

- ... I had an issue with this for quite some time. When we book these appointments and they get a reminder call and on that reminder call it says please press 2 if you want to cancel your appointment, there are many patients that do cancel their appointment because they can't make it and it doesn't go thru system and that appointment still says and now we have no-shows. We call the patients and we tell them about the missed appointment and they say well I canceled that. But it's not showing up in the system.

- I think it's kind of interesting that you lead access to care with this question because while we provide a quality product with what we have you have to take into account that the furlough slowed down civilian hiring so the reason we are suffering is because there was ... such a withdrawal from civilian staff ... because people were leaving, the uncertainty of temporary positions versus permanent positions so people are finding permanent jobs elsewhere and the military has been trying its best to make up with whatever they have left. So this question of our access to care yeah our access to care is insane right now but we are doing the best we can with what we have. And it is because of the furlough and because there are bigger things going on in the world right now and we have to take that into account and what we are truly doing. We are doing the best we can with what we have. I see permanent positions opening up where I am ... But right now, we are scrambling to find office space for these new people coming in for our access to care but it is an unfair question to lead into with quality first and then how is your access to care

- Fill empty employee billets that are currently gapped

- Hiring process requires that, even when we know someone is leaving we need to wait until they are gone before we can post. No overlap is a problem. Need to hire into a hot seat. Leaves a gap otherwise...

- Make it easier to fire civilian employees

- [Give] better feedback to clinics with accountability for customer service/patient flow-through

- In regards to access to care, I had a [condition] in June and I can't get an MRI till middle of July.

- Compare patient load to appointment slots available by doctor (i.e., why is OB/GYN not filling slots) ...

Question to Audience: How often do you book each type of these types of appointments prior to a patient leaving the MTF? Follow-up, PCM to a specialty clinic, office visit, outpatient procedures. Comments?

Responses from Audience:
- ... I had my OB care here at the hospital. I never left my appointment without my next appointment being booked and them telling me exactly where I had to go, the labs, the follow up, everything was extremely processed. I may have had to wait 30 minutes to see my provider, but I did see the provider. And I always left happy.

- ... I have never had a problem getting any appointment that I needed here and then I called a couple of weeks ago because I had [an issue] and I wasn't sure what it was and they said nothing, I'm getting old, that's all it is. For a follow-up appointment, when I see the PCM, he says I'm going to put you in for a consult with this place or that place and they call me to tell me my scheduled appointment time. So, I don't see a problem.

- For inpatient booking appointments, I can tell you it is part of our discharge criteria that when they leave here, they have an appointment. The inpatients do not leave without making a follow-up appointment. Actually, I can tell you that those physicians make the follow-up appointment themselves.

- For the specialties, you can't really do it. It's kind of equivalent to making a promise that you can't really keep. I mean 6 weeks out for peds, PCP, but typically for specialists, you typically don't have a 2 week follow up. We usually have like a 3 month follow up and even if that. So that being the case, you ask patient to go to the front of desk, and you say go ahead and make an appointment with them to make apt 3 months amount.

Questions Related to Patient Safety

Question to Audience: Safety: how do you report a safety issue or concern?

Responses from Audience:
- For patient safety, we have event reporting on front page of internet, we have good catch [Catch of the day?], the safety hotline, I mean it's almost like everywhere. We are looking or anywhere with a safety issue.

Question to Audience: What do you do when you see problem? Do you see problem? What types of problems do you see?

Responses from Audience:

- Duplicative records kept.

- I have noticed they have wheelchairs available like at parking but here no wheelchairs so an elderly wife bringing in her elderly husband has to walk, try to find a wheelchair has to walk halfway across the parking structure leaving her husband in the car.

- To address that, now they do have concierge at traffic circle and wheelchairs there and they do advertise that but we patient safety need to do a better job, they are trying safety begins with culture of safety. A culture where you don't have to wait. The command has embraced the culture of safety. We talk about TeamSTEPPS®, all eyes, all ears, all voices empowered, all encouraged to speak up about issue or concern. So that is definitely something that has been an issue. It is more and more important to report. If you are in the OR, in the case, you speak up if you are suffering in silence a lot of patients are suffering in silence too. You say if you are a new tech, you are a new tech student, we can say sir I'm not sure that this is the right next step. And my role as a ... [provider] is to say thank you for making me aware of that. There is culture where there is no bias or fear of retaliation or concern that you may be wrong.

- So I'm on the low life but I am directly connected to patients and quality side by side. As far as STEPPS, it is by far the most vast improvement where anyone can challenge once, can challenge twice and then cuss at you because that is the culture. And as far as safety goes, you can't walk here on this campus without hitting 300 people looking at you that would remind us of your appointment. It is a very safe place.

Open discussion: Audience was invited to provide comments

Responses from Audience:

- ... it has been a great hour... in the end it is patients who determine our success and I think most of the command knows this but when you ask our patients, 19000 responses in 12 months, our overall satisfaction is 96%. You can't get 96% of people in this room to agree that this is a bottle of water. That is with 19000 patients. And there is a metric called met-promoter so 96% of our patients would recommend our services to family and friends and availability of appointments is at 92% from 19000 responses and that is the best in the business.

- One of the concerns that I have is one of the parts we do, for example we do pap smears, or lung cancer screening, we do not have a centralized database to prevent people from falling through the cracks. We do a really good job with notifying providers but that provider may get deployed next week or transferred I think we need to have a centralized database. We do a great job finding stuff but we have patients that fall through cracks.

- ... [MRI] ... just one of those clinics in high demand ... It is unfortunate that right now it is at 28 days to get an appointment. The problem ... is that ... [patients are] schedule[d]

24 7, 7 days a week, some people just don't show up and unfortunately the no shows could have been given to someone else …

- Training is suffering because we are asked to do it during leave – and the system doesn't pay for as much training anymore.

Site 2 Beneficiary Town Hall Questions and Answers

The following text reproduces the Town Hall facilitator questions and audience responses, transcribed as close to verbatim as possible during the session. It also includes, in a separate section, comments from two individuals who replied to the MTF's Public Affairs Officer's invitation that attendees send further comments to the MTF web site, and from one individual who provided written comments to a site visit team member after the event. Information that could potentially identify individual participants has been omitted for privacy purposes.

Approximately 210 people attended this Town Hall meeting.

Questions Related to Quality of Care

Question to the Audience: Do you think you get quality care here at [this MTF] and if you think you get good quality care here at [this MTF] tell us why?

Responses from the Audience:
- Yes I believe we get quality care and the care has improved over the past several years. Having said that RelayHealth has been a tremendous asset in improving the overall care of the patients here who have internet access. In 2002 [this MTF] was a pioneer and early adapter in tracking records through [a web-based system]. On RelayHealth they have a link to [the previous system] except I believe [this MTF] at some time has eliminated [that system] where you would access all of your records and now patients must get their own record which causes a great amount of extra work for [this MTF]. It interferes with quality of time for [this MTF's] patients and refers to paper records which I believe is dinosaur. Thank you!

- Ok, so mine is more of a personal example, but as far as quality care … [personal information omitted] we are assigned to [a specific] medical home which is very convenient access wise and location wise. My son was recently diagnosed with [personal information omitted] … we were seen at [the medical home] and immediately referred here to [this MTF's] [specialty surgeon] … It wasn't anything that they could treat but we were given the diagnostic test very quickly. The MRI, x-rays, everything that we needed and then put in touch with [a hospital outside the MTF] to the [specialty surgeon] who has seen this condition and was able to treat it so from diagnosis to him actually having surgery … if it had not been done so quickly the prognosis would not have been as good as it is. So I have been nothing but pleased.

- I went into the breast pathways system … [personal information omitted] and I can't say enough about it. For women who have breast cancer … I read in the paper this morning that there is concern that women are not getting enough treatment in the military hospitals of the VA. To me it has been outstanding. I have had fabulous doctors that have track me over the years and I can't say enough about how grateful I am because I have had friends who have gone through the civilian system that didn't have near the level of care that I have had.

- I have to congratulate [this MTF] on everything that they do. I have had personal experience with [personal information omitted] [multiple surgeries] ... Now I am having trouble with [personal information omitted] ... and I have had this since the last week of February and have not been able to get a hold of anybody to see me until tomorrow. Between the MRI and now it has been almost a month and a half.

- ... [Personal information omitted] ... I have never gotten better care than I have had here at [this MTF]. I cannot say that the care is better anywhere. I have been so pleased whether it has been operating room intensive care. My husband was medevac'd here with [personal information omitted] ... and the staff was just fantastic.

- I have to say that my care from the specialist and sub specialist here has been very good but I have some serious concerns about my primary care....

- ... I have been very disappointed in being able to access breast care... [personal information omitted] ... I couldn't even get a mammogram here and I work here. [personal information omitted] ... when I went to see my primary care provider she would only look at [personal information omitted] ... which is part of the process and told me to go see my civilian provider who could not get an appointment within 8 weeks and she did nothing including not reviewing records or talking to other specialist. This is my third primary care provider in [my time] at [this MTF] and none of them has put my condition together.

Question to the Audience: How many of you have gone out into the network for care? Among those who have done that, tell me how quality compares out of the network as opposed to [this MTF].

Responses from the Audience:
- ... I need to compliment [this MTF]. [Relative] [personal information omitted] ... went to a civilian provider [and] he was told he needed surgery. It would have taken him six weeks to get surgery he needed on the outside. He came to [this MTF] and he was seen on Friday in the Acute Care Clinic. He was sent to neurosurgery the very same day for evaluation. He was asked to come back on Monday and was moved into surgery that day and he walked home the next day. I have had excellent primary care providers. I have had one for [over 10] years and one for [over 5] years. Now I have a new provider for the past 6 months and I have tried several times to make appointments and have been unsuccessful in [this MTF]. I always have to meet with someone else.

- ... I have seen changes in primary care ... we have seen a lot of issues with patients who have seen mid-level providers never getting to see an actual doctor. Or, if you see a doctor you get a 25 min time slot which is useless maybe even less. Also when we move from doctor to doctor there are no transitions of care from your past provider to your new provider unless you have one of those very good providers and that is a small percentage. There is no hand over of you from one provider to the next.

- ... I have been a patient at [this MTF] for a long time .... From [this MTF] they have referred me to the outside. I have been referred for [personal information omitted] ... When I had [personal information omitted] ... I was referred outside ... very excellent care and that's why I can't understand why everyone cannot get that same level of care when I am not special. I am just like you guys. The care is there and your primary care doctor needs to refer you if you cannot be seen here.

- ... we have the best cancer care all the way through the different sections. From the doctors explaining problems through the chemo and the radiation. I don't think you find anything better around here.

Question to the Audience: How should [this MTF] improve the quality of care here?

Responses from the Audience:
- My husband has had several issues and he has been referred outside and inside and I have to say that I think it comes down to the doctors themselves. My husband has said that he has been in every department or division except OBGYN. [Audience laughed] The one doctor who said we are rolling out the [treatment], he went over to the vascular clinic and talked to the doctor there and his cardiologist. To me that is a great doctor. It would be nice if the doctors could get together and go over that person's issues. That makes you feel good that you are getting quality care.

- My wife and myself have had excellent care here. We have had excellent care outside but the problem that we have both run into is when we've been referred outside then we come back our primary care doctor can't seem to get information from the doctors outside the doctors that need to be seen later if you need to see a specialist. I ended up having to hand carry the information. I had to go outside, get it from the doctor, bring it here. They have sent it several times and it has gotten lost. There seems to be a lack of ability for [this MTF] as a whole for [this MTF] to communicate once they send you out of their system.

- [Personal information omitted]... We are a mixed group and I love us because we need us because we are skilled and our staff is skilled. There once was time when we had a committee which was a requirement called the Healthcare Consumer Advisory Council which I attended for a number of years. It has dissolved. It was a requirement to meet once a month. Can you all look into that please? Thank you.

- Get one system for the pharmacy and stick to it! Every time we come around there is a new system. It is ridiculous. And to sit and wait for 2 hours for a prescription is nuts! Please fix the system, one system. Let the staff know that we are here because we are sick not because we want to argue with you. That's my biggest gripe.

- I want to echo the comment about the pharmacy. I don't know who came up with the system. You get one number so they can identify you then they tell you to have a seat then when your name comes up you get another number and they tell you to come back in 3 hours. If you live 30 minutes away and you come to get a prescription, what do you do for 3 hours. If you miss it you start all over again. It's the worst system!

Questions Related to Access to Care

Question to the Audience: How easy is it for you schedule an appointment at [this MTF]?

Responses from the Audience:
- I would like to say that [this MTF] needs to synchronize medical records. They do it well at the VA, probably better than here. For the prescriptions especially you need to have the same information on both ends of the system.

- It is not very difficult. It depends a lot on the clinic. I have no trouble trying to get in [this MTF] or trying to reach my doctor. If I need to get a hold of him, I can go online.... [personal information omitted] I had several operations and I got excellent care from the providers at [this MTF]. I probably would not be here if it were not for them.

- This is an outstanding place. I have been around the world [several] times and [this MTF] is very good. Just like everything else, nothing is perfect. It's not easy to get an appointment. I call to set one up and they tell me there is no availability can you call back. Then when I call back they still can't setup an appointment. So what I do ma'am is walk right in tell them I need to see a doctor and you know what try it, it works

- ... I don't know what the reason is .... I have had to wait over six weeks to go to one of the clinics and I have been able to bypass that by going directly to that clinic and getting an appointment that way. I have been satisfied with [this MTF] but as of late it has been more difficult than before.

- I have gone to [this MTF] ... [personal information omitted] and have had excellent care here, however I have fallen through the cracks. The majority of my care is good. Until there was RelayHealth, I had a difficult time getting in touch with my doctor but now I am very happy with this and at least I am getting feedback. ... [personal information omitted]... I would like to live until I am in my 90s. I just need to be listened to.

- Hello, I am an active service member and we are in the system all of the time and one of the things that I have noticed that it is difficult to get that access without having a primary care manager who is managing the system on which providers you go to and getting feedback. It is difficult to see that with people who are not more vocal.

- Some of the people who have retired, it seem to be a bit easier. I'm am active duty and it's difficult. I went to one of the department couple of weeks ago and they told me that I have to wait until August. I will probably go and see the provider if they are available and then reschedule another appointment because the initial one is just to see what's wrong with you. Quality is not that good for active duty service members because most of the time they assume that there is not a whole lot wrong with you and that we are just trying to get out of duty. My commander got involved somehow and he bullied my care provider around and told him that there was nothing wrong with me. …

- … I have been referred out because I am on TRICARE+. Recently my wife and I have been having trouble getting referrals out since we have had a change in health care providers. We cannot get a referral out and TRICARE is telling us that we have to start the process all over again by getting a primary care provider and then we are being told that if we get a primary care provider outside of the military system that we get unenrolled in TRICARE+. I just want to bring this problem up because it is happening to me and to my wife.

Question to the Audience: How does getting an appointment in the network compare to getting an appointment at [this MTF]?

Responses from the Audience:
- I think [this MTF] is wonderful. Most of the time my provider calls me before I call them. We cannot lose the fact that this is an active duty [Service member] hospital and they should be receiving first service. The rest of us are just along for the ride. This is their hospital.

- Communication with outside including the VA has got to be improved considerably so everyone is on the same sheet of music. Calling to make an appointment is like spitting into a hurricane. So there is some frustration. You sit in the pharmacy and you start collecting spider webs because you don't move.

- One of the things that I really enjoy is RelayHealth. I use it consistently. Last week I needed lab work done. I emailed my doctor; she scheduled it and I got the results back in 2 days. I have had several [procedures] and the care has been wonderful. In [a different state] I was misdiagnosed several times and if I had stayed I would not be here today.

- Since January I have had three different providers and how I find out about is through a message in RelayHealth and then I have to go through the whole process again. Some doctors are not even in the system to be added so we can communicate with them.

- I have had an easy time getting appointments for myself and my kids. If they happen to be full we have received referrals to urgent care that same day. The TRICARE system in general is not that good. I had to call them four times to get an appointment. They kept telling me that they didn't have anything available in a particular time frame and I ended calling the specialty clinic myself and got an appointment the very next week.

- Is there any way to add the health care system outsourced to other hospitals because we were told that we couldn't go outside of the system and we had to use [this MTF] however we live in [a different city] and I don't have problem with the care here at [this MTF] but travel wise we have to come a long distance. There have been times when the traffic is horrible and I have missed appointments.

- TRICARE online and RelayHealth has been excellent. I have been able to get appointment within a day or two of a request. It has been wonderful for my family and I.

Question to the Audience: How satisfied are you with respect to getting appointments?

Responses from the Audience:
- I think there is a glitch in the system. They want us to give up our primary care provider here to get one outside. There is something wrong here. I had to go to the ER to be admitted and that is ass backwards to me.

- My wife and I have had excellent care here at [this MTF]. I have a practical recommendation. I get medication from the Veteran's Administration and it comes through the mail every 90 days. If something like that could be implemented at [this MTF] that would go a long way. It would take a great deal of stress off of the pharmacy.

- If I can I would like to tell you how my entire month has gone. I was able to get an immediate appointment of my yearly checkup. I got a [procedure]… done today without a problem. I am having a … [procedure] on Friday here. I have absolutely no problems and no complaints with [this MTF]. It is fantastic here. From A to Z and back again.

- Every time … I go to make an appointment it's, "No I'm sorry we don't have anything for 4-6 weeks." I could go to the emergency room but I would like to have my appointment before 4-6 weeks.

- Yes, I have a foot in both doors. Both [this MTF] and the VA. VA will manage all of the medication from [this MTF]. The pharmacies are talking to each other. Otherwise, [this MTF] and [another location] [are] so far ahead of everyone else.

- I can never get in to specialty clinics and I see a lot of specialty clinics. It is always a two month minimum. I can't tell you how many times I will make an appointment at a clinic and TRICARE will call and tell me to that it was cancelled and to start all over again. Not quite sure why they do that.

Questions Related to Patient Safety

Question to the Audience: Do you feel that the care that you get at [this MTF] is safe?

Responses from the Audience:
- I have had excellent care in the specialty clinics that I have been to but if you call TRICARE to book an appointment they say that we don't have our calendar up you'll have to call back. By the time you call back on the first day of the month they won't have the month's calendar so you can't book an appointment. That's very annoying.

- In a specialty clinic, the doctor was afraid that I may have [condition] so I was referred out and I can't be seen until the end of July, which is two and a half months. That's a long time.

- I had a conversation with a doctor via email to get an idea of whether or not my medication will be changed and all she said to me is that it won't change. And that response was not good enough for me. I want detailed responses because I want to be involved in my health care not treated like a child.

- I have a worry that something may be taken away. Is there anything coming that I should know about?

- Safe care is keeping the patient and the doctor safe. Half the people here are not sure if they should unsheathe, touch, not touch. When in doubt ask them what they're doing. The providers have a responsibility to keep us safe from previous patient they have seen and being honest about my health. I am very conscientious about new providers with a lack of experience. When in doubt stop and ask questions.

- I feel safe here and I feel like I am getting safe care from my provider.

Question to the Audience: If you have a concern about safety, quality, or access, how have you expressed your concerns?

Responses from the Audience:
- Realizing that it is a training hospital, sometime it nags me. I was recently diagnosed with [personal information omitted] … and I have had a lot of blood work done. I like the fact that when I go to the lab I go to the same person. I like the fact that when I have concerns about my health I get my questions answered. However there was an incident when a technician took out a pair of scissors and cut a lollipop for my daughter and she popped it right in her mouth. I addressed it head and asked him why he did it and where have those scissors been. I feel safe because I use my voice.

- My main problems have been with interns. There was one instance when they gave me a shot in my nerve instead of the right place. Another time a doctor misdiagnosed a … [personal information omitted] ….

- When I first came here it far exceeded anybody, it has gone downhill so badly. Some doctors are doing their own things. Some doctors refuse to see any patient outside of their panel. I heard of RNs verbally abusing the LPNs and not being reprimanded. The problem is the system and people are not being held accountable for their bad actions.

- [Personal information omitted] ... I know that here at [this MTF], they are concerned with your safety. I have been twice now told in the pharmacy that one medication that I am taking does not interact well with another medication that I have been prescribed. They have caught that mistake and pointed out to me. You also need to be your own advocate with it comes to your safety. Make sure they ask your name and label things.

Additional Beneficiary Comments Submitted after the Town Hall Meeting via the MTF's Public Affairs Office Website and Written Comments Provided to a Site Visit Team Member:

- When I asked [my provider] ... to renew the Handicapped Parking tag the civilian doctor had given me, [the provider] ... refused because "I don't know anything about your [condition]" (I had provided records) and "there are lots of people worse than you."

- ... [At the outpatient unit where I go] ... There is no check in/sign in desk and if you take a seat in what appears to be the waiting area, every office person who walks by very pointedly will not make eye contact and acknowledge your presence...

- There is no transparency or explanation to patients for policies at [this MTF]. I believe even the PCMs may not have correct information. It seems to me that there must be some kind of quota (number of patients seen which somehow equates to dollars they receive) that is more important than the timely access to first level quality care at [this MTF].

- RelayHealth is being used effectively by my [providers]. I feel comfortable asking a question or requesting an appointment because I get a response within 24 hours (not an appointment necessarily, but a response that, at the least, acknowledges my request). I also like the informative messages I get such as the schedule for flu shots, the change in the pharmacy hours, and events such as the Town Hall Meeting.

- TRICARE appointments phone line cannot make appointments beyond the end of the current calendar month. Repeated calls near the end of the month tell me there are no openings for the following month. How am I supposed to schedule a follow up appointment for 6 weeks from my last visit? This is true even for surgical follow up appointments. Four years ago I could get appointments at TRICARE Online, but that is not the case now. There are never any appointments

- [Specialty clinic] ... puts me on a wait list every year for my annual follow up. They call me to schedule the appointment directly rather than through TRICARE ... For follow up appointments in less than a year but beyond the current month, my doctors keep their own appointment calendars, pencil in an upcoming appointment, and I receive a confirmation call as soon as it is entered into the computer system. If interim issues arise, I am always encouraged to call the clinic directly and immediately.

- I asked for an outside referral to a nearby civilian [provider] I had previously used for back pain. [This MTF] refused to send me outside the MTF, but could not give me an appointment in less than 6 weeks ... [personal information omitted] ... I then called my civilian [provider], and got an appointment in 1 week

- ... and I wonder if $13.00 for a three month prescription through Express Scripts is worth the wait, especially considering travel costs. The problem is that [this MTF's] providers cannot (easily) get a Rx to Express Scripts. With civilian e-prescribing, the patient can have the Rx sent to literally any pharmacy he desires at the mere strike of a computer key, yet the only option for [this MTF's] prescribers is to send Rx to a pharmacy in the system. I think everyone would benefit if [this MTF's] providers could send the Rx electronically not only within the system but to Express scripts or even civilian pharmacies.

- There appears to be a disconnect between the TRICARE appointment system and the actual availability of appointments in specialty clinics. Several times TRICARE has told us nothing available and their schedule only goes out for two weeks (or a month), but standing at the clinic's desk one is likely to miraculously find numerous appts available, same day, next day, etc. Why is that?

- I appreciate the regular notifications I receive from [this MTF] about general health and wellness services. Annual flu shots, nutritional counseling, and other services are ... available

- Pharmacy services ... [have been] a bit challenging during the past few months because of wait time ... [but] are easy to utilize

- ... my treatment could not have been better managed than at [this MTF]. [My provider] and nursing staff supported me ... physically, emotionally, and spiritually. [Procedures] ... were thoroughly explained ... and scheduled ... to ensure I could balance treatment ... and other commitments

- ... [this MTF] is ... an effective, caring institution

- My primary care physician ... maintains excellent communication with me via electronic mailings ... I always have a record of our discussions and decisions

- Scheduling appointments poses no barrier – I am often able to see [my provider] within 2-3 days of making a call. He has full copies of my medical history ...

- I am a full partner in my care [and am] often asked for my opinion and input

August 29, 2014 — Appendix 1. Introduction

Site 2 Staff Town Hall Questions and Answers

The following text reproduces the Town Hall facilitator questions and audience responses, transcribed as close to verbatim as possible during the session. It also includes, in a separate section, comments from two individuals who provided a handwritten note to the Facilitator immediately following the event. Information that could potentially identify individual participants has been omitted for privacy purposes.

Approximately 60 people attended this Town Hall meeting.

Questions Related to Quality of Care

Question to Audience: Is quality a priority here? And if it is, what do you see and experience? If not, what is it that you're seeing that it is not?

Responses from Audience:
- I think the goal of the people who work here is to have quality health care. I've been floating here … [around] multiple departments but there's not a lot of time due to … training that I have to take … and quality suffers. I can [provide care] … but [I am not] [as effective as I could be] … since I'm constantly being pulled and aside from vital signs changing stations … [I am a provider who] wants to give care, that's my perspective, but I don't know what I'm doing.

- … As far as in [inpatient unit] … I know clinically what to do … but to facilitate a new birthing mom, I'm not the right person to do this.

- … Quality is excellent especially compared to the outside. Doctors or the nurses in the VA are pressured to see so many patients per hour … [this MTF] compared to the other providers or doctors outside [this MTF] – just like at the VA are pressured to see many patients per hour but quality in [this MTF] has not been affected

Question to the Audience: How in your view does quality at [this MTF] compare to quality out in the network?

Responses from the Audience:
- … Support staff is so overloaded on what they should do … It all comes down to the specialty care clinic and the PCP (Primary Care Physician). There are no standards given by the clinics for a CNA (Certified Nurse's Assistant). There are no formal trainings and it's all word of mouth, as to what [CNAs are] … supposed to do.

- … [there is] …no standard operating procedure or no set rules or guidelines. Seems that there's no structure … because [when the] [leadership] changes the rules change too

- You get frustrated what you're supposed to do from this team to [the next] … team – You get frustrated when you're moved from one team to another … You are pressured to learn all the changes and this is a big issue

Question to Audience: What barriers or challenges do you face in implementing quality improvement initiatives?

Responses from the Audience:
- [As a patient here] ... I have been unhappy ... nurses are phenomenal, friendly and helpful ... [but] doctors look at their screen – didn't look at me – and stayed on [the] screen... [for] four months, I've [seen 6 doctors] ... and I was [mis]diagnosed ... I think that's substandard

- I was seen by Family Medicine and came back because I was able to get a slot

- Going along with the work overload and the lack of training: We are feast or famine, we are burnt out ... We have call outs ... we don't have staffing to support it ... We have patients who require one nurse to two patients. Because of the work overload, they get two patients for half a nurse (half of the nurse's time – or better yet four patients to one nurse) ...

- ... As a ... [health care provider], whenever a patient doesn't get a sponge bath, I get complaints.
  ... I give up breaks a lot, my lunch breaks ... We will not turn [anyone] ... away. I'm dancing around and doing scanning and calling, things that I'm not supposed to be doing. We lost a lot of support. Running the hall for keys to the cabinet is such a waste of my time so quality suffers

- [Supervisors say] we want to see more of you or you will lose your job.

- Quality is suffering. You are making me use a template that I don't have time to edit, so [I have] ... to choose to either make a splint or make a copy ... We are hitting breaking point.

- [We are being told] ... we need you to double up ... We need you to do 2.5 patients ... I don't know where success is, do your job, keep your head down ... At the end of the day you just keep on going (audience clapped)
- ... the providers are not entering the orders in the computer ...

- There are 20-30-50 people in the waiting room and three clerks are checking them in and we still get the things that we need to be done.

- I work in the ... [specialty clinic] ... and [I think] that [with] the emphasis to decrease [people going to the] ... network we sacrifice quality of care patient ...we have the skill but ... we don't have the set up to effectively manage it... guidance on [base] is that we [shouldn't] ... push anyone off [base] to purchased care. So the quality of care is sacrificed.

- We do everything and this is from staff trainings, to equipment orientation and the clinic's appointment time … the system has a lot of redundancy, this creates extra work

- Training is an issue – takes out a lot of time

- … Patients come through pre-op, [get] paper work, then come back – same paper work lost … then when it's time for the appointment [paperwork is lost and must be re-done] …

- Staff that we have – we have to do whatever is needed

- Listening [to] what was touched on, we are here and our hearts are in the same place – teamwork is what works, phenomenal staff – Saturday nights, we work, its true I float and that I'm all over the place but there's needs to be someone in the room with patients

- We do work well as the team … we are so short staffed that there is no way you can do it on your own

Questions Related to Access to Care

Question to Audience: Do your appointment templates and schedules meet appointment demand?

Responses from Audience:
- … we encounter roadblocks. Providers/doctors/PAs are having problems with the template and scheduling. We get sick calls and we send them to the patient care since they have medical homes. [There aren't enough providers/ doctors/PAs for the 800 enrolled in the medical home program].

- There is a template and it's not a joke but at the start of the day it's 10 and by the end of the day, it's 30. There's no flexibility might need 20 – TRICARE [is a problem for us]

- TRICARE cannot ascertain level of complexity – [they have] never seen our process. They (TRICARE call center) cannot figure out accuracy and honestly, at the end of the day, you still see a full list.

- TRICARE hotline, they always miss bookings on specialty care and follow up

- You have to scroll on multiple screens

- Patients call TRICARE call center, the likelihood is better than getting someone on the front desk, there's not enough staff

- … It took me 6 months to get seen here because I'm registered in [another location] … Is there a way I can be registered to both here and [that location] that would be great.

- ... we had to cap employee hiring and because of that staff has gone down ... and there's not enough staff to do the things we have to do

- ... Our hearts are there, and [in order not to] cut corners ... we end up staying longer and cut lunch breaks. We need enough staff to (help / assist) our [Service members'] needs

- ... a lot has changed [since speaker has been with this MTF] ... [this MTF] [is known] for change. Increased flow of patient care. TRICARE is in the middle of it. Family practice appointments have to go thru TRICARE call center and this is not updated

- Communication is a [problem] ... [doctors are] distracted and it's disappointing and I'm trying to get the trust of [this MTF]. Let's go back to the old days

- ... [The scheduling branch] has a certain amount [limited] of staff ... [they] ... care and ... also miss breaks. ... [The scheduling branch] build[s] your templates ... and ... hear a lot of bashing. If you call at 6, that clinic has those appointments frozen and they have not released them ... Clinics have control and misuse it ... Clinics need to look at the criteria ... If you take a look at your criteria anyone can decipher any stipulation that you put in these appointments, not [the scheduling branch's] decision.

- ... we just talked about follow up – what was said, we mostly have newborns and they are not enrolled. So another thing is that access to care.

- We pull the tracker every hour and recapture some of those referrals and pull them back in [pull every half hour]. [They fill in their track/template every hour and recapture some of the referrals inputted. They pull them every half hour instead of the hourly since they change very often.]

Question to the Audience: How often does your clinic respond to secure messaging from patients within the time requirements as directed by policy/guidance?

Responses from the Audience:
- Is that the same as RelayHealth? ... secure messaging is predominantly a nurse or medical telephone consult and they return my calls within 72 hours from the time I leave a message. We get an answer from the provider and somebody will get back with them.

- I use secure messaging for my husband. Family medicine emailed me back within 30 – 60 minutes. No issues with it.

- We use secure messaging with results from pathology reports, internal medicine with orders, [but we have] ... no idea how others are doing theirs.

- We use the secure network and it works real [well]; I can't say anything bad about it.

Question to the Audience: What do you do if you are unable to meet the patient's desired appointment timeline?

Responses from the Audience:
- If there are no appointments, we get them through the charge nurse and they will give them the desired time.

- ... I have investigated the number of patients seen by the provider, [she's stating that the clinic appointments are not – frozen] ... someone needs to supervise the supervisor ...

What is "freezing the system?" Freezing the templates are blocking the appointment system and no one can input/add/delete the appointments made in the template and they are considered locked. The lady who spoke was sharing that the majority think that the system is frozen and she said that she sees it and that it's not frozen and thinks that someone needs to supervise the supervisor

Question to Audience: If you are unable to meet the patient's desired appointment timeline, what do you do to make the patient happy?

Responses from Audience:
- ... The 28 day standard rule of providing access to an appointment with a specialty is not possible ... they send the patient to the network. This is a problem with [specialty department]. [This MTF] has the [specialist] but since they (call center) have control of the appointment, they can't assist with the patient. We have set up processes to internally make that appointment and we even can squeeze them (the patients) in for an appointment but the patient will only be seen for five minutes

Questions Related to Patient Safety

Question to Audience: How do you report a safety issue or concern?

Responses from Audience:
- The PSR (Patient Safety Report) is reviewed and is provided to our direct supervisor/boss. They are available online and that's what they use to provide their supervisors to address a safety issue or concern.

Question to Audience: When you are concerned with patient safety, how does the process work?

Responses from Audience:
- Depends on where you're at ... I ended up receiving retaliation so I left the clinic because of it.

- I've never had retaliation but we do have the PSR (Patient Safety Report), we go to the supervisor or the patient safety office.

- [In my department my main issue is how patient visits are conducted and documented] and how people are trained [for these] ... I've seen instances where [patient records do not accurately depict the care they have gotten or should get] ... I'm afraid of retaliation ... [a lot of time this is a function of the time we get] ... Standard is not being maintained ... depends on the individuals ...

- Sometimes, there are road blocks, but we can carry it on.

- There are mechanisms in place, there are also a lot of resources available.

- ... If the concern is with patient information, I send them to the patient services, and then follow-up on what happened to what I submitted. I never found anyone who's not satisfied with the patient services.

- I do review those under the PST (Patient Safety Team) in every clinic. We stay concerned with PSRs and wait for them. We see them and take care of the issues with the PST.

- ... I have a concerning issue that I know I have submitted personally and I have not seen anything that anyone has taken care of this issue I know is happening. I want to see where they go, when will they take action and make changes.
- It's scary, because the PSR is going to be in the report and there's no follow-up on the issue I reported.

- I'm from ... [specialty] department and I see safety issues. We do give a number of grievances to safety and access to care. Some of it is hidden like I'm saying we do get complaints with specialty and these grievances are shared with the boss.

Question to the Audience: Was there any question that was not asked or ideas you have that you would like to address?

Responses from the Audience:
- Customer service training – [patient satisfaction survey] scores are rated. There are complaints about the phone service that patients can't get through to the clinics. They track them through [the patient satisfaction survey] but do not train when there is a customer service issue.

- I take my badge off and I'm standing in line at the desk, [and the clerk] she sees me and will not lift her head up and I timed her...

- ... I think the care begins when a bad experience with the front desk – whether the doctor is nice or not

Additional Staff Comments Submitted to the Facilitator Immediately following the Town Hall Meeting via a Handwritten Note:

- [Enlisted medical personnel] are underutilized in the hospital setting. They are limited to the scope of a CNA taking vitals and delivering patients. They can be trained and have had the training and experience to work in a broader scope. If their competencies are validated and they receive the continuing education to broaden they could provide a lot more care to a lot more people. The [enlisted medical personnel] are motivated for the most part to do this. It will require a checks and balances and a validation process. It should be compared to their responsibility on a line unit to that of a hospital setting.

Site 3 Beneficiary Town Hall Questions and Answers

The following text reproduces the Town Hall facilitator questions and audience responses, transcribed as close to verbatim as possible during the session. Information that could potentially identify individual participants has been omitted for privacy purposes.

Approximately 35 people attended this Town Hall meeting.

Questions Related to Quality of Care

Question to Audience: Tell us about the quality of care you're getting. Are you getting quality of care here and if you are, how do you know? What is the indicator that you are getting it based on your experience?

Responses from Audience:
- The quality of care that is the most efficient and proficient organization that I've ever run into is the lab in the hospital. I've seen people out there and no one ever has to wait. I tip my hat to them.

- The website that we have now for feedback is excellent because that stops me from re-calling and re-calling and re-calling over days and days trying to get a hold of the doctor. It gives me feedback in a day or two. So, I think the website is a good idea.

- I'm very pleased with having the opportunity to able to correspond with my doctors and medical staff through the [secure messaging] system. Whenever I need a renewal on a prescription or referrals, a renewal or referral, then I can go on my laptop and be able to send that to them and they quickly get back with me with the information that I need. So I haven't had to come in here for [some time] … so I'm thankful for that.

- [Personal information omitted] … I have been very impressed by the quality of care at this facility and I've been here enough and seen enough doctors come and go and really doesn't matter whether they come and go or not because the next group that come in are always professional. I echo the comments about the lab, always have good treatment there, always efficient. The pharmacy is always efficient … [Personal information omitted] … the pediatric department is super. And if there is some unusual need that …

the MTF can't handle, they are good at farming us off to a local county or [other hospital] ... to take care of it. So, overall, I have been exceptionally pleased with the quality of care that I've gotten since I've retired. It's been every bit as good since I've been on active duty.

Question to Audience: How many have gone into the network for care outside of this hospital? Tell us about how the quality of care compares between the care you get at this hospital as opposed to what you get out in the network?

Responses from Audience:
- We are new to TRICARE, just this fall. We've had maybe two contacts with the medical care here at this base. If I had to rate it on a scale of 1-10, I would give it a 4 or 5. We were very disappointed. We were new to this doctor that we saw and he didn't really seem to have much time for us. He kept saying okay, okay, okay. He didn't really spend a whole lot of time with us.

- To give you an idea, my first contact, it was my physical. He checked my ears, nose, and throat, listened to my heart, listened to my chest and we were done. In the civilian world, they check everything. You name it and they check it. That didn't happen. And I just thought for a doctor seeing me for the very first time, a physical, that would be a really great place to start but that didn't happen. We're going back outside the network...

- [Personal information omitted] ... I had [a physical] ... and it was not as comprehensive as my active duty here but it was almost the same quality physical. A complete check of every part of me ... I'm sorry that you didn't receive proper care but I've received excellent care.

- [Personal information omitted]... the care that I've received here ... at [this MTF] has been excellent. Overall, I'd give it an A+ ... [but] ... when I went to the civilian facility, there was a considerable amount of information that they had not absorbed even though it had been given to them. When I came back to follow up [at this MTF] ... my PA ... did a very good job but it was obvious to me that when we discussed some of these things, it was because, let me put it this way, because of the way she attacked the problem, I believe that she went through very carefully everything that I had given her. It was obvious to me that something things had dropped through the cracks. The practitioner that I saw I think did a really good job. I don't know how the system works as far as how communication flows.

- [Personal information omitted] ... generally good quality. I did have one case where the doctor here in Family Practice didn't seem to have that much time for me... [personal information omitted] I wanted to get some advice or get an appointment or what not and there were no appointments and this is kind of getting into access of care and it was on a weekend but they said if it was bad enough, I should go the emergency room but it wasn't bad enough, I just wanted to check something. Part of this is also, I noticed the different in quality...they put me in the [specific clinic] here, I think it is and they have longer appointment times [here at this MTF] and I think I had the same doctor ... and he moved over to [specific clinic] and [there] ... is more time to go over results and my experience at the [specific clinic] was better.

- [Personal information omitted]... We've been in the hospital in [specific department] ... and all other aspects of this hospital. In all instances, the continuity has been there and we have never experienced a problem and we have also experienced the outside and we always experienced a problem. Okay. We have never experienced a problem at this hospital. They care about the patient and they go out of their way to ensure you get quality care, you get the safety of the hospital.

Questions Related to Access to Care

Question to the Audience: Tell us about your experience scheduling appointments.

Responses from the Audience:
- ... I spent 6 hours for two days trying to see a doctor for an immediate need and finally the only way I got in to see a doctor at the end of the second day was talking to a triage nurse who was able to get me an appointment.

- We talked to the appointment line where you dial to get the same day appointment. We could not get a same day appointment calling in from 6 in the morning two days in a row. I called to talk to the Nurse Access line. I tried talking to the family practice clinic. I tried to talk to everyone I could possibly talk to just to get in to see a doctor for a [medical] ... appointment need. Couldn't get an appointment to save my life till I got to a triage nurse.

- I have to hand it to the internal medicine clinic. They are superb. They are great. The people will go out of their way. [Specific clinic], those guys are great. They will go out of their way ... You can't look at the [MTF] as a whole, you gotta break it down a little bit. Family Practice has had some issues. This is where the initial quality of care is a problem ... it came from a lack of oversight ... The other clinics ... [and lab are also] ... superb. That truly needs to be looked at.

- ... I think we have lost a TRICARE Kiosk ... here at [this MTF]. I don't remember a reason why that happened. Maybe someone can answer that for me. I'm not sure why. The TRICARE Kiosk or office where we walk into. We want it back. Why did the [Service] do that? Because I believe in face to face. I'm old fashioned. Exactly, face to face. I'll jump on the computer to communicate with people on [secure messaging system] but I do that all the time. I want to communicate with people on TRICARE.

- [Personal information omitted] ... What are the criteria on who can stay on base and who quote unquote gets kicked off. When we got kicked off and went into the Medicare system, it's taking 7 weeks to get an appointment for a new patient appointment. Between those 7 weeks, there are prescriptions that you know come up that need to be provided.

So, I guess the primary question is very little transparency when you turn 65 on who gets to stay in the facility and who gets kicked off base.

- I just wanted to make a comment about the quality and also about access. I think you're looking at the quality for me regarding the comment about the lab but also continuity. [Personal information omitted] ... I have had the same provider and to me that's quality. I don't have to start over with giving my history or someone that doesn't know my overall health. And we can just pick right back up. So with that quality perspective, that continuity of provider makes such a big difference, at least for me ... I do agree with someone over there ... having some issues with Family Practice ... you may not get the same access [across all departments] ... where some providers don't do a full assessment on the initial visit and some do, so maybe standardizing some of that on the initial visit would make sense.

Question to Audience: When you come to this hospital for a doctor's visit, before you leave are you asked to make an appointment for the next time? Do you get appointments for when you want it and how far out are you able to make your appointments?

Responses from Audience:
- When I was trying to get an appointment and I agree with a lot of these people. The lab is fantastic. They are on top of everything. They did a great job.

- The first thing I was trying to get an appointment and I was like okay, you don't have anything today? No ma'am. Okay what about tomorrow? You gotta call back at 6 o'clock in the morning and try and make a same day appointment. You don't have anything open tomorrow? No ma'am. So, if they could have told me that I could come two days later, I would have been there. But I couldn't get one. I would call 6 in the morning and they still didn't have anything.

- [Personal information omitted] ... [could not get the treatment I wanted so] ... Thank goodness for [other medical facility] being here. [A leader] ... called me that morning of my appointment and said you need to go to the ER. I said TRICARE doesn't work like that ... [He said] ... just go to the ER just because you have [personal information omitted] ... I hadn't even seen my primary care physician because he was out of town. He had sent me through TRICARE and that's where they had sent me. Well he said you need to go there. He told me to go [to the other medical facility] so he could be at the ER because of my [omitted] ... problem also ...

- I was just making the comment that the [MTF] that we discussed, well a lot of problems with access to care and quality care come from not the [MTF] but from TRICARE and [managed care support contractor] and the policies that they are bringing up because I can echo with the lady back here ... [personal information omitted] ... I can tell you multiple stories of trying to get access to just talk to somebody at TRICARE and now that they have closed the office, you're at the mercy of the phone... Well under the current

TRICARE /[managed care support contractor] plan, if it's not a cookie cutter stamp of this is what you have to do, they don't know how to do it ...

Question to Audience: TRICARE's standard is 24 hours for urgent care, 7 days for routine care and 28 days for wellness visits and specialty care. How well are these standards being met?

Responses from Audience:
- [Personal information omitted] ... [unable to] get an appointment within 7 days for routine exams. She sees a civilian doctor for routine care. She doesn't even try here at the clinic. But I do know that she never gets an appointment within 7 days.

- My husband waited 22 days to get an appointment at the clinic, that's follow up to a test that he had done ... But we've been happy with our care but it just takes a while to get an appointment.

- ... We were told when we signed up for TRICARE at the TRICARE office that if you want to see a doctor in this facility, you had to be TRICARE prime. If you were TRICARE standard, you would be seen by a civilian doctor or go to urgent care because they don't even take TRICARE standard here. They don't have the capacity. So, they told us if you want to see a doctor here, you need to have TRICARE Prime. Whether or not that's true, I don't know. Standard doesn't even occur here.

- ... When you think TRICARE, you're thinking of the contractor, [managed care support contractor] and military veterans so trying to get an appointment in the network with TRICARE, that's kind of one aspect. And then trying to get an appointment at the clinic, there is a military and GS contractor type of cell that does this appointment scheduling. They are technically kind of TRICARE, but they are more with the military. So, that's what some of the folks here are thinking. Even though the entire system is TRICARE, it's still kind of with the military. So when you want to get an appointment off base, you will coordinate with TRICARE and directly with the actual clinic whether it's primary or specialty, i.e. standard or prime. So, that's why it's kind of confusing for me too ... If you're talking about this facility here, yes, I've been able to get the urgent care appointments that I need or if not, get the referrals off base and the routine and wells, they are within those standards.

- ... we were told by a nurse at the clinic, her suggestion was that we go to TRICARE standard, get a doctor off base because they were pulling an extra 1300 more people, active duty and stuff back into this clinic so she said that access it going to get worse and worse and worse when this happens.

- ... the very TRICARE office that used to be in [this MTF] ... one of the technicians ... told me that if you sign up for dual enrollment when you turn 65 you can go both places. You can go off into the network or you can stay here. That's the comment I had but it's kind of confusing if it's not true...

Questions Related to Patient Safety

Question to Audience: With respect to the care that you get here at this hospital, do you feel the care you're getting is safe? Do you feel comfortable asking questions?

Responses from Audience:
- [Thumbs up].

- [Thumbs up].

- ... taking away the emergency room or reducing the pharmacy hours of the community to Monday-Friday, these things look good to a commander but they are never reversed and so the commander moves on and the rest of us are here with the remainder of what's left. So, I just don't know how to make that statement or who to make it to.

- ... Yeah, she just triggered a thing I remember. The pharmacy hours at the community center used to be open on Saturday mornings and every time I went there, there were people there. And then one day I went there, they had all these notices up saying well due to not many, they weren't busy on Saturdays, that's why they were closing on Saturdays ... when I found out they closed, I thought man, this is bad. And also when the emergency room left here, that was bad also.

Question to Audience: During your visit with a provider, do you feel comfortable asking questions? Do you get the information you need and do you feel comfortable asking?

Responses from Audience:
- [Thumbs up].

- ... When I have an ... appointment, the one thing I'm wondering is that every time you go in there and you get the little notepad with the information sheet and you fill out the same information over and over again. Every single visit. It's just a piece of paper with my name, my address, and I know that information is sitting right in front of them on the computer. It seems like they could streamline that process so that I understand if there are changes to my medical condition, I'd be glad to given that to them because they need that but every single visit, is a waste of time.

Question to Audience: If you were to have a safety concern, how would you express it or whom would you go to?

Responses from Audience:
- I'd like to back up to your other safety question... I am not much of a computer guy and computers kind of scare me sometimes, and they put all of my stuff on the computer and the only safety concern I've ever had in the military is where does that stuff really go, really who has access to it, and when they started this thing the other day and they sent

- me an email that said I could access my records. I don't know but from a safety aspect, I'm wondering who else can access them?

- You had asked what would do you if you had a safety issue … , me, I would go to the patient advocate. I have not had any safety issues. I have not seen many safety issues…

- … Every time you made an appointment, they asked if you feel safe at home so they usually try and take care of the outside thing…

Question to Audience: Any other comments?

Responses from Audience:
- …. one thing that I have noticed when I was sent to [other MTF] … they would send me a specific appointment on a specific doctor that I would have seen. I have never seen that done here at [this MTF] … gave you the opportunity, if you want to say something "bad" to voice your opinion. But I've never seen that done here at [this MTF].

- … [other MTF] does good surveys. The other thing [the other MTF] does and civilian doctors, they give you a reminder call sometimes automated and sometimes in person. I never get them here.

Site 3 Staff Town Hall Questions and Answers

The following text reproduces the Town Hall facilitator questions and audience responses, transcribed as close to verbatim as possible during the session. Information that could potentially identify individual participants has been omitted for privacy purposes.

Approximately 75 people attended this Town Hall meeting.

Questions Related to Quality of Care

Question to Audience: To what extent is quality a priority here and to the extent that it is or is not a priority what are some indicators?

Responses from Audience:
- … The group of individuals at the [specialty clinic] … is so awesome. How they treat the patient at all levels is simply amazing. When I think about quality, I am so proud to be in their midst. The … guys that I work with are fantastic…

- … going to quality classes and TeamSTEPPS® and even on your desktop there is a link to put in a patient safety report. They really educate us and try to make it as easy as possible to incorporate a culture of quality.

- The demands for quantity especially in primary care comes at the expense of quality sometimes, so that there is less critical thinking and more referrals to specialists without taking initial steps to provide initial evaluation or treatment prior to going to a specialist. The demands that are placed on primary care for quantity is at the expense for quality.

- ... [at my previous station] all of our printers and scanners were all new and it surprises me here that the equipment that we use is so outdated and they are not connected to the network.

Question to Audience: What are some other challenges with respect to giving quality care?

Responses from Audience:
- ... we are not able to use a lot of the equipment because it does not interface with AHLTA. ... with all the changes in regards to bringing 50% more prescriptions from [outside the MTF] back to the military facilities and we are losing 30% of our "manning" with contract being renewed and people getting kicked out. With us we are seeing an increase in the wait times for patients. You only have 8 people to handle 200-300 prescriptions a day. Sometimes I think that we put too much emphasis on making the patient happy with short waiting times and not enough time to do things correctly.

- I think we suffer from too much central management and not enough freedom of the MTFs. Having the freedom to make more hiring decisions. For example we could do a ton more [specialty exams] if we had more techs. We have the doctors, [the equipment, and] we have the rooms. We just aren't able to do that and we are sending patients [outside the MTF]. [We may have a certain piece of equipment but don't have the staff /staff trained to use it ...] [Likewise] we also have the [trained staff to operate] ... a certain piece of equipment which [could]... save us a lot of money but we have no budget [to purchase that equipment] ... that as well.

- I am worried about the HAIMS (software system used for patient appointment scheduling) which is the system where we get scans and results from outside consultants. But the issue is that they are attaching it to a telephone consult and they are not labeling them so if you look at past medical records they won't have notes attached to them and you would have no idea what they are. We are burying the information and in the future when we go to look back at these documents it won't be accessible.

Questions Related to Access to Care

Question to Audience: Do your appointment templates and schedules meet appointment demand?

Responses from Audience:
- ... our [specialist was] ... just PCS'd and we do not have an inbound [replacement] that we know of. Anyone who needs any kind of [specialty] care, whether is it routine or specialized, everyone is being referred to the network. From our clinic there is nothing we can do to keep them. So that is a huge loss of [procedures] for us from our standpoint.

We are doing the best we can with what we have. Unfortunately we do not have answers for these patients.

- ... in a specialty clinic ... [staff can] ... make ... [their] ... own templates, which is great because [they] ... have the flexibility to have patients in, and cover for other providers when one [person] ... is out. So [they] ... do meet the demands of our patients. We have good access in my opinion and we are always able to get people in which other clinics may not be able to do since they have a fixed template.

- ... we've got 14 providers and this week we have 7 of us here. Tomorrow is in-processing ... so we are down ... appointment days and there is absolutely no way that we can meet the demand and that hasn't changed since 1986. In the past we have tried to get reservists sent from other bases or assistance which helped a lot but we can't get any now.

- One big challenge is to match department demands to the demands of outpatients. We ... are tasked out quite a bit for additional duties which reduces the access for our patients. It's a constant balance between having that availability for patients and meeting all other demands.

- ... If you look at the nurse and medical tech staffing, there are so many things that they are doing besides providing direct care that they are tasked and pulled to do between trainings and medical readiness.

- It's not just trainings. We have [specialty clinic] ... techs running the front desk.

- At this base in particular we have to have guys parking cars for [events] which takes away from their job duties.

Question to Audience: When do you release appointments for booking?

Responses from Audience:
- In my clinic we only have two appointment types: established and acutes. Anyone can be seen for anything. Our appointments are open at least a month in advance. 4 to 6 weeks is what we are hoping for.

- ... we are a specialty clinic. We open our books for our providers 45 days in advance ... we also have technician book appointments that I can only open 30 days in advance because I need to know what kind of training they are doing and if they are being tasked to do something.

Question to Audience: How often do you book each type of appointment prior to the patient leaving the hospital: follow up visits, referral to a specialty clinic for an initial visit, and outpatient procedures?

Responses from Audience:
- ... we try to schedule those the same day before the patient leaves the clinic.

- ... we try to schedule what follow ups we can ... if we have an open slot we will schedule them that day. For [procedures] we go back and schedule them during the week or two to three weeks out when the [procedure] schedule is open.

- ... if it is a follow up we will book them that same day. If it is for referrals or an ASAP if it is routine we will put it in the system and book it later. If it is within the MTF we have very good access with our MTF specialist. The only challenge we have is that fewer and fewer specialists are [working with the managed care support contractor] due to poor compensation. [Specialty] ... takes longer and longer because there a fewer and fewer specialists that we can refer them to in the local area.

Question to Audience: How often does your clinic respond to secure messaging from patients within time requirements as directed by policy?

Responses from Audience:
- I think we do meet the standards which is a response within 72 hours. We have a good system of our techs pre-screening for our providers as well as for the team box of incoming messages and distributing them as needed. The requirement that we have is that we take this secure message and convert it to a "TCON" to generate the workload then it has to be circulated to the provider, then closed out in AHLTA, then closed out in [the secure messaging system]. It makes the process lengthy but we meet the standards.

- I think secure messaging is a phenomenal idea. The implementation is going to be highly dependent from MTF to MTF. The concept is a great idea but the problem comes in mainly in the duplication of works within telephone consoles. It has potential to be very effective.

Question to Audience: What do you do if you can't schedule someone for an appointment?

Responses from Audience:
- I know in [specialty clinic] ... we do have issues scheduling patients. We go very close to the 28 day mark. We tell our patient to give us a couple of weeks and we should have something available. We went from have three providers to having two so we have been very close. It is a policy issue.

- Sometimes in the clinic I can schedule out as far as I want to go but because management might want a meeting or a commander's call, something shows up on the radar under 30 days. For me, I am already booked out. In terms of policy they probably don't want us booking appointments any further out because that limits their flexibility.

Questions Related to Patient Safety

Question to Audience: How do you go about reporting a patient safety issue?

Responses from Audience:
- In [specialty clinic] ... they have had just a couple of near misses on labeling specimens and they came up with a great program to ensure that all of the labels were printed beforehand and it has now been over a year since we have had any misses.

- In the [specialty area] ... they have installed a new process where you cannot move or treat a patient until a timeout/huddle has been conducted (patient has to say their name, etc.).

- We have a pretty open policy in the [inpatient service]... but we do Patient Safety Reports (PSR) which is an icon on the computer screen were you can fill out pertinent information and that gets forwarded up to safety management where it gets handled ... [specific example given] ... this past week and we had to fill out a certain form based on policies that we have set in place. That goes into the PSR and gets escalated accordingly.

- This is the first clinic that I have been in where everybody attends TeamSTEPPS® as part of in-processing. If you are witnessing something occur, you are given the tools to address the situation. You can express your concerns and you can escalate it if the particular issue continues.

Question to Audience: If you have concerns regarding quality, access or safety, how do you report it?

Responses from Audience:
- I work in [specialty clinic] ... and my chain of command has an open door policy in case you have any questions or concerns. With us it is open line of communication with our chain of command.

Question to Audience: I would like to open up the floor for you all to voice any concerns, challenges, issues you have in terms of quality, access, and/or safety.

Responses from Audience:
- There are two major issues I have encountered. [The managed care support contractor] is horrible. It's been a complete disaster since it has started. It is a barrier for our patients in getting the care they need. It's driving patients away from seeing our providers. Wait times for specialists are climbing higher and higher. It's turning nurses into referral managers. We also lost the referral management desk (TRICARE service center) so there is no one to talk to. The centralization of our admin people is another issue. They are very separated from our clinic and we have no control over them.

- Whenever you had a computer or electronic issue, we used to have people who were in-house who could take care of the situation. Now you have to put in requests and it may be 48 hours before you get any assistance. You spend an hour on the phone while your patients are piling up and that has a terrible effect on quality and access.

- Referral paperwork is also far behind in terms of scanning into the system. ... even if [staff] ... spend the entire day scanning [they] ... will only be able to input a fraction of the overall paperwork. It's becoming a patient safety issue. It's a staffing issue.

- One other issue that effects quality is that there is a policy that if you reach out to a patient 3 times without talking to them you book them anyway without having a conversation and then a letter is sent to them with their appointment information which creates a ton of no shows. Instead a letter should be sent stating for that patient to call us because we can't reach you. Then it becomes a spot that is occupied that you cannot fill with other patients.

- We don't have the staff to see patients.

- The key issue comes down to the inoperability of our systems. None of them communicate with each other. It is discouraging because with the amount of interoperability that is capable. Lag time is also an issue. It becomes a day to day challenge. We are measured on quantity and not the quality it takes to support the quantity.

Site 4 Beneficiary Town Hall Questions and Answers

The following text reproduces the Town Hall facilitator questions and audience responses, transcribed as close to verbatim as possible during the session. Information that could potentially identify individual participants has been omitted for privacy purposes.

Approximately 70 people attended this Town Hall meeting.

Questions Related to Quality of Care

Question to Audience: Tell us about the quality of care you're getting. Are you getting quality of care here and if you are, how do you know? What is the indicator that you are getting it based on your experience?

Responses from Audience:
- I think it really depends on the doctor and the clinic. I know personally with my PCM right now, I only go in for referrals. I went in [month] ... and I got 3 referrals and I haven't been back since. I will only come in for referrals out into the network. I go to [three specialty care clinics] ... I will not go in for care, especially after the multiple times I have had to call the office [for test results]. Not after repeatedly asking for my numbers and being told they are in the normal range. But where in the normal range? What specifically are my numbers? [regarding test results] I have also been told that

specific locations don't particularly care what your exact numbers are. So far I am more satisfied with the care I have been getting in the network. It is different with my kids. So far I am happy with the treatment they've received.

- I had a problem that started back in [month] ... The physician that I was assigned to at the time would not see me for that condition ... I finally got a physician to see me through an ICE complaint. Then they did not do all of the testing that was required. I was referred out and that doctor said, "Why didn't they do this blood work..." Now the problem has been diagnosed, I am going to another specialist in the network, in [city] ... That was back in [month] ... and I don't get to see him until the end of [month]. That is the first ICE complaint that I have had answered relating to this hospital.

- I went into see my PCM and it has turned into a referral service. I am looking around and I don't see many in active duty. But when I call in the morning, they end up referring me to the [specific clinic]. I don't need that. And when you go to the [specific clinic]and it is a situation that your PCM can't handle, they end up referring you to a specialist. It turns into a chain of referrals and it keeps getting put off.

Question to Audience: How does the quality of care that you receive out in the network compare to the quality of care that you receive here at [this MTF]?

Responses from Audience:
- ... The outside providers are far superior to the providers here at [this MTF]. The care is so much better when you are seeing a civilian doctor. There are shorter wait times, there's better treatment and an understanding when you go into the facility. They listen more; they are more attentive to your needs. It is a totally different animal outside of the military care system.

- We went out into the network because of an issue here at [this MTF] ... [personal information omitted] ... instead of trying to determine what was causing [the] ... pain... it turned into maybe you're just seeking drugs. That is how we felt. ... [Personal information omitted] ... You are seeing a [group] of providers to get the right care and you have to keep answering the same questions over and over again.

- I have had mixed results. I have seen both military here and civilian out in the network. One local provider that I saw in the network was awful. I actually got two referrals, one here at [this MTF] and the other in the network. First I went to see the civilian because I was able to schedule that appointment earlier. He was so terrible. Next I came into [this MTF] to be seen and the doctor was the best. The care was excellent. They couldn't provide the [procedure] ... here ... They sent me to another military doctor who did the [procedure] ... The care was excellent ... Some of the service is not so great but other times it can be very, very good.

- ... I have never received anything but the best care ... [personal information omitted] ... I never had nasty care. I have gotten the best care as a [Service member] here and as a civilian. I'm sure there are individual issues but overall I am happy with my care. If you want to talk about down-side sometimes it takes a while to get in to see a physician. I understand that we don't have enough doctors to do everything that needs to be done.

- Quality and access are the two biggest issues in terms of medical care.

- ... [Personal information omitted] ... [I have] ... had to argue with a provider. I knew that I needed to be hospitalized ... [personal information omitted] ... That was the only bad treatment that I had here .... Recently I have had problems ... [personal information omitted] ... can no longer come here. That's my biggest gripe now. ... was referred all over the place ... was seen by one doctor for five minutes who didn't do anything and now Medicare is going to get billed for it. My main thing is [people] ... should not be turned away from medical care because we are over the age of 65.

- ... [Personal information omitted] ... Most of my care has been good. What I have found is that you have to call at 6:30 to get an appointment. If you call at 6:31 you will be on the phone for a long time. Call at 6:30 AM and you can get an appointment that same day. I have had good care.

Question to Audience: If you have an issue with the quality of care that you receive, how do you express your concerns?

Responses from Audience:
- I would talk to a supervisor but sometimes that is not the best way to work my complaint up the chain.

- Sometimes we get surveys which are mailed to beneficiaries to fill out.

- I have a comment about the quality of care as well ... [personal information omitted] ... received great care in [specialty clinic] ... no one really knows about RelayHealth. My particular provider uses it and uses it well. If I need a referral, I send her an email and that day she will put an appointment in the system. [Personal information omitted] ... when ... [we] ... need an appointment I will send an email for that. It is an excellent system. I really hope more people start using it.

Questions Related to Access to Care

Question to Audience: Do any of you use RelayHealth for secure messaging and how many have had success using it?

Responses from Audience:
- Yes! *(Many in audience)*

- My biggest concern is how different the hospitals are. I think in terms of access to care they are different across the board. We came from a base in [personal information omitted] ... and the access to care there was different than it is at [this MTF]. The doctor

I saw here for my [personal information omitted] ... prescribed the standard [medications] ... without performing any lab tests. I tried to get another appointment for my [personal information omitted] ... and they said to call back at 6:30 AM to get a same day appointment or they could set something up for next week. I thought that was unacceptable. So I called a patient advocate and she was able to get me an appointment on the next day ... Pediatrics is fabulous. I love the doctors there.

- I have only had a couple issues here [personal information omitted] ... see several doctors. I can honestly say that they are very good here in terms of making appointments and transitioning ... records.

Question to Audience: Other thoughts on getting appointments when you need to be seen?

Responses from Audience:
- TRICARE has an online system and I have been arguing with the hospital ... because whenever I go in to use that system to schedule a same day, same week appointment, nothing is open or available for any of my family members. I went through the same situation last year just to get my family members listed. Nothing in the system in terms of available appointments ...

- I recently had a very rough time getting an appointment for my ... [child] ... and they told me to call back in 28 days to see if there is available appointment. I went to a patient advocate and had a discussion but nothing came of it. I had to go to [leadership] ... and was then able to get in front of someone [personal information omitted] ...

- I've had two situations where I have needed to get a same day appointment ... [for my child] ... I had to call in [personal information omitted] ... and the person told me to keep trying back at 6:30. I didn't know about making appointments online.

- Quality in terms of my clinical experience was excellent. Sometimes however, the customer service support staff are miserable to deal with. When you come in to any clinic they are not friendly and they don't want to help you ... [personal information omitted]

- [Personal information omitted] ... Making an appointment [for my children] is absolutely the most horrific thing that I have had to deal with. For instance, my PCM has changed. We are supposed to be notified when our PCM has changed. I was never notified until I called to make an appointment. I called [on a certain day] and my PCM doesn't even have a schedule so as far as continuity, this gentleman [here in the Town Hall] said that you don't have one doctor but an entire group, that is absolutely true. I have not seen my PCM and if I don't ever see them, it will be too soon. If I need to schedule an appointment ... why am I being told to go to the emergency room?

- I do use RelayHealth and I have been able to go there to schedule an appointment. I would like to make my comment in reference to quality of care ... [Personal information omitted] ... I have seen many health care facilities and I am very satisfied with my care here at [this MTF]. I have been treated on the outside as a dollar bill. I appreciate [this MTF]. Keep doing what you are doing!

- ... I am satisfied with the care. There are good doctors here and on the outside. We do our best to schedule appointments. We are serving all of the military dependents all over the world and they come in and get an appointment. We try but you have to understand that every department has regulations that they have to go by and there is only a certain number of appointments that we can make in a day. I do feel that customer service reps are compassionate if you are pregnant or sick. I have been fine with the service I have received here at [this MTF]. I have one doctor that was mean and yelled at me but he soon came to me and apologized. I think it has to do with the personality of the person you are dealing with.

- My TRICARE is all messed up. Sometimes I am TRICARE Plus and sometimes Standard. I called in because I was sick and I really needed to see someone. The person who I spoke with really hurt me because they said I have TRICARE Standard and cannot be seen. I feel as though whether I am TRICARE Plus or not, I deserve to be seen.

- I have had them call me and tell me that I need to come in to look at test results but then I have to call the customer service line at 6:30 AM to make an appointment. It doesn't make any sense when you are calling me to make an appointment and there are no appointments available ... [personal information omitted] ...

- ... [we] ... had been calling trying to get ... medication renewed. No one called ... back. ... Left a message for the nurse to call ... Long story short, we kept going around and around. And we could not reach them to renew ... [the] medication. This lady from the call center took time out to talk to me and told me to call in the morning at 6:30 AM. I forgot about making the 6:30 call and the young lady I spoke with called me back and made an appointment for [us] ... later on that day. Every time I call the call center I always get someone nice even if they do not tell you what you want to hear.

Question to Audience: At the end of your appointment, how often are you asked by the scheduling clerk to arrange for your next appointment?

Responses from Audience:
- ... I have a phone number for my doctor's nurse. I can call her. At 6:30 I can get her but for the rest of the day it is hit or miss. She is very responsive. I have [regular] check-ups where I have to do labs so she will put that in. Going through the call center I get all types of excuses. I did have one exceptional doctor that I have seen and I can't say enough about her but as far as a same day appointment, forget it.

- [Personal information omitted] ... I have been satisfied with my care. I have only been sent off of base twice in ... [personal information omitted]. The service here is fantastic and I have never had a problem getting an appointment. Wait until you go to another base with a small medical center you will have major problems there. I have never had a problem at [this MTF].

- There are issues with follow up appointments as well. [Personal information omitted] ... I was unable to get an appointment [in pediatrics] when [my pediatric provider] ... recommended so [nurse] told me to walk in at 7:45 and ask to see me. That was the only way I was able to get the appointment on time. So it is not just same day appointments that are difficult to book, the same goes for follow-up appointments. I feel like the military should have some standardized system that depending on your condition you should automatically get a follow up appointment instead of calling at 6:30 AM on a business day to try to get an appointment. I have been to some hospitals where they automatically give you a follow up appointment in the ER, but here they do not and that is disconcerting to me.

Question to Audience: TRICARE standards are 24 hours for urgent care, 7 days for routine care, and 28 days for wellness visits. Are these standards being met?

Responses from Audience:
- Not at all. Here you are told to call at 6:30 AM when every other facility automatically schedules you for follow up visits. If you call at 6:35 AM the appointments are gone. As far as 7 days for a routine, that doesn't happen. Like I said my PCM doesn't even have a schedule. So I see his team of people which is ok but it is never within 7 days. The follow-ups are never in a 24-48 hour period.

- [Personal information omitted] ... told me to go to the emergency room and tell them that you want ... acute care. I got seen in 30 days.

- As far as follow up [personal information omitted] ... We went to the emergency room here [to get] ... treated. When I called to make a follow-up appointment they told me that [if you are] ... 65 [you] ... can't make an appointment until 10:30 AM. At 6:32 AM all the appointments are gone ... You just can't get an appointment down here unless it is emergency care.

Questions Related to Patient Safety

Question to Audience: Do you feel like you receive safe care at [this MTF]?

Responses from Audience:
- When it comes to OB ... appointments [personal information omitted] ... well we don't have any appointments for two weeks. What am I supposed to do? They should block out appointments for people who are pregnant ... and get them scheduled ...

- I have had good care so far. [Personal information omitted] ... I feel that the care I received [from OB] was very safe. Everyone on my care team up until I delivered was great. I felt like everything was great according to my experience. Being able to have conversation with folks and their gentle care, made me feel safe.

- I think the safety here is excellent. I had orthopedic surgery and they sent me to physical therapy ... [they] made sure I had the correct medication and provided lessons on how to use your crutches before you had your surgery. I think that was very proactive of them and very excellent.

Question to Audience: Do you feel comfortable when you are with your provider at [this MTF]? Do you feel comfortable asking questions about your care?

Responses from Audience:
- [Personal information omitted] ... and I took [my child] to pediatrics. We had to wait six weeks to see a [specialty] doctor just to get a renewal of ... medication. [Personal information omitted] ... Now I have to go to patient advocacy because they don't have a specialist that knows anything about [personal information omitted] ... We go to [a different city] for my [child's needs] ... I would rather drive four hours than come here.

- As far as a safety issue, my [personal information omitted] ... was dealing with a [personal information omitted] ... issue and ... hadn't seen a specialist for three months. [Personal information omitted] ... For some reason [s/he] slipped through the cracks and nobody knew what was going on.

- [Personal information omitted] ... I went to the pharmacy to pick up my prescription and they said here is another drug, we no longer carry the one you were looking for. My doctors never told me. I don't understand how that was not addressed through RelayHealth, in the mail, or on a phone call. I would have to go out of pocket for it or take the generic.

Question to Audience: If you have a safety concern where do you take it?

Responses from Audience:
- You could go to the pharmacy and there could be 5 people sitting there and you are waiting for an hour. You sit and you sit and you sit. In some places you can leave the ER with your prescription in hand. Here, when you eventually get your prescription you have to go to a [civilian pharmacy] to fill your prescription and you are paying out of pocket for it since there is no 24 hour pharmacy here.

- On the whole, [this MTF] has always been wonderful. When there are problems, there are problems in every installation that you go to. Could customer service be better? Yes. Most of the people who are answering those phones, you can't do anything about it. They have got those jobs and it is locked, so you have to do your best in dealing with them. The ER has a quality problem because it depends on who sees you. Some will read your file and some won't even pay attention to if you are allergic to anything ... [personal information omitted] ... Also [this MTF] and TRICARE are not talking.

- [Personal information omitted] ... I have always had those [specialty tests] done here. Why all of a sudden I have to go offsite? On top of that I went to my scheduled appointment and was told that I had to go see another to doctor to get the treatment.

- If I have had health problems, I go in and sit down with my provider to have a conversation. I am not someone who takes medication because you told me to take it. I ask for explanations. I haven't had any problems. [Personal information omitted] ... I went to the [specific department] ... The only thing is that I went to the [specific department] ... and they took a little too long [personal information omitted] ... When I left I had my medication and had my next day appointment. It depends on who you talk to. I believe that leadership need to be more in touch to what is going on and then I think we will see an improvement. We all know that with the military, they tell you to hurry up and wait all day.

- ... I think there needs to be a quicker turnaround time. I have also heard that this hospital is going to be turned in an outpatient clinic. I would like for that to be reevaluated. There are a lot of people who depend on this hospital. Also I was told that the system does not allow you to make appointments after a certain point or on a certain day of the month. I don't know why they are not aware of openings three months in advance. It should be a lot easier for individuals looking for care to get care

Question to Audience: How does patient safety compare here to out in the network?

Responses from Audience:
- First of all [this MTF] is a great hospital to be a part of but I think the main problem is that they do not have enough staff. In the [specific department] ... they have so many people waiting there and it takes so long to be seen. It is obvious to me that they do not have enough staff.

- One issue that I would like to address is [personal information omitted] ... went in at 7 in the morning and did not have [procedure] ... until 7:30 that night.

Question to Audience: Who haven't we heard from that would like to speak?

Responses from Audience:
- We have had wonderful care here. RelayHealth is wonderful however TRICARE is terrible as far as retirees are concerned.

- As far as the access in the system, I was referred out for a mammogram. After I had my mammogram done it was an additional 30 days to wait for my results. I continue to have problems getting care here however sometimes. I have been able to get my mammogram result back the same day which was great. As far as civilian care goes, I was [personal information omitted] ... and here, it didn't feel like it was done. I would definitely come here before I go out to the network.

- [Personal information omitted] ... it has been hard to get the inside medical care providers to accept the diagnoses from the people who diagnosed [the patient] ... in the first place... it is difficult to transfer care from [other location] to [this MTF] because they have a separate section of medical care. It is hard to communicate with providers. It doesn't get shared well.

- [Personal information omitted] ... as far as availability goes, it has pretty much been terrible the entire time ... [we] ... will not go TRICARE Prime because the fact that [we] ... had problems with medical care providers ... [personal information omitted] ... I wish I can get some availability here instead of driving two hours to get an MRI. There needs to be more synergy here at [this MTF].

- My main concern with TRICARE is that little by little they are taking our medical care away. After 65 you can't be seen. [Personal information omitted] ... DoD is increasing our costs. If they would take care of the excess expenditures and not increase what we have to pay ... Stop charging the retirees. We went to war and fought for the country. Stop taking our benefits away.

Question to Audience: If you were running this, what is one solution that you would implement?

Responses from Audience:
- Honor promises made

- Standardize the record keeping process because from one facility to another you don't have any records available when you go to get treatment elsewhere.

- I think the leadership for the hospital need to have more sessions. I think they need to have more private sessions with the people who actually do the work. They could then probably fix a lot of the problems. That's number one. So number two, I think they need to get rid of their union and have more leadership presence.

- Yes ma'am. Electronic medical records. [Personal information omitted] ... When I came here, I had to tell them the same information over and over again. If I do not talk they are not going to know.

- Process Improvements. Have a step by step process for everything that they need to do. They should automate who needs to go to MRI or ER so people do not have to wait as long. Just to cut down on the wait time.

- I think the staff is grumpy because they are overworked and understaffed. Patients are grumpy because they see it as a simple solution to hire more staff.

- Make sure that all the departments communicate with each other. They are not on the same page.

- Standardizing education training requirements. Document procedures that are outside of the normal scope so that there is something to follow.

- Standardize things like emergency care and ortho safety issues across the hospital. It should not vary from hospital to hospital.

- Why are we on a 30 day window? Why not go to a three month window?

- [Personal information omitted] ... as a civilian you ... schedule an appointment and see your physician [on your] way out. If you wanted to change your appointment you would not have to wait an extended amount of time. The system of scheduling appointments needs to be fixed.

Site 4 Staff Town Hall Questions and Answers

The following text reproduces the Town Hall facilitator questions and audience responses, transcribed as close to verbatim as possible during the session. Information that could potentially identify individual participants has been omitted for privacy purposes.

Approximately 35 people attended this Town Hall meeting.

Questions Related to Quality of Care

Question to Audience: Is quality of care a priority for your facility? How do you know if it is or if it isn't?

Responses from Audience:
- ... At one point ... I trusted the quality. I trusted the doctors and anyone they sent me to. But at one point, I cannot say that they could have prevented my [personal information omitted] ... but had they just listened a little closer to me as a patient and not looked at me as an employee, look at me as a patient, and I asked which is in my history that I explained very deeply, very highly. I was told what I thought all along. I was told it was just a [personal information omitted] ... and go home. Put a warm compress. I listened to my doctor, paid attention and even said during my examination, please don't let this turn into anything that is going to cause any problems later. I was told don't worry about it. ... I'm hurt because ... I felt they didn't treat me the way I should have been. It's not that they could have prevented this but ... I believe that possibly it could have been [less difficult for me] ... instead of what I went through. And I am not angry, I am truly hurt by who I am employed by. ...

- ... I believe every provider wants to provide quality care and the correct diagnosis the first time but we are no different than any other industry and quality suffers at times especially when we have to produce more and more and more. Number one, when the patient waits a long time to come in, they have more to discuss, more than a 20 minute appointment. The provider is not just trying to diagnose the patient, but oh yeah, we have to answer questions, oh yeah, there may be other patients waiting, and oh yeah, we have to provide refill prescriptions. On top of it, all of the training requirements, let me calculate in my head, almost four weeks of training hours in one calendar year that we have to accomplish, so anyways, my point is that quality suffers I think because the quantity has to be pushed through. We don't mean for quality to go down but unfortunately, it is a side effect so yes, unfortunately it suffers. But to answer your question, quality is expressed by the commander, by everyone.

- The training in my area and I know our providers have a lot on our plate with seeing patients and doing notes, and all the meetings they have to attend … I know at [one time] … on [a certain day each week] the hospital would … close down for a little bit for training and everyone would catch up on their training and providers would catch up on their notes for things like that. Some sections of hospital still do that but majority of the sections don't especially for civilians. So that, I think if that could still happen, it would really help and it would be a little better. We would know what's going on. The training would be caught [up] on, I believe, the training would be caught [up] on and providers would have more time to do other things. A lot of things are pushed on providers not just the staff here at the hospital, a lot of things are pushed, but I understand why when I ask we can't do certain things because it is a business and I understand it's a business but there is such thing as burn out. If you don't give a person time to catch up on the things they need to do, you give them more and more things, you're going to have a lot of problems.

- I work with [specific department] … and it is so true, we are bogged down with all our training and other things, and on the other side we try really hard to do quality of care. The problem is too that we have so many requirements and everything that when we do shut down, the one place that does stay open is the ER. And everybody comes to the ER and the command does look for good quality and we try really hard. The requirement is that that we want patients to be happy and when they can't get into their provider, they come to the ER especially because it is a hard stress area and no one is happy when they wait 4 or 5 hours in the ER and their expectation is that it is a drive-thru ER. You come, you get seen, and you leave. Why should I wait in an ER? I can't see my provider so I am going to the ER. So quality is pushed and we try very hard, and I know the command does I agree with you that the command does come down very hard. But the reality is these patients have no place to go so they come to ER. They are cutting down. They don't want patients to go to the urgent care facilities on the weekends that's been cut too… There is one place, [specific clinics], that's where active duty [Service members] have their providers. The patients go to [these clinics] in the mornings and they are told that there is no appointment for them for three weeks. Well, that doesn't sit well with them, they go to the ER. It's kind of hard, it's a double edge sword. You want to provide good quality for them but they can't get in, they can't get seen. But they do push quality of care but it is difficult. They have so many requirements for everyone to come down. There is just not enough access to care. There are not enough providers for people to get seen. Unfortunately, we are a big one we see a lot of patients coming through the ER.

- ... one of the things we all come in when working in health care ... [is] ... wanting to take care of patients and being the best. Part of that is being able to see how well we impact them. So when our quantity is hyped up so much, you don't feel that type of impact that you are looking for as a provider. And that really truly impacts the way that I feel about coming to work. I feel stressed coming to work every day. I feel anxiety every day coming into work ... I feel like that when I come in and I feel anxious and one side they say you are very important to the organization but it is a business. But on the other side, they say we actually care. You can't say it both ways. If you treat us like whatever you do, you have to take care of all these patients, and all this training and oh by the way, you have to do all this training in the middle of patient care. I mean if you have multiple tasks, you are not going to be able to do any task efficiently or to the quality that you are wanting to. And that gives you feedback about your work and you can't sustain that type of environment. You just can't.

- Too little staff. And the staff we do have are not being used effectively or efficiently. I am looking for help at the clinic and where are the [Service members], they are looking out to see those that parked in the wrong area in the parking lot or some area. I get all the training but there is such thing as overkill. We are doing a lot with a lot less, a lot less time, a lot less in terms of funding and equipment that we need. And in personnel, it's just like you said. It's just very difficult. I actually and not everyone can say this, I love what I do, I do. And I like to enjoy coming to work. But lately I have not been given such satisfaction because of the additional stress that is put on not just on myself but the place as a whole where I work. And it affects quality of your life, and you don't feel like just like you say the impact or being able to provide the care on a daily basis. You are bogged down with so many additional responsibilities but some of them are not even priorities. But it seems to change depending on who is in charge at the time. If I can't do what I need to do for my patient or to complete my training because I have no assistance because you're out doing something that's very ridiculous.

- ... we have had quite a bit of turnover and I understand what you mean by they are not able to access, actually it's probably more than the access, the quality does suffer because in [specific departments] ... we don't have any ancillary staff and I do help out with [specific department] ... does quite a bit so I have a lot of additional duties. A lot of the problems [are] the referrals that we do get, so we are a referral clinic so we are getting patients from all of the other [specific clinics] ... the quality of referral that we are getting is kind of bogging us down as well. They are not being evaluated at the [specific clinic] so when we get them, first we had no studies done, no eval done and that is kind of cutting our time, doctor's time significantly.

- ... I would recommend them to find providers and those providers get patients every 30 seconds, you are trying to get patients in and out and in and out. You don't have time to sit with patients and really get into their medical care and really making a difference because by the time you get one in, there are already two waiting ... [Providers] ... get 30 minute spots and before they can get a good history on them, it's time to leave so they can see another patient and they still don't have time to do the documentation.

Question to Audience: Has something changed recently? Was it always like this? I'm hearing that "now I'm feeling stressed." I'm wondering, were you feeling stressed before? Or has something changed?

Responses from Audience:
- ... I've seen a gradual increase in those extra demands, the extra and the extra. Somebody had a priority in Congress or DHA or DoD and they said we need to do this type of training. For example, human trafficking is one. But my personal favorite was a couple years ago when they added the Constitution Day training that we had to go online to answer a quiz about the Constitution. That's several weeks' worth of training. When you don't drop any but simply add to it and over time, it simply becomes this massive quantity of mandatory stuff. A couple years ago, one of the department chiefs did try to prioritize it. And they said we are going to call this Tier 1 – you have to do, Tier 2 – do it by no later than this time, Tier 3 – do it if you can because it reached that point when they had to make a local decision but at the same time, by the letter, it is still mandatory. So, you still have those meeting demands. There is the question, what is the priority of the day. How can we allocate our time? How can we get from where we are at now to where we want to get.

- ... We've got several weeks of mandatory training and maybe 5 percent relates to direct patient care. There is very little time or resources allocated for continuing professional education. Whether you're an RN, LPN, and the implications for the professional here in the hospital is that you go get that stuff with your own money and your own time on the internet. Most people can't afford a good course say at like Duke or Harvard with that kind of money. It is a system-wide problem trying to save some money so they cut professional education funding but long-term it is going to hurt us and we are going to have great difficulty recruiting and keeping good people.

- And then when we don't complete the training, we get reported for our evaluations and then we get performance evaluations that reflect that. So daily I get emails that let me know "oh in addition to the fact that you have to see your patients and chart on them and do the training, oh by the way, you're also up for [training]." ... you try to do good patient care and you continue to get evaluations that you're terrible, you're terrible, and you're terrible.

- ... My issue is I think the problem with this hospital or MTF starts at the top ... people need to be held accountable. And ... the manager set[s] the tone. There is no tone set at [this MTF]. Managers to me aren't always held accountable. My issue is that when are our chief or our manager, when are they held accountable? You want to chastise us for things that we have been telling you going on for years but when are they held accountable. That's my issue. I mean training, I can only do what I can do. If I can't do it, it's just not going to get done but allot me time like what most employers do.

- I can honestly say I work with a wonderful team. We keep working with what we have. We've had times where we have had to share 1 ream of paper between like 40 people so the supplies are like so sparse, we can't cut anymore ... We've had furloughs and hiring freezes. So, we have just in the last two months, we've had hiring freeze open back up so it was like we're finally going to have people, everything is going to be perfect. ... [but] from the time he did his paperwork and the time the person was notified, it was like four weeks. Well by that time, the person had already taken another job. If you interview for a job and you don't hear anything for four weeks, you just assume you don't have the job. As a result, they went to the alternative person but that person had taken another job and now they are back to square one. So, I'm thinking not only is the funding an issue but hiring process needs to be looked at.

- ... you talk about staffing and supplies, the thing is that you see a lot of civilians retiring, you are short-staff, burned out, resiliency, where is it, not here. Then you have management up here coming down on middle management and the people on the bottom are lost, gone. Careers are starting to be ruined. I just feel like everything is such a ... access of care, patients not being able to get in, calling the nursing staff and you want to help them and emotionally you feel drained but you can't help them.

Question to Audience: Do you see successes anywhere, do you see something that *is* working anywhere and what do you think should change, what our some solutions that come to mind that you wish someone would hear?

Responses from Audience:
- ... What I can say is that what is working is the PCMH model to an extent. It's Patient Centered Medical Home. It's a model we went to several years ago. It's actually within a few clinics but they are trying to disperse it through the military system. The morning huddles allow you time to address with your colleagues while patients who are coming in, problem areas that can be addressed so that does help to an extent. Morning huddles do help. It helps the staff be prepared for what's coming in for that day. But it also gives you actual time to coordinate with your colleagues for the morning and get started for the day. What could be better is what used to be about what we've already said about training. There was time allotted for us to train, sharpen our skills within a clinical setting. And also if you expect us to give good patient quality care, you gotta take care of your employees. You gotta to allow time to build back up again within the organization. What recently happened in the [specific clinic] ... time out was called for about 5-10 minutes and it actually gave us great life skills to reduce our high-stress levels. One last comment I want to say is this – what could be better. We cannot assume that every patient is right because they are not. And right now they always assume that every complaint is always correct, but I'm sorry that is an error. It's a business sense of doing things and it's not right, it's really not right. So, when a patient is claiming to be correct about a medication, or about a staff, it needs to be investigated. But they always assume that everybody is always doing the wrong thing.

- What is working ... is that we care for these [Service members] and we continue to assist them up in the circumstances. So that is working. What could be better? I just don't see how management can supervise you and rate you when they don't know anything about what you do or the program ... how can you evaluate me if you don't know the program? The good thing is that we have continued to assist these [Service members].

- The emphasis is always on the patient being right. Sometimes the patient needs to hear something different than what they are coming in here wanting to hear. So, then you have that extra stressor of do I tell this patient what they need to hear or worry about what my [satisfaction survey] scorecard is going to reflect. The patient comes in here and wants an MRI, you don't need one right now. If that patient gets that survey and they go fill it out, did you get the care you felt you needed to receive. No, I did not. And then you get counseled on why your patient satisfaction survey was low.

- I just want to say I think what is working is us as a team. What could be better is that when we have sessions like this and it's taken back to management, that they are held accountable to address the issues. That's what needs to be done, is for them to actually take their employees and say we got their back and how can we work this out as a team. That's a team. That's never done. You take issues after issues to them to the point that I don't even trust you anymore. I'm here for my patients but for my supervisors, it's out the window. And that's not a good atmosphere to work in. So, if they are held accountable for what you take back to them and they address it, until that's done, it's going to continue to go down the drain, which is bad for our community and our co-workers.

Questions Related to Access to Care

Question to Audience: Do your appointment templates and schedules meet appointment demand?

Responses from Audience:
- No, we have [Service members] that are PCSing July 10, August 10. July is next week. August is one month away. We don't have our overseas screening till the end of July. So, you have a lot of [Service members] that are not going to meet their appointment dates. Some of these [Service members] have turned in their lease to their houses and things of that nature and they have to stay at hotels and have actually made arrangements up to the point that they leave. So, to answer your question, no.

- ... in some ways we have enough appointments if we would manage expectations better. ...the example of the low back pain and the patient wants an MRI, that same person may walk in the door and say, I just sprained my back doing sit-ups. I need to be seen now. Well, we have an appointment at 1500 now. And they don't like [that option] ... so they go to the ER office. And then we see all that administrative turn-around to manage the patient expectation which I believe is already difficult to manage. So, I think following up on what a couple of people have already said, manage the expectation better for both patients and the staff, I think we are going to see better access because we are going to manage our necessary appointments, which will help us manage things overall.

Question to Audience: Manage expectations. What's an example of how you would do that? Give me a specific example to manage expectations?

Responses from Audience:
- And that is a daily fight that we have to try and figure out a practical way to do that and frequently it turns out to be on the active duty side when you're dealing with the active duty [Service members]. Frequently it turns out to be that the PA who works for that unit consistently has the same type of treatment for the [Service member]. [Service member] 1 talks to [Service member] 2 and says you know what, the VA is going to see you today for this type of appointment. You walk in for the sniffles that you got four hours ago. They are not going to see you for your cold today. They will probably see you in a few days if you try some over the counter med and it doesn't work. But they're probably not going to drop everything.

- ... Access to care has been a scary, scary phrase for me because we are a specialty clinic, we have 28 days to get a patient in from the time they get a consult. So, I've added in so many days without editing days. We get penalized for patients that don't get in or if they are a no-show. So, we have to add in all these patients. So, my providers don't have time to go to the bathroom sometimes, they are eating lunch. And at times, they end up doing charts while eating lunch, which is nasty. They don't have time to go, or I understand. If we do get them an appointment and the patient don't want to come in [because that appointment time is not convenient for them], we get penalized. We have to hear that our numbers [are] not meeting the standards.

- I think you hit on it too. I think it's an issue in our clinic. We pretty much all of us are referral clinics are held to the same standard and everything is kind of odd. We get in trouble for the breaks that we do get in the schedule. They are asking us, why is your schedule cleared for this block of time or why are you not seeing patients during this block of time. Why aren't you seeing patients all the time? You know my doctors ... actually go off [base] to do ... procedures. Why doesn't this doctor have four days of clinic? It is hard.

Question to Audience: When do you release appointments for booking?

Responses from Audience:
- ... technically all appointment slots should be open at least 45 days out. I believe that this access to care issue can be resolved. Nothing is unfixable if you work together as a cohesive unit, every single department. But it seems like everybody has their own agenda. There is not unity. So, rather than pursue the mission, which we all are called to do when we join the [Service], we don't do that. I don't see anything where there is access to care standards. Regards to the templates, I don't see anything where we adhere to access to care standards.

Question to Audience: Are you saying it's different in different parts of [this MTF]?

Responses from Audience:
- … in specialty based clinics, they do specs and in certain circumstances, they do acute. In primary care, [they] … have … routine [and] … acute. Very rarely are there … routine appointment[s] because normally the patients demand to be seen. Yes, I want to be seen. They have up to 7 days to be seen but they want to be seen right away.

- … With access to care, there is a problem when you call to get an appointment and at 7:30 in the morning, they are all gone. We are sending some of our providers to other [bases] when we have a shortage here. That doesn't make sense to so I don't understand that. I don't understand why we would send out providers when we have a shortage of providers ourselves. We are a generation where a 99.9 fever they are running to the ER.

Question to Audience: Talk about how you educate patients. Who is supposed to do that and what is it supposed to look like?

Responses from Audience:
- One of the things we hit around is the concept of the access to care standards that we work with and when schedules are open. There are two critical pieces of guidance that come from the core above at this hospital and I think it's the Surgeon General's office that actually published the standards that we have to meet. So, if that is the published standards, we also have a published standard that says how far out we have to create our appointment schedules and our templates. If we are only and I hear it routinely from [scheduling staff] throughout the organization in lots of different things, "I can't book that appointment on that day because it's more than 28 days". If that is the case, why do we create templates for more than 28 days out? That makes no sense. There is no reason to create the template only to leave the appointment slot open for weeks on end.

- … I remember at some point, you used to get self-care books. That you had a class that you would take so when you did come up with the sniffles or you know you when you did come up with something, you would know to try this first instead of running into a clinic to get a cold pack, which by the way is sold over the counter.

- … I just wanted to comment on who is responsible for educating patients. Every provider has been in contact with that patient on a daily basis, ensuring that there is no medication error. You have to communicate with the patient. In the [specific department] … patients come up to me with really unrealistic expectations. No one educated them down there in the clinic when they spoke to them about the [procedure] … They get to me and their expectation is that they are going to [have the procedure] … the same day. On a daily basis, my coworkers and I have to constantly apologizing for the wait time, we're constantly getting called out of our name or put in a type of predicament where we are accountable for someone else's lack.

- [The previous speaker] ... was talking about the self-help initiative. That initiative was back in the early 1998s, 99s, around there. Those were classes taught by the TRICARE department and they gave out the books and the cards, one part for the pharmacy. There is so much emphasis on training, we have gotten away from the basics of just taking care of yourself. I mean the only way to get things done is to take it over, tell the patient that we are having training, the PA sits down and tells them, this is how you go to the doctor, this is when you go to the doctor till someone is down there in their units.

Question to Audience: How often does your clinic respond to secure messaging from patients within the time requirements, as directed by policy and guidance?

Responses from Audience:
- ... we are missing the mark with access to care. The biggest problem I see right now ... the responsibility by the service chief because he/she is not paying attention to the schedules that are not open with 45 days. They are not approving whether a manager can talk up to a front-line supervisor and say, don't book any of my appointments so there is no one protecting the [scheduling staff] because everyone is looking the other way to see how often that provider is adjusting their schedule ... our reconfiguration [system means we can] ... adjust to a routine or adjust to acute slot so that we don't go un-booked ... why do we have so many un-booked spots? ... [we] can pull the data and tell the providers who is not working.

- Just to piggy back off of what [they were] saying ... We have to make money to use money. We are not generating that much funds. There are some providers that actually do the work. And there are others, they leave early, they are in meetings.

Questions Related to Patient Safety

Question to Audience: How do you report a patient safety report or issue?

Responses from Audience:
- I just report to my NCOIC – Non-Commissioned Officer in Charge.

- PSR, it's automatic.

- We're probably going to have a problem sitting in here – some of us. Seriously. Some of us may have a problem sitting in here ... When you bring people or hire people off the street that have no knowledge of what you hired them for but you hired them because that is the husband of this person or that husband. People suffer. They didn't hire her when she didn't know all that with her numbers. She has been here for years. Each commander comes in with a different flavor of Kool-Aid. ... Those doctors should sit at the front desk and make those appointments in the privacy where no one else gets in because they were afraid.

- Patient safety ... I guess it goes back to not having enough personnel.

- ... We do all sorts of reporting, processes to ensure we are not overlooking anything but it happens so it is providers.

- We have them here at this hospital – complex medical patients. Providers don't have time to stop and take care of them. Mid-management, [staff] ... don't understand the complexities it takes to take care of these patients. So, when you don't have the numbers saying that you took care of a massive number of these [Service members], they don't want to hear how it really is, it is their way or the highway. They don't want to hear why something is so complex. So, the problem is that they want you to divide yourself but that one person that is critically sick that needs you the most, you can't stop and take care of it and push forward for all the things they need.

- ...I just want to pass on a comment from a gentleman that had to leave. [Specific department] ... is where he is coming from. He said a lot of times they have complex appointments because a [Service member] will be scheduled to come into the clinic and they will be told by their chain of command or their [senior enlisted] that they need to cancel their appointment, which creates a snow-ball effect.

Site 5 Beneficiary Town Hall Questions and Answers

The following text reproduces the Town Hall facilitator questions and audience responses, transcribed as close to verbatim as possible during the session. Information that could potentially identify individual participants has been omitted for privacy purposes.

Approximately 120 people attended this Town Hall meeting.

Questions Related to Quality of Care

Question to Audience: Do you think you get good care here and how do you know?

Responses from Audience:
- I come here for [care] ... and last year I was diagnosed with [personal information omitted] ... They treat the patient not the numbers. ... I was [ok] until a few months ago then when the symptoms kicked in and I saw [multiple specialists] ... and the very same day I got pulled into [treatment] ... The quality, the reaction, the people I have seen are professional, all the way from the [enlisted medical personnel] ... right up to the Commander. I always feel like I am the only person there because of the attention they give.

- Before I was assigned to [this MTF] I was constantly asking to see someone who could talk to me about [procedure] ... and it was brushed off until I came here. I saw my PCM who immediately took my information and recommended a specialist for me to see. I went to see the doctor and had the best care I have ever had. Every appointment went so smoothly. I am just so grateful.

- [Personal information omitted] ... I just want to say that the care here is incredible. I am your biggest cheerleader. I have only wonderful things to say whether it is PCM checkups to emergency surgery, emergency care. They are great all around.

- [Personal information omitted] ... [came to this MTF for care] ... they decided that they could not see [the person] ... The reason I was given was that they didn't have bed space. On the way out [I was ...] told ... that bed space was not the case. The reason they could not see [personal information omitted] ... was because they didn't have the doctors. [We went] ... to [another location] [personal information omitted]... it was the trauma of having [a procedure] ... and moving from place to place that caused [the person] to pass away. It was excessive. Where are the doctors?

- Bottom line, this is top notch, professional care. If you need to see someone off of the base, they will make sure that happens too. They will find the help that you need.

Question to Audience: How does quality care here compare to quality in purchased care?

Responses from Audience:
- I worked for [personal information omitted] ... and my job was to see patients. I have perspective on quality of care. After serving two or three hundred patients, I don't think I saw one that wasn't highly appreciative of the work done here at [this MTF]. That has been the perspective of several patients. I have been referred out and I think the care here is wonderful. It think it is very personal and everything else.

- I have nothing but accolades as well. From primary care to physical therapy I have had extremely good care. My question is, my husband has just turned 65 and is now on Medicare and was told he had to leave the system. Why is that? I am hoping that changes before I get there.

- I must say that I have had a mixed reaction here. I have had everything from great to not good at all care. If I compare this to the outside system that I have been referred to, there are many ways I can see the outside care being better. They gave me better feedback. They gave me better information on anyone that I needed to get in touch with.

- In many ways the care is equivalent. I have had [procedure] here in the Emergency Room and the care was fantastic. The doctor saved my life. In some cases, the military does not cover what I think should be basic. You have a lot of people who do manual work and chiropractor treatment is not covered. I think that is kind of strange.

- It was very hard to get an appointment and outpatient behavioral health pediatrics was closed down which was very frustrating. It took me eight weeks to find outpatient behavioral health pediatrics ... for [personal information omitted] ... Once we found the provider it was not a very good experience. The provider was understaffed and he had a large workload. What I found since then is that in outpatient behavioral health pediatrics

... there is a huge need for providers. I tried to go through the system and still could not find a provider [personal information omitted] ...

- [Personal information omitted] ... after several years of living there that primary care is nothing like it is here. People here think there are problems getting in [to see a provider] but [they] haven't seen anything. The care is rushed and the treatment is not the same [there]. What I have noticed here is that a chair is moved and I am sitting with the doctor as she goes over my x-ray. Not that I understand it but at least I am looking at it and she is talking with me about it.

- I'm a patient and I come here for treatment as a result of wounds [in theater] ... This hospital gave me my life back. My body was not performing correctly and ... I got the best treatment. The people here just did everything for us.

- I had an experience where I could contrast care inside the hospital and outside the hospital. I was treated for [personal information omitted] ... and all of my questions were answered, everything was explained to me, and I felt that it was very thorough. At the time of the government shutdown I was referred to outside for [personal information omitted] ... and I felt like it was just a revolving door. It was very quick. Things were not explained and I did not have a feeling of confidence. I felt like one of their jobs was to have me get as many add-ons so that the government would pay for it. They constantly offered me things that I didn't need. I was almost directing my own care as oppose to them directing my care.

- ... I came to this hospital on a routine visit. I had some tests done and never got any of the results back. [Personal information omitted] ... The lack of communication could have put my life in danger. I soon after got a specialist on the outside and the care has been great.

Question to Audience: If you have a concern about the quality of care that you receive here, how do you let someone know?

Responses from Audience:
- It should be a requirement of the MHS that when they refer a patient out, whoever receives the TRICARE money needs to be required to gather personal health records. We need to improve communication through file sharing.

- The hospital has comment cards and I write emails with the subject heading "Mystery Shopper" to give feedback when I see something that isn't right. I send it to Patient advocacy office.

- Whenever I am dissatisfied, I make it known immediately and I pick out someone that I believe will do something about it. [Personal information omitted] ... I follow the chain of command and the last place you stop when you don't like something, is the hospital commander. In terms of things being wrong, I no longer come to the pharmacy in the hospital because I got so tired of witnessing an inefficient operation. I don't know who worked out the system down here. I came when they opened and after a few months I got tired of going there. I have received good care here for the most part. In the neighborhood that I live in, there are residents with a lot of [personal information omitted] and those people are seldom satisfied with their care. Pediatric care is very difficult. This hospital does not do a very good job of taking care of small children.

- [Personal information omitted] ... I talk to anyone who will listen. I talk to the patients in the waiting room, nurses, and doctors. I do the comment cards. I am not sure that I have seen any changes but I have gotten feedback via telephone. I have not seen any changes in regards to my comments.

Question to Audience: What should [this MTF] do to improve quality?

Responses from Audience:
- More doctors, more doctors, more doctors! I have had excellent medical for [personal information omitted] ... Right now primary care concerns would be MORE DOCTORS!

Questions Related to Access to Care

Question to Audience: How easy or difficult is it for you to schedule appointments at this medical facility?

Responses from Audience:
- I am very happy that you all are receiving excellent care. [Personal information omitted] ... I needed to see someone, they told me to go to emergency. To me emergency is broken bones and blood. I went to the ER but I also asked to see my PCM [personal information omitted] ... The first appointment I could make was two weeks later. I went in for my appointment to see my PCM but it was not my PCM. The doctor only checked me out for one issue instead of all three issues I was having. They referred me to therapy ... appointment for a month later for [personal information omitted] ... This doctor also did not give me a follow up appointment. This is just one little story. I am having good luck with the pharmacy.

- I have received excellent health care but sometimes I wonder about the coordination between the doctors. There is a big gap there. Most of the time, when I go to schedule an appointment, I hear that my doctor doesn't have an opening for another month, so I then get referred to another doctor. There is a big gap in care there. As far as same day appointments, [personal information omitted] ... and the customer service rep that I spoke to [personal information omitted] ... ended up telling me that I would have to wait a week to be seen. This facility has issues with access to care.

- I would like to see all of the providers on RelayHealth. There are so many providers you have not subscribed to it and it ends up being harder to communicate with them.

- [Personal information omitted] …. I often have to anticipate … so that I can call right at 7 AM to get an appointment. If not I am advised to go to the ER. I have been told by ER doctor that, "Our job is to assess whether you are going to die." I feel hesitant to go in there sometimes because I know [personal information omitted] … is not going to die. So the access to pediatrics has been very frustrating to us …. If I call and have my referral it is 28 days before the next appointment. If I can't go because I am out of town that day I will try back the day after and it is not 28 days from the last time I called, it is 28 until the next available appointment. That is very frustrating because it is months down the road before I feel like I have been properly assessed.

- Same thing for me. I call in and they tell me that they cannot see me for a couple of weeks. That means it is going to be a couple weeks before I stop having [personal information omitted] … that is just to determine what the problem is, not to see if they can do anything about it. RelayHealth is awesome. Don't like coming to the doctor so I wait until I have 3 or 4 things wrong. Then I come in and they say that they can only treat one … [personal information omitted] … The ER is great …

Question to Audience: How does this facility compare with getting appointments in the purchased care network?

Responses from Audience:
- I can always get an appointment outside if you get a referral.

- [Personal information omitted] … I used primarily treatment in the purchased care network. When I call [personal information omitted] pediatrician I always get a same day appointment. [When] I call [the] … specialty care provider to ask a question, I always get a same day reply. In terms of comparison I can provide the perspective from a family who seeks care in the civilian purchased care network. I always get an appointment if it is an urgent care matter.

- We switched to TRICARE Standard because of the lack of access to urgent care appointments in pediatrics. Ever since doing that we have never had a problem getting a same day appointment.

- [Personal information omitted] … Access to behavioral health care under TRICARE is extremely problematic. … [Personal information omitted]

- [Personal information omitted] … Getting an appointment now is better than it was at [another location]. I think it is wonderful because I can easily get a referral however the referral is never for this facility. I always have to travel and that is very frustrating from a facility that is this large that I have to travel [over 50] miles round trip to see a doctor… [Personal information omitted]

- There is no instruction on how to use the medical home and RelayHealth. There is a button on the top of the website but if you are not aware it doesn't help. I also want to address IT. Often when I come to this facility the computers are out and your provider can't access your medical records. One day I tried to do a walk in for [personal information omitted] ... and I could not do it because the computers were out again. For a [facility of this type] the IT is very poor.

- When I call for a same day appointment I cannot get one. ... my next option is to take the first available appointment which may be two to three weeks down the road. You could call every day and due to cancellations you may get an earlier appointment. Eventually I can usually call in on one of those days and get a same day appointment. Access is extremely frustrating for me.

Question to Audience: TRICARE's standard is 24 hours for urgent care, 7 days for routine care, and 28 days for wellness visits and specialty care. In your view, how are these standards being met?

Responses from Audience:
- Nonexistent. They do not meet the standards unless you are active military. The standard response is "are you active military" and if you are not you are pushed to the back of the line.

- Same. Nonexistent. You can call at 6:30 AM and all of the appointments are gone. My experience I can never schedule an appointment. I am always told that my doctor's schedule is booked. [Personal information omitted] ...

- One thing I would like to highlight, is what are contractors doing to recruit and retain providers in the network. I think that is a big question. Pediatrics specialty care is problematic.

- [Personal information omitted] ... has yet to fail in getting a same day appointment...

- [Personal information omitted]... I have had no complaints. Whenever I have a question or need help, I always get an answer. I don't always see my doctor but I always get what I need.

Questions Related to Patient Safety

Question to Audience: Do you feel that you get safe care here at [this MTF]?

Responses from Audience:
- There was an article relating to this in the NY Times yesterday making the point that we need transparency as well as informed consent. (*Beneficiary reads statistics directly from the NY Times article in regards to comparisons with civilian clinics and access to information*)

- [Personal information omitted] ... they have a policy that pertains to [staffing] ... that changes shift. Before they do so they give detailed briefs on the patients they are treating. Because of the procedure I was able to hear them talk and interject when they misremembered the medication I was taking. That procedure improves safety of care.

- [Personal information omitted] ... there was a [staff] ... shift change report which I was able to participate in and ask questions and listen to what they were handing off.

Question to Audience: When you are with your provider at [this MTF], do you feel comfortable asking questions? And are you getting answers?

Responses from Audience:
- I feel very comfortable when I am with my provider. When I have to have tests done with someone else, that is when I get uncomfortable ... [personal information omitted] ... [equipment used to conduct the test broke down] ... The knowledge level of the people who were conducting the test was questionable. That is my concern.

- We do have concerns about safety. I want to know that what we have spoken about today [is] going to be taken seriously and not just going to be incorporated in a poster or a program. We need improvement processes to actually work.

- I noticed in the past month or so that they have moved all of the refills from the pharmacy over to the other side of [this MTF]. I don't think that is the right way to do it. Put all the prescriptions, if you are getting a new one or a refill, in the same place. At the new place you have to stand until they get to you. There is nowhere to sit down.

- [Personal information omitted] ... [we] had the test done here at [this MTF]. We went to [another location] and the doctor could not access the information. I thought this was supposed to be a single system which the doctors in [another location] could access all of your information on the system. That is not the case.

- My biggest concern is that now that we have gone through this dialog, how are we going to find out if this was useful. I noticed that everyone took time away from their day to come here and I see it as us being pushed. There is only an hour and we can only say so much. Anytime I have gone to a forum of that nature, we don't get any feedback.

- The problem [is] that ... retirees [personal information omitted] ... are an issue. Getting an appointment within the system is very difficult. [Patients] ... on Medicare [are expected] to find doctors on the outside. In this part of the community there aren't that many available doctors who will take Medicare patients. So [people] ... go on in a circle trying to find care and many times ... [must] wait months to get a problem addressed...

- [Personal information omitted] ... am really disappointed that I have not received any kind of explanation of what to expect when [Medicare kicks in] ...

- Does this clinic have an Ombudsman to bring questions to so we can receive feedback from the front office?

Site 5 Staff Town Hall Questions and Answers

The following text reproduces the Town Hall facilitator questions and audience responses, transcribed as close to verbatim as possible during the session. Information that could potentially identify individual participants has been omitted for privacy purposes.

Approximately 65 people attended this Town Hall meeting.

Questions Related to Quality of Care

Question to Audience: Is quality of care a priority for your facility? How do you know if it is or if it isn't?

Responses from Audience:
- Yes, it is. Of course, I mean quality of care in terms of patients, customer service, patient satisfaction as well as evidence-based treatments.

- I am not located in [specific department] ... anymore ... one marker that I saw was that people didn't leave until the work was done. We moan and groan when people show up late but if it was urgent or emergent, it definitely got done and people took the time to make sure that it was in fact urgent so they didn't just automatically immediately just say oh no you have to go to the ER. I'd say that sometimes the systems, we worked on improving the systems so they would work better so we would have less of that last minute stuff but I never saw a nurse, MA or LPN, or doctor leave if something really needed to be done that day, really needed to be done that day.

- Through developing policies and procedures that more than adequately serve our patients; standardizing services that we provide, and continually reevaluating so that we can continue to improve, process improvement providing as much as we can to our patients, identifying the needs as they arise and meeting them. It is a dynamic situation. I'm a [specialist] ... here and so you know we may say okay, when a patient leaves we are going to make sure we provide this appointment or that appointment, we may find another appointment is more important ... Providing alternative [approaches] ... so being open to new ideas and not only open to them but implementing them.

Question to Audience: What are some examples of successes you've seen here in terms of quality?

Responses from Audience:
- We have been able to offer an evidence-based training for PTSD via training here for about 70 individuals over three days.

- I think that the hospital education department goes above and beyond and out of its way to accommodate people ... Don't see that everywhere ... That is flexibility. So, I would say the hospital and department [do] a good job.

- [This MTF] has won a couple of awards on labs and use of "VOSERA" to decrease reaction time in the case of emergency events. I forgot the lab document that they were working on but they have won a couple of awards for it.

- I work in the [specific department] ... we take the patients [from all outlying clinics] and we deliver great care. Whether we get upset or not, we put our patients first. We should be applauded for that.

- So we also measure quality metrics like other MTFs like the HEDIS measures [specific department] ... they measure compliance with wellness exams, pap smears, colonoscopies and things of that nature.

- A couple of things that come to mind [are] the baby friendly initiative at this hospital. It has gone command-wide so everybody here should be able to answer a few questions on it. Also, for our wounded warrior care, we have a dedicated ... team, that's our primary mission is to go and bring those patients from ... other facilities in the area. Baby friendly initiative is ... focusing more on baby to make sure that all the needs it has are met.

- I work in the [specific department] ... and as far as safety issues/concerns, when we bring about any issues concerning safety ... [in our department] our leadership is very open and works hard on safety issues. But unfortunately, when I worked here in the [specific department] ... that was not the case. When safety issues or concerns were brought up, there was a lot of retaliation from leadership and even hospital administration that did not want to hear or address any of the issues that were brought about previously. ... We had a lot of safety issues in the [specific department] ... We always ran out of equipment, we always ran out of gloves ... A lot of issues of safety. Not sure if issues have been resolved since I don't work there anymore.

- Like the other team member said, where I am now ... quality is definitely being adhered to. But when I was assigned to the [same department noted by previous speaker] ... I did not see that. I felt like the staff that provided quality of care was not valued by leadership and if they spoke up, they were reprised against by leadership. And that greatly impacted quality and that was the [specific department] ...

- I just want to mention some examples of quality. We focus here on transitions of care and it's important to do that to help our admission rates. [Staff] ... call patients after surgery [and after they have been discharged]... [and] counsel [patients] when they leaving [to ensure] they are able to reiterate what the discharge instructions were that were given to them.

- I have another example of quality process improvement which is we really wanted to make sure that the providers that would be working with the patients prior to the admission, we stay in loop with them with everything that was going on so we started letting them know immediately when their patient was admitted, when we have the discharge meeting, and we have that with everyone, that they would be invited either by telephone or in person so that they could know exactly what was going on with the patient so when the patient returns to them that it was a seamless transition. So, we implemented that over the last six months.

Question to Audience: Talk to me about challenges? A couple ladies up here were talking about issues in the [specific department] ... Anybody else?

Responses from Audience:
- ... I've noticed that people care about their patients. Providers are very good here. We really care about the patients that we see. What I find frustrating here are the roadblocks and the inefficiencies that we are faced with as providers. So, for example this is a silly example that you would think would have fixed because it takes up so much time. It's a patient safety issue for the patient, it's an infectious control issue for other patients. But I thought, why are we having this problem. This is not that hard to fix. We have a patient come in, we know they are leaving, they have had [procedure] ... We know they are going to need a [equipment] ... when they go home ... why can't we have the [equipment] ... delivered to the hospital instead of the home. Oh well, I guess apparently some of the vendors have been double billing if it goes to the hospital. So, now it has to go to the patient's house, somebody may or may not be there to sign for it. Meanwhile, they are here, they are discharged, there is no [equipment] ... for them to go home. They get discharged in the morning and guess what, 3:00 in the afternoon the [equipment] ... is supposed to show up. This is not safe for the patient ... So, we are sending them out with no [equipment] ... [Staff] ... to their credit want that patient to go home safely so [equipment is given to the patient and the patient is asked to return the equipment next time] ... I think that's a big infectious control issue because now patients had it in their home, you gotta make sure it's clean but why is this so hard. Why can't we at least, everywhere I've been, we give them [the equipment they need] ... it is not asking the people that take care of the patient "what is good for your patients?" This is ineffective, it is inefficient but again we have no power to change that. So we spend an inordinate amount of time trying to get them something to go home with.

Question to Audience: What kinds of barriers are getting in the way from your perspective, if anything, in terms of delivering quality care? What are some of the barriers that you are seeing?

Responses from Audience:
- The high turnover of leadership. I'm not talking about the change over after every 2-3 years but I'm talking about every few months or every year ... we have a lot of turnover.

Question to Audience: What is the impact [of leadership turnover]? What does it actually do to your ability to implement quality improvement initiatives?

Responses from Audience:
- Most new leaders want to make an impact and want to make a change so they come in, let us know what changes they want, and as they are trying to develop their processes, they leave. So, the staff adhere to this new policy that's been changed and a new leader comes in and wants to implement new policies. And many policies and procedures, they aren't best practices but rather [they have] taken something from previous clinics and want to implement here.

- I think it's the toxic leaders that impact the quality. Leaders that do not lead by example. They do not display the [Service core] values. When leaders speak up they reprise against other leaders.

- … [elsewhere where I have worked] if I ask 10 [personnel] … what is the process for doing something, they can tell me "this is how you do it." Here … there have been many times where you'll hear from a [staff person] … "this is how you do it on our floor" or "this is how you do it on our floor." I've gone to the educators and said that okay we can't have [personnel] … doing it differently on [each of] their floor[s]. It all has to be the same. They say, "yeah I see there is a problem" but you hear nothing else about it.

- I believe that when you're considering quality of care and the delivery of that care, I think you need to take a look at our documentation. Since this hospital has opened, our documentation, for me it would be something like the [specific department process] … has changed several times and in my opinion, it is not getting any better and I have been doing this for a very long [time] … both in the military system … as well as in the civilian world. The documentation does not seem to collect what is pertinent to the patient's care. Allowing us to individualize prompts that ask specific questions do not necessarily pertain to why that patient is here. We have a set of care plans that do not collect the data in a fashion that care plans were intended to collect. It has to be patient-specific. It has to be in a certain timeframe.

Question to Audience: What needs to change?

Responses from Audience:
- I've always said I like to leave it to the professional. And there are people that are very skilled at setting up the type of documentation with our input, the type of documentation that we need to ensure that across the board in this hospital as the patient moves elsewhere that that person's needs are communicated.

- One of the things that I think is a challenge for me is that I really like the area that I work in but I think we do a good job but I think we could do an exceptional job if the communication was better. I don't like this model where the decisions are made up here but it is not communicated down. Okay? So, somehow we are supposed to gather from the air that this is a new initiative. For instance, I was making referrals to outlying clinics and for whatever reason, they couldn't accept the referral and so they asked, so what about this initiative to recapture all the people. I just sat there and asked we have the initiative to recapture all the people, apparently the DoD is trying to bring in dependents and vets if they have openings. And so there are no meetings. In my area, everyone is in a silo. You're just in a silo and you do your job and no one comes together. That's where you get all the good ideas from, from the people that are working for you, not from up here. You have to listen to the people below in order to make improvements. But that's not how it works around here at least from my experience. You get your direction either through an email or you're passing a person in the hall.

Question to Audience: If you have a quality concern here at [this MTF], where do you take it? How do you address it? If you have an issue around quality, where do you take it?

Responses from Audience:
- ... [The previous speaker]... has touched on something that I've noticed since starting to work here [in the] [specific department] ... the constant change in leadership turnover and how it impacts the quality of care. The constant turnover in leadership – what it does is interrupt the continuity of care for patients. So many of our patients that come in become more and more complex each day and I'm sure when we start seeing VA patients, they will be even more complex. But when your main providers are constantly deployed and there is a new face every few months, the providers themselves have a hard time keeping up with what is going on with the patients. Patients will say I saw so and so and he told me this but then I saw this guy and he told me that I don't have that. Oh wow, maybe I need to get another opinion then. I think that how patients perceive good care really comes from the providers that they see and continuation of their health care needs from what they are being told, new studies, new diagnostics, or providers that know what diagnostic studies were done so when the results come back, patients can say this is what I have and this is what I have. But often times, patients will come out and say yeah wow that's not even what I came in for. But to me, it's not so much that the provider was wrong or the patient was wrong, it's that they are looking at it from a different perspective and the patients are getting confused in the process. Same thing with staff people who are working with providers. You get this patient ready for something and they come out and it's something different. So, the continuity of care issue is huge when your main providers are constantly deployed and there is no formal handoff process and even if there was a handoff, and the other guy who is getting the handoff is not there on time, they don't get a handoff.

Question to Audience: Are there documented health records? Are they effective?

Responses from Audience:
- Yes, of course there is. Sometimes they are down and sometimes, depending on the time of month it is, they are available. So there are times when patients come in and there is no record whatsoever to go by because the system is out. That is a constant factor. So, yeah there is but I can't speak for the providers. Those are some things I get told from patients and then same thing with leadership. So you know you have your leadership constantly, so when the leadership goes on deployment and someone else takes over, there is no

continuity, here's the vision and mission and this is how we are going to carry out things. It's gone and this new person will try to do something else but this person has 100 good things on the plate. So, it's never really addressed. So whether there is quality issue, it really depends. The leadership is tied up to a ranking system because it's a military facility, they can't go any further than a certain point, so it gets tossed around. I'm not really sure. I don't really know one particular place I would go to for quality issues.

Questions Related to Access to Care

Question to Audience: Do your appointment templates and schedules meet demand?

Responses from Audience:
- [The appointment management system] is misery ... when we were at [specific department in another location] ... [and] scheduled patients and we did better. I can only speak for that department. I'm sort of out of that department now but that's the one I've worked for. And I am just writing down here mostly responses to what other people have said, the [equipment] ... issue you brought up. I feel like going around good-will and picking up all the [equipment] ... in good shape and bring them back to you all here to look at to see if they can replace the ones that walked out and never came back. Because letting someone go without [the proper equipment] ... that has been adjusted to their [needs] ... is a safety issue. Another question that somebody brought up, this lady here, [staff] ... change of shift, I ask you does that have to do with problems with Essentris® issue.

- Documentation for us and inpatient services is found on Essentris®. So yes, it is an Essentris® issue.

- This is an issue that has happened repeatedly. And that is the lack of communication with [the appointment management system] or TRICARE and booking patients. Patients have been told that [there are no] ... appointments available on [the] ... schedule. And that is for ... [the] August schedule and September. The schedule has not even been opened yet. Patients were furious calling back to their doctor that meant it took sometimes 3-4 hours in order to resolve the issue. [Staff don't] ... know where they are getting their information but they are not communicating ... and they are not taking the time to communicate with [staff].... .

Question from an Audience Member to Another: Do you know if it's a problem with the Essentris® program?

Responses to the Question:
- I don't know if it's the program itself because you know there are folks that put information into the program so the data that is being input into the program so we can chart on it.

- I personally feel it doesn't. I myself was trying to get a [specialty] ... appointment and I had to be referred out and it was like more than two months and then we are scheduling our [other] ... appointments, they were supposed to have been done with all the list schedules but there are some that have clinics that have lists instead of putting the appointments into the CHCS.

- I work in [specific department] ... I feel as though at times, the templates are not there for the patients but for the providers so they should make it accessible for the patients more. For example, don't stop your clinic at 2:00 in the afternoon and push it back to 3:00 PM in the afternoon and maybe don't start your clinic at 8:30 in the morning, start it at 7:00-7:30 in the morning like everyone else so to be on the same page.

Question to Audience: Do different clinics have different hours?

Responses from Audience:
- Yes, they do.

- It could be when a provider wants to come in early so they can leave early. So then when you have a clinic that works from 7 to 2, another one down here that works 8 to 3, and everybody at different times, even though they have the same rehab department or something like that.

- I was approached by a military member ... who had called in to the specialty clinic and they [said] ... "we can't see you here for 2 months but we can get you in next week at such and such facility." [The patient] ... called [a] ... provider who is a friend ... and he [said] ... "my schedule is clear for tomorrow. I have nothing." So, [the patient] ... had to go the back way... to get an appointment [and] ... was seen at this facility by going the back way. [The patient] ... called into the access line and [said] ... she could be seen at another facility but not here.

- Maybe that provider who got his friend in was on admin so that he did her a favor and told her to come in – so we get a lot of that too.

Question to Audience: When do you release appointments for booking?

Responses from Audience:
- Again as providers, we all know this changes constantly. First it was 30 days out, now it's 60 days out, now I heard a rumor again, a rumor mill, 8 weeks out. But what we are finding when we release those appointments, especially those that are booked through [the appointment management system], we do a lot of proactive bookings for [specialty clinic] ... and we get dinged for it because we have a lot of provider only book on the slots; however, we book those appointments. If we let [the appointment management system] book those appointments, if it's more than 2 or 3 weeks beyond, so a month or six months, you know what usually happens, they start to feel better and we have a high no-show rate on spec and why book with [the appointment management system] when

it's two or three weeks out. So, when we book them ourselves, we get them in sooner when they are having the problem. We book and people show up. So that's the frustration as well.

- ... and as we start to have this conversation, I would like some of you to wonder where these patients end up when they can't get an appointment. Patients are going to turn up in the Emergency Department. No matter if it's a rash, back pain, or something. So at the end of the day, they sign up, no wait times cause they can't get an appointment. I'm going to give an example ... [recently there was]... a patient [who came] ... in and it was her 5th visit to the Emergency Department in one week because she couldn't get any access to health care for the last month. So, these are my questions. Any talk of a copay for any patient that misuses the ED? Any talk of financial penalties for access of care outside of the military health system? Monitoring usage of the emergency department?

Question to Audience: How often do you book these types of appointments prior to the patient leaving [this MTF]? Follow-up appointments or PCH appointments for an initial visit?

Responses from Audience:
- For all situations. They are usually booked 2-4 number of visits. And if they need a joint visit with the physician, then we book that at the same time. And the patients are extremely grateful.

- We always book appointments, whatever appointments the patient needs, no matter what it is, before the patient leaves the hospital.

- I think some of the patients at some of the clinics get their appointments before leaving but a lot of them do not. So, there is no continuity or it's not consistent. My concern is assisting a patient. You have a [Service member] who has [health issue] ... and what's really slow is that they are not assigned a new PCM so they're trying to get in to see someone, they don't have a PCM to see...

- About new [Service members] coming to the area and not being assigned a PCM, it also affects the patient. Even if they are MTF, we've talked to many patients – it takes 24-48 hours before they can pick up any medication, which hinders them being able to if it's something they have to take otherwise they will end up in the ER, we can't do anything because they aren't assigned a PCM ... a specialty clinic ... can't touch them until a referral is sent ... which means they are not to get any medication, which is when we have to talk to them to tell them that they must talk to the other clinic from where they are coming from and put it into Walgreens and I'm not sure they get paid for it. So all that hassle that you would think wouldn't happen since they are coming from one MTF and going to another MTF, actually does happen.

- I think what happened is that the process is they are assigned a PCM but that PCM is not there so you can't book them for the PC so it's just not happening but I can't say why it is happening but it is happening a lot, I mean really, really a lot. So, if you have complicated patient and you have to see a PCM and you call and say hey I got this patient and he's got Dr. Smith and Dr. Smith is gone and no one can give you answers and you try to get them help but no one has any answers and they ask you to call TRICARE and TRICARE can't help.

- It is a TRICARE issue.

- I'm not sure it's just a TRICARE issue. I think it's a clinic and TRICARE issue.

- I work in [specific clinic] ... and this is the clinic you may be referring to. We lose about one-fourth of our providers each year. So, they rotate through here because it's used as training. So, we lose a chunk at the same time. People are not assigned new PCMs right away.

Question to Audience: How often does your clinic respond to secure messaging from patients as directed by policies and guidance?

Responses from Audience:
- ... We aren't one of them. I don't know why they decided who has access. So what we end up doing, we do a lot of work-arounds for our patients. We do, I give them my card with my email on it. I tell them if you have any issues, concerns, problems, drop me a line. And so of course, they drop me a line and I have to call them. So unfortunately it's a big hindrance to the clinics because I don't know how many there are, but not all of us have that secure messaging system.

- Well, like some providers don't even want to do the Relay messaging. Like I have someone that does not want to do Relay messaging.

- The reason I am in here is because I have a lot to say. It's that leadership expects too much from RelayHealth. Used in a smaller, controlled fashion, like [specialty clinic]... has developed, it's narrowed down its use and it's functional. The web visits are in my opinion ridiculous and bad medicine. So, even though the word is that RelayHealth is wonderful, it will replace all these visits and you can do all these wonderful things, I think each department has to figure out how they are going to use it and how it's going to help them. I talked to [specialty clinic]... and for them, it is extraordinarily difficult.

Question to Audience: What do you do if you are unable to meet the patient's desired appointment time?

Responses from Audience:
- ... From where I stand and where I've stood in the past, the system that requires them to be seen within a specific period of time, sometimes it is 2 weeks, sometimes it's 28 days, sometimes it is longer so they have to put it out longer. If they put it out longer to meet the patient's desire to want to be seen further out, it's a hit against the provider for putting

them out. So, they want to meet the patient's demands but they get dinged for putting it out so far in advance.

Questions Related to Patient Safety

Question to Audience: How do you report a patient safety concern that you see something that is a problem?

Responses from Audience:
- Well, we have our PSR system and it's a great system but the problem I see is that a lot of us [staff] ... will put a PSR in but they will never hear back about it. No follow-up. You know some feedback would help.

- We do use a PSR system; however it's a cumbersome system and we're probably not using it as much as we could. There is a lot of data on there that could be auto-generated from the fact that the user is putting the data into the computer here. It ought to know my location and my information, my designation. Five or six boxes that I had to do. It would make it much easier and user-friendly and probably get a lot more reporting done.

Question to Audience: When you are concerned, how does the process work? So, when you see something, what is the process by which you can let someone know that it's a safety issue?

Responses from Audience:
- So, if it's beside the PSR, it is important to determine how critical the patient is. ... I had a patient and I could not get on them as fast as I wish I had. From what a computer was telling me, it's an issue that should have been taken care of. Did I do anything about it? No because things in place that should have happened but just didn't happen so there are processes, processes and processes. Why bother making another process? Let's cut down on our plate to do and actually do the things that are already working. ... The operating room [has a] ... timeout, the World Health Organization checklist, there is another checklist for fire safety. If you keep bringing more checklists, people start to forget to do things. They are worried about getting more checklists instead of taking care of patients. It's a military thing. It's a knee-jerk reaction. Joint Commission is coming, we're up for Joint Commission but they forget about patient care – that gets lost.

- I feel that whenever there [are] safety issues and concerns, I think if we foster a hostile environment, it is very difficult to bring about any patient safety concerns, or say anything. A lot of people were always afraid to say anything due to reprisal. I just [saw] everybody else getting reprised again. All the people that left before me, even those that left after me, they are afraid to say anything because of the reprisal.

- I worked in other MTFs and a lot more focus on the ... culture, training and implementing. That process for guidance and I think I have never seen that here at [this MTF].

Question to Audience: Any further comments?

Responses from Audience:
- Just speaking for myself in relation to quality, patient safety, and access, I think we have a communication issue, we have a consistency issue, and we have an accountability issue here at [this MTF]. A lot of the times it is do as I say and not what you see me do. I think that in the process of standardizing across the board, there has been a lot of things that have occurred and a lot of things that have been missed. Standardization is not the be-all end all. Standardization is good for some things but not all. A good example is the CAG notes. We are having CAG notes done by people not really referring to subject matter experts. CAG – clinical action group. So not just with CAG notes, but a lot of things, processes, but we are not referring to the subject matter experts, we just have people who are doing these processes who do not have much of a clue on what to do.

Site 6 Beneficiary Town Hall Questions and Answers

The following text reproduces the Town Hall facilitator questions and audience responses, transcribed as close to verbatim as possible during the session. Information that could potentially identify individual participants has been omitted for privacy purposes.

Approximately 50 people attended this Town Hall meeting.

Questions Related to Quality of Care

Question to Audience: Do you think you get quality health care here? How do you know?

Responses from Audience:
- [Personal information omitted] ... The quality of care is so good that we drive an hour to come to this facility. Even when they're understaffed which they've gone through multiple times. They have had exceptional attitudes and have been helpful.

- I agree with everything she just said

- Absolutely

- I disagree. I had an experience with the hospital ... [personal information omitted] ... So that [we] had to drive to [other city] to get appropriate care. Called multiple people expressing that this was a problem. Tried to switch doctors but ... [*Facilitator: What I hear you saying is that you came here, you didn't feel satisfied with the advice that you got, you couldn't get a referral outside the network. So you went back to [other city] ... to stay within the MHS system ... Am I understanding that correctly?*] Correct.

- [Personal information omitted] ... I've had absolutely exquisite experience both [of us] ... No problems with referrals to specialties [in] [another location]. No problems.

- [Personal information omitted] ... was trying to get a [procedure] ... 2 months out they told her they couldn't get her in ... She was stationed here and they got her in, at her own convenience and she drove all the way here from [location over an hour away] to get her [procedure] ...

- For myself personally I've had great health care. I can't complain. Every time I call they usually get me in. I've had quality care. [Personal information omitted] ... I was seeing a doctor out of town but it was taking too much time to go see him ... [personal information omitted] ...

- I want to say first of all I'm very pleased with the care. [Personal information omitted] [Staff are] ... professional, efficient, and friendly. The problem I have is the provider turnover. A lot of people in this room, we're not leaving every 2-3 years. So to an active duty person and their family they might not notice the provider turnover. Every time we go in we see a different provider. Fortunately ... we don't have complicated medical issues but it's still a pain in the butt to establish that rapport [with] a new provider every time we go in. Why don't they get a provider that's dedicated to seeing the retirees and their families and that way we have continuity.

- I agree with everything everyone has said and I urge you to not give up on the clinic ... [Personal information omitted] ... They have pulled all the specialty care. They have tried to get contractors. I don't think they are paying people enough. It's hard to get people to move to this ... area. So it's hard for them to fill the contractor's spots. The military allows too many gaps, sometimes four months or more between active duty doctors. [Personal information omitted] ... I haven't had problems with referrals ... [staff] ... are under supported, understaffed, can't get people to move into this area to support how many people are in this area.

Question to Audience: How many of you go out into purchased care? How many of you have been referred out? Do you go?

Responses from Audience:
- *Crowd:* Yes, yes

Question to Audience: When you do go out into the purchased care world, how is the quality there compared to the quality here?

Responses from Audience:
- I would say that's not an apples to apples question. Your primary care [provider] is the gatekeeper. So you can't really say my care here is better than the specialty. To answer your question the referrals I have gone to have been excellent. I haven't had any problems.

- Just to amplify on what he's saying. When we come here, they're referral writers. They give us the specialty care we need. The problem is access to the primary care managers.

The problem is getting an appointment. It's not satisfactory. [Personal information omitted] ... [we] ... can't get in because there's no appointment. In the last two months 50% of the time care has not been available. They tell you to call in the morning. They tell you to [go] ... to urgent care or the emergency room and that's unsatisfactory.

Questions Related to Access to Care

Question to Audience: Let's shift gears a little bit to access of care. How difficult or easy is it for you to book appointments?

Responses from Audience:
- When it comes to continuity of care that is a lot of the issue. Whether it's trying to see our same PCM. When you do need a same day appointment, they try to squeeze you in but it's not with the same PCM that you've been seeing.

- I've had three PCMs in the last year. You have to spend the first 15 minutes explaining your issues.

Facilitator: So it's not in the records somewhere?

Responses from Audience:
- It is but they either don't have time to go that far back to review it. It is but they don't have time.

- There's not enough time because they're backed up. The problem is getting in and understanding who my PCM is.

- I'm a little different. I chose to see someone off base because of what I'm hearing ... [Personal information omitted] ... I can't come in and see someone different every single time, and go over my history every time and can't get my refills in a timely manner, or they can't see me when I need an appointment. So I stayed off base.

- I totally agree with changing PCM so quickly. [When] I came here ... my PCM was fantastic. When she got here I was miserable. She was willing to sit down and understand what was going on. Really make sure I am being her patient. For the last year I keep getting messages every couple of weeks that my PCM changed. I don't know who my PCM is anymore. About a month ago I had [personal information omitted] ... and I was concerned [personal information omitted] ... This [new] physician couldn't have cared less ... So I said if this is my PCM I want out now.

- I have called in for dermatology ... I called for my referral and got it easy. If they can't see me, they will refill my meds until they can see me.

- [Personal information omitted] ... I had a great PCM [this PCM] ... was phenomenal. When I was reassigned, I complained because I did not want to start over with someone else when my PCM is still in the building. [Personal information omitted] ... The problem is not a lack of wanting to help but the red tape. Staff is overworked severely underpaid. So it's unfortunate for us in the military ... to see [my PCM] leave was horrible. This base did a huge injustice in letting [this PCM] ... get away.

- Patient population is [within a certain region] and the pot of the pool of specialty resources outside the gate is small. Clinic has basically no specialties. [Other locations] are booked out for a month. If we get booked out of town it still could be a couple of weeks. I have travelled as far as [over an hour away].

- I actually would rather see a doctor out of town.

Question to Audience: TRICARE standard is 24 hours for urgent care, 7 days for routine care and 28 days for wellness and specialty care. How well are these being upheld?

Responses from Audience:
- ... [Personal information omitted] ... if I [go] ... to emergency room or urgent care, I meet that standard because I received care within 24 hours. But the access to our clinic. You get triaged in ER and spend 6 hours waiting for an earache. They probably think that they met it but it doesn't meet the standard.

- ... They can write a referral for us to see a specialist but that's about a month and a half wait unless you're lucky enough at 7:02 in the morning to get an acute visit scheduled. The problem with urgent care and the emergency department is that you can't get the referral you need and you're likely to come home with something worse ... [personal information omitted] ... we need to be able to be seen in our clinic.

Facilitator: When you are unable to make an appointment do you call and cancel or no show?

Responses from Audience:
- *Crowd:* Call and cancel

- I really have a problem with people not showing up here and I think based on my experience with other clinics they have a policy for no shows and this clinic does not. I think they should implement this and it would help make it functional.

Facilitator: What would be the penalty?

Responses from Audience:
- A fine. That's what they do out of town.

- If you miss your appointment you pay the office.

- If you miss 3 or more appointments they dismiss your care.

- I want to ask a quick question. There's not a lot of active duty here anymore but retirees staff most of the area. More and more seniors seem to keep coming to this base. [This MTF] [has downsized its capabilities] …

- The base population is [mostly contractor and GS]. Many are retirees. Base services are based on military population.

- The commissary is here for active duties but retirees have privileges as well. We are overwhelming the clinic because there are [many fewer active duty members than the number of people who] … technically have access to care.

- Maybe we're using the wrong method to determine the size that the clinic should be.

- I sympathize with the hospital. The types of services are continually declining.

- I agree with that. There is a decline in services and men overall.

Questions Related to Patient Safety

Question to Audience: Do you feel that you get safe care here?

Responses from Audience:
- Yes

- I hate to be a broken record. Access to the same provider is lacking which is a breach of safety. Lack of continuity speaks to safety.

- We're often educating our physicians

- I'm very comfortable

- I agree in the confidence and abilities. Overworking anyone will generate mistakes and mistakes affect safety. We like the people that … deal with us here but there are not enough of them and that is a cause of all the problems that every person addressed today.

- When you have only 4 minutes to see a patient, there is a safety issue. These people are overworked … [personal information omitted] …

Question to Audience: If you were king of quality improvement, what would you do differently other than adding staff?

Responses from Audience:
- I would like to see the appointment time being longer. The appointments should be longer than 15 minutes.

- I would like my whole family to have the same PCM

- Work on the IT system. Every time I go there the system is down. They can never access it and can never give me electronic referrals. The pharmacist is always out of my prescription.

- The building is so old. In the triage, the equipment is outdated.

- Long phone waits

- PCM doesn't get any breaks or lunches

- Bring the specialists back that used to visit

- Pay civilian provider staff more so we can retain them

Question to Audience: Would anyone else like to say something?

Responses from Audience:
- [Personal information omitted] ... The care is declining on the base. The whole thing is confusing.

- Are we going to support retirees or active duties? We need to know because no one is saying it.

- I think the days are gone when doctors remember when the kids were born and growing up. I think we just have to be our own advocate for our health and our families.

- When they closed the TRICARE service center it did affect quality because you can't get service from an 800 number when you have to wait for 25 minutes. [Personal information omitted] ... with TRICARE I never walked into the center and walk out without being treated and getting everything I needed in a fast and professional manner. And I am not experiencing that on the website or 800 number.

Site 6 Staff Town Hall Questions and Answers

The following text reproduces the Town Hall facilitator questions and audience responses, transcribed as close to verbatim as possible during the session. Information that could potentially identify individual participants has been omitted for privacy purposes.

Approximately 25 people attended this Town Hall meeting.

Questions Related to Quality of Care

Question to Audience: Is quality a priority here at [this MTF]? If it is, how do you know? And if it isn't, what makes you think that?

Responses from the Audience:
- I think it is. I mean I've seen from my perspective several process improvement schemes to provide better patient care overall. We have a few in our department and I know several other departments as well; I'm not entirely sure what they are. I know what they are in my department just not in other departments…

- … We have patients that become no show. We have put in place a policy or procedure that if patients are no-show, we make sure that we assess those cases so we have a list of high risk patients. If one of those patients is on that high-risk list, we make sure we follow certain protocols. We don't just leave it as a no-show. We follow up … So, I think … the front desk has to do some of that, but as a provider, I will ultimately do the assessment but he will be the one calling and following up. This process is in writing and everyone does buy into it. We review the list weekly.

- The … leadership, they are all about process improvement and they make it known that nothing is set in stone. That it can change. That if it doesn't work, we will improvise it. And the [leadership] even made customer service one of our strategic goals. He is very customer focused. He wants feedback. We have implemented so many ways for customer feedback, which then allows us to change our processes and procedures but yes, quality is number one and I feel leadership is very, very customer focused.

Facilitator: What are some examples of the customer feedback mechanisms that you've put into place?

Responses from the Audience:
- We have … online feedback. It's called ICE and … it stands for interactive customer evaluation. And then we have the monitored database, which [headquarters] sends out patient surveys. And then when the customer fills it out and sends it back, it gets input there. And we have customer comment cards for each department. We have town hall meetings. We have the patient family advisory council.

- … That is our number one customer complaint area basically because of the wait times. So, they did implement [a window] which is strictly for refill pickups.

Question to Audience: So, you've already started answering the next question, which is: tell us about some of the successes that you've observed. Tell us about the patient family advisory council.

Responses from Audience:
- It took the place of what is called Healthcare Consumer Council.

- Quality is a very broad term. It has to be defined. There has to be a lot in place to achieve that. For example, when we don't have providers, right, so patients can't see their PCM on a consistent basis for, say chronic illness such as diabetes, quality is impacted so you're missing those components. That's the problem. So, you can't say quality is good maybe individually but not for the patients because they are not getting the follow ups that are necessary. The end result can't be quality. There isn't enough time for doctors and nurses to discuss the patient and the work that needs to be done to provide the care that is required for there to be high quality.

Question to Audience: Other thoughts in terms of successes or challenges you face with respect to quality?

Responses from Audience:
- A challenge within [specific department] … we don't have a [specialist provider] … but they are very limited within the community … A lot of our active duty patients have to travel [to other locations]. Sometimes, [a particular location] but they are having staffing issues so they can't [be] as open to our patients. Certainly some of our PCMs can handle some of our patients but we have a lot of complicated patients and if that patient really needs to be handled by a [specialist provider] … we have people having to travel … there and they are late for appointments because of traffic or travel issues … a drive [to another location] is just adding to the frustration. I mean I think leadership is aware of that, it is an ongoing issue for our department but I do think it does affect other departments within the clinic.

- The lack of specialists that we have and the accessibility. We used to have specialists that would come down. It was very educational for the providers as well as the access for the patients. But that has really dwindled since we are no longer falling under [another location]. And so in a lot of avenues, we have to send our patients out to the network for radiographic studies, MRIs, mammograms, we have to send them out for CT scans because we don't have that availability. If we had a local unit that would even come down here and see you know for one or two days even a month for MRIs, it would cut down a lot of our expenses …

- I think that sometimes there is a sense that people are not sure on how to make a change happen. I think there are times when there is a lot of change or there is a lot of good talk and conversation about making changes happen, make things work and progress, seeing improvements made. Sometimes it is put back in the deck plate to make those changes happen but sometimes people are lost it seems on how to make those changes happen. And I think there is not always good direction on how to make change happen. Not to say there isn't strong influence, positivity and encouragement to do things, sometimes that message gets lost on how to make change happen.

- I think it touches on the training that we've all gone through. … If we implement TeamSTEPPS® into our daily lives, then it would answer your question that you just asked. The thing is that TeamSTEPPS® is inherent to us. I think that every question in this town hall today can be addressed with TeamSTEPPS®.

- TeamSTEPPS® is great for what it represents and what it is about and what it is supposed to do, and yes it is inherent to us. But one challenge I see is that if a certain number of people are trained up on TeamSTEPPS®, somewhere along the way that message or training will be drained or diluted down. So if everyone is not sort of hearing me or seeing a process or how it works and participate in the training, then those members may not get the full breadth of the message. So, I think it's great but I think everyone needs to see and understand it and participate.

- It's not my understanding that everyone does [participate in TeamSTEPPS®]. And part of that reason is access to utilization. So, it's almost like you don't want to cut the right arm so it's hard to balance with the challenges that we have with utilization and access. Not shutting the clinic down completely but at the same time, having everyone understand the process would help. That's just my two cents.

- This just came to me to dovetail off of what you were saying, the forward momentum going and … I think the nature of the, not just this clinic, but the nature of other clinics when those people at the upper echelon are all changing every two to three years, this start stop ratchet movement in a forward motion and it becomes difficult to continue in the same direction. Good people come in, they have to get up to speed, understand the nature of the clinic they are at, understand the dynamic nature of the people, the job that you do, the barriers. That takes time. Then they have their agenda on what is going to work and what they have to implement it and then they are gone. And then to do that every two or three years, it is very difficult. There is no continuity, there is no thread of continuity so I think and that is not inherent to this clinic. I think it makes for a very difficult forward progress and moving forward. Everyone is different on what they think it important and they want to move forward on that piece. Well then, a new leadership is going to come in and say no, I think this is really important. So you have this very ratchet flow of your command.

- One of the things we don't have here in [this Service's medical structure] is a civilian in upper management to hold that continuity whereas there is a [leader] who is GS so that you can continue on instead of start in a new direction each time …

- Those are my thoughts and have been for a long time. We get started, have a goal and everyone is on board, so they let everybody know because we have new leadership and then everything changes due to a new leadership after that. I think for the most we are an agreeable group of employees but it gets, it becomes, it is unproductive. That's not to say that what we are doing is wrong and we should change, I think that is always a reason, it's just something of concern.

- … when we think we are understanding what the change is all about, bam, everything changes again. So, now you have a new focus and everything changes. We do have focus on patient care but how we go about it, that changes all the time. So quality assurance, it is difficult.

Question to Audience: If you ever had a concern about quality, how do you manage that? Who do you talk to? What is the process to handle that concern?

Responses from Audience:
- It's called the chain of command. That's hard wired into all of us. Multi-service. Use your chain of command. And if you feel fear or repercussions, then there is a chain of command above that.

- I would address it with the person providing the poor quality. And then we also have a PSR [patient safety reporting] system, a patient safety report. I don't think we have shy group of folks and I think we would go to that person.

- It should not matter [if the person a staff person had to confront is above them in rank]. That is what TeamSTEPPS® teaches us.

- We have had lots of training that it should not matter. And we should speak up and rank does not matter.

- But realistically, I think people will speak up. I don't think that the situation will be corrected. I think that nothing gets done when you take up the chain of command. The tools are in place but nothing gets done. Here is the problem I see here, here is my solution. Can we try to implement this? They will think about it, think about it, and nothing gets done.

- We have the tools in place but executing them, using them, but what happens after that, nothing. We check the box and that's it.

- [To address this managers would] … need to have confidence in the ones doing the job. Supervisors need to have confidence in the work that we do. They have no confidence in the work that we do. We are the ones doing the work. They are sitting behind the desk.

- It depends on the supervisor you have. But then your supervisor takes what you do up the chain, and then you're still criticized or whatever, or so they don't implement it. The solution is I don't know.

Facilitator: What is a fix you would like to see happen?

Responses from Audience:
- Fire them all.

- It's not them because they do change. But things don't change.

- It would be nice to have some continuity. Say if the [leadership] was a civilian or maybe have a comptroller that's a civilian so it didn't have to change everything, they could train people. That way you keep going forward

- We are great at creating and developing different boards and committees to address certain things but I don't speak for a lot of people and maybe some people think that all the boards and the committees is another meeting to be had. But there is not much traction that has gained within that committee. So, maybe a process that would help that, maybe some program or tool to keep it accountable. So, maybe if we have a facility where we needed something done, it would get documented in there. Maybe if someone saw a process that needed to be improved, you could document in the system that someone has to be accountable to.

Questions Related to Access to Care

Question to Audience: Do your appointment templates and schedules meet appointment demand?

Responses from Audience:
- No.

- I know for a fact [staff are] …on the phone every morning at 7 AM and … put the schedules and templates in … [they] … are switching acute appointments just to get people in in the 28 days. And it doesn't do any good to say anything because they consider that acceptable access. How is it accessible if you are using sick appointments to book a physical and [staff] … were told … to send [patients] out into town, they are accessible. We are not going to send them [outside of the MTF] for a physical. We could get in trouble for that.

Facilitator: So, let me understand. If I'm sick and this lady needs a physical and you don't have any room, you bump me and send me to the network so you could do the physical and you do that because physicals have to occur within 28 days and you can't send them out?

Responses from Audience:
- I didn't know we could send them out. I was told we couldn't send them out for physicals.

- I was going to say perhaps you should have more appointments. I mean if I'm sick and I call you one time and you say sorry I can't see you, do you really think I'm going to bother calling you again? I'm going to go around where I can be seen so you're putting yourself out and I understand what you're dealing with but maybe you need to look at and say you know this, I don't go to this facility here but I know if I call in the morning at a certain time, I will get seen today. It's either going to be at this hour or this hour and I pick.

- But if they would look at the numbers in the last month, just how many they sent out to urgent care because we have no sick appointments. We start out some mornings with one appointment that we can book a sick appointment with. One.

- If you don't have a provider, there are no providers because they are fully booked, how can you squeeze more out of it.

- The same thing happened with the VA. They didn't have providers. The problem is they have to resort to waitlists to cover up the problem. We don't have to do that. We send them [outside of the MTF] to see urgent care or somebody in town. Or they go to the emergency room.

Question to Audience: When do you release appointments for booking?

Responses from Audience:
- They are out there 6 weeks in advance. [Staff is] ... about to book to the 28 days. [They've] ... had to schedule for up to 6 weeks at a time. They open at 7 AM every morning but ... can book a sick appointment 24 hours. But unfortunately, they are being put on waitlists basically because they are using them up. But I know they have to.

- I just think this clinic, we are used to doing more with less here and so it is overwhelming everybody. We all love our jobs but we need our resources, we need providers, the staff in order to help the patient. You know we are all getting stressed out and upset. And tired and frustrated, you know. And we are feeling unappreciated for all that we do. And it doesn't seem to be any resolution. I think this is what all of this is saying. I'm just trying to sum it up.

- We are a doctor's office, if we have no doctors, how long do you think this circle is going to be moving. You know the primary purpose is being tainted. I can't imagine and I don't know I don't think every doctor walked in here one day and said okay, I don't think I'm going to be in here anymore. And now we're at a point where we don't have any doctors, we don't have anybody. What are you doing to fix it? This is the question because you're never going to have enough appointments because you don't have anybody to see them.

Question to Audience: How often do you book each of these types of appointments prior to the patient leaving [this MTF]: follow-up appointments? PCM visits to the specialty clinics or initial visits? and outpatient procedures before that patient leaves?

Responses from Audience:
- In [specific department] ... we book them before they leave our office. And if they don't book before they leave the office, it's usually because they don't know what their schedule looks like and then we follow-up within 24 to 48 hours.

- I've noticed a lot of times lately and it all has to do with not enough doctors, going through schedules and actually canceling appointments that are follow-ups. Like the [staff] ... can call to avoid them from coming in because they need the appointment slot. We have to cancel it, the [staff] ... calls them. So it's very frightening because you're going back to the problem with no doctor.

Question to Audience: How often does your clinic respond to secure messaging or in some places called Relay messaging from the time you received it, as directed by policy and guidance?

Responses from Audience:
- Daily basis.

- It's another place to log on to. It's okay for certain things and not for other things.

- It's good for providing results. You can copy and paste. So, test results for example.

- [It is good for] ... refills because you can just call and leave a message. I don't have to open it. I can just address it right there in the system.

- I've heard pretty good feedback from patients that I see regarding the system. Maybe something that would be helpful is a kiosk that they can actually say not only that they are interested in registering and/or enrolling but a system to complete the process because sometimes they will fill out the little inquiry form and leave and never confirm their registration and come back on subsequent visits and still not be on the system. So, if you have a designated station asking them to complete the registration process and that way, we can send them the welcome and whatever else.

Question to Audience: What do you do if you are unable to meet the patient's desired appointment time line?

Responses from Audience:
- If they are looking for ... a physical and [staff] ... don't have anything within the 28 days, [staff] ... steal acute appointments to book their appointment. Because they might have their medications expire and they have to be seen for their physicals. PAPs, at one time [were] ... postpone[d] ... for a couple of months because [many patients] ... want just a female [provider] and we have only one. So she pretty much is always busy.

- Or [in specific department] ... [if] someone comes in [for] ... an initial [visit] ... and we can't get them in within 28 days or more, we have actually been using a colleague in the interim given some continuity of care to come in and see us. That way we get a little bit more information and they still get that continuity here ...

- It is not our first choice but ultimately, you want to make sure the patient is seen.

Questions Related to Patient Safety

Question to Audience: How do you report a safety issue or concern?

Responses from Audience:
- Patient Safety Reporting – PSR.

- Yes. If you have an incident, you enter as much information as you can and it goes to our patient safety authority and he will do a follow up with the person reporting it, the person involved. If it was another employee involved, he will do a complete follow-through and educate us. What we could have done, what that person could have done to prevent this from happening. It's not, you're not in trouble for anything that's happening. He makes that clear. It's strictly learning how we can avoid this from happening again.

- You have that option to hear or get a response back.

- You can go to the safety officer.

- We are hardwired to do a PSR.

Question to Audience: Do you have any other comments or ideas you would like to share?

Responses from Audience:
- I got an issue with the TRICARE system, I guess. It's not really TRICARE but TRICARE Prime and how they are received on base. Right now I work at [specific position] … [Patients prefer] … to get seen by a doctor. … It's taking appointments away from people who actually really need [a doctor] … this is one accessibility technique that they are missing out on. My solution was to have at least co-pays for TRICARE Prime members, not military members but to civilians, dependents, and retired veterans. Accessibility to care for patients wanting to see their primary care physicians for acute issues …

- The entitlement feeling that I think a lot of patients have that they expect they can call in and be seen today even though they have a cough that started this morning and they haven't done anything for it. So, they will be seen and given over the counter medications instead of by prescription so they don't have to pay for it. And they will ask for that chest x-ray from the provider and if they don't get it, they will complain and go up the chain. So, I think some of it is entitlement by the patient that they don't feel like showing up for an appointment, it's not a problem because it's free for them.

- That's not going to change.

- Well, it may change. They will be a no show in the morning and they will go to the ER in the afternoon.

- They don't want [patient education materials] … They have a degree at Google University.

- As far as no-show policies ... there are really no repercussions. For active duty, yeah you can tell their command. But for civilians there is no repercussion in the system for no-shows.

- Letters do go out to those people that show a pattern [of no shows].

- [The] ... on-site finance office [is co-located] ... with the VA department in the same building ... [there is] no security. People [are] coming in and out all day. Sometimes [people are] just walking around there because VA reps are there and so there is no one stopping them when they come back. There is a sign that says Only Authorized Personnel so [MHS staff are] ... sitting so far in the back and VA in the front that we can't hear what's going on ... security is needed.

Site 7 Beneficiary Town Hall Questions and Answers

The following text reproduces the Town Hall facilitator questions and audience responses, transcribed as close to verbatim as possible during the session. Information that could potentially identify individual participants has been omitted for privacy purposes.

Approximately 60 people attended this Town Hall meeting.

Questions Related to Quality of Care

Question to Audience: Do you think you get good care here and how do you know?

Responses from Audience:
- ... I'm a [personal information omitted] ... having gone through medical at [one of the Services] and [another location], received nothing but the best care, outstanding care. Received a second opinion from a top person in [another location] who has said [this MTF] was the best and spot on and is very proactive [personal information omitted] ...

- Recovering from serious illness. Years later, came back and got follow-up check. I got very good care and great follow-up from treatment years later. Very good across the board.

- I'm glad to hear that our retirees are having good experience. I'm [personal information omitted] ... and I have to say we're getting very poor care ... [personal information omitted] ... I think our experience here has been characterized by a lack of continuity with doctors who don't pay a great deal of attention to our patient histories, who don't actually give attention to the remarks we're giving and aren't willing to actually hear our feedback on medications that we're assigned. So yeah ... Our care has not been quite as good as some of the care we have received at places like [other facilities] and places where it has been good, it has been barely good.

- [Personal information omitted] ... I gotta agree with him on this one. It was really poor. I don't think the doctors communicate with each other. Mostly hit and miss. I also think they just want to get you out of the door. For example, it's like I went to pain management doctor and I don't think they ever talked back and forth between the doctors because it's like I went back to my primary care manager and he didn't have any idea what I was talking about that the pain management person brought up. [Personal information omitted] ... it felt like they were trying to get me out of the door like I was a bad [personal information omitted] ... trying to get out of the PT test.

- [Personal information omitted] ... My ... doctor told me he was tired of dealing with whiny dependents. My doctor that I was sent to, the OB/Gyn told me that she couldn't be bothered with me [personal information omitted] ... they were doing an exercise and I am on the phone with a doctor who said I'm sorry I'm in an exercise room and hung up on me. That is not a standard of care. [Personal information omitted] ... We deal with a lot. Having my medical professional tell me that they just don't want to deal with dependents and I'm like I'm not the only one who hears this constantly. I'm tired of being sick and told that I can't see a doctor. Last Friday I was told "well what you need is a specialist but we don't have one and TRICARE won't ever pay for you to see one."

- [Personal information omitted] ... our experience here has been very mixed. When we first got here, I went to the doctor for some routine item. I don't know who it was. And I got yelled at for the whole time from the doctor because they inadvertently scheduled me during the time that was supposed to be active duty. I had no control of the time they scheduled me and I had no idea about that. [Personal information omitted] ... retiree[s are] ... often ... told to go off base ... [personal information omitted] ... I went to the ER for the injury and was not X-rayed until I went the second time. They didn't do an MRI ... [until] ... later. I finally had surgery ... and ... the surgeon was remarkable ... [Personal information omitted] ... now my biggest concern is that I may have a disability for the rest of my life to some degree because [of the delay I experienced] ...

- [Personal information omitted] ... I have dealt extensively with the hospital. And I must say that from my perspective ... [personal information omitted] ... not only did the people here deal with [personal information omitted] ... but they also coordinated with [off-base health care] to make sure [we] ... had the proper treatment ... [Personal information omitted] ... from my point of view, they were fantastic and I'm sad to hear about these other things but me personally, I just felt I had to say that.

- [Personal information omitted] ... during [a diagnostic procedure]... [the patient experienced an unrelated issue] ... the doctor didn't stop straight away but continued because [they were] ... near the end of it. And we were left ... [to] make our own appointment to see a [specialist out in the network] and that procedure cost us [over $10000], which we had to pay up front

- My experience is that routine care is great. I needed specialty care, and that wasn't provided on base. And unfortunately no one knew how to get connected with [off-base health care] or was willing to tell me how to connect until I made several calls and visits, got in touch with someone there, the ... TRICARE office and ... she told me straightway how to get in touch with [off-base health care] and get services from them. And it got resolved but there was quite a delay because I kept getting put off by providers here.

Question to Audience: Tell us a little bit about how being referred out into the network for purchased care compares with the quality of care you are getting here at [this MTF].

Responses from Audience:
- [Personal information omitted] ... We have had 4 outside referrals. One was for an unnecessary test that we knew our insurance wouldn't cover [personal information omitted] ... They wanted [over $5000] up front before they would even see [the person] ... [personal information omitted] ... [we are trying to see] ... other specialists [but they do not] ... accept our insurance or accept a referral from [this MTF]. And so we've been stalled since December in trying to get ... the care that [is needed] ***So you have been referred but the physicians that you have been referred to are not accepting your referral?*** Right or they want us to pay them [over $5000] up front in the hopes of being reimbursed by insurance ... ***Follow-up: What happens when you take that experience back to [this MTF]?*** We get the same answer every time: "We don't know what to tell you."

- I just like to add that I got hurt [personal information omitted] ... and it took them 8 months to basically say what was wrong but I went to the VA ... and they figured out what was wrong with me in 3 days [personal information omitted] ...

- With the basics, like if you need physical therapy or something, that seems to be very quick and streamlined but ... for every referral that I needed off-base, the doctor kept saying we will not give you a referral because TRICARE won't approve it so there is no point wasting our time.

- I have had a number of referrals this past year and it got bad enough, I contacted to complain about the ... claims office. They don't understand their own claim forms. They filled them out wrong. They don't understand here ... You don't see anybody in person. And they don't understand that and I tried to relay that back to them to explain that this is how broken the system is and I didn't even, the referral care management office here at the hospital is 4 times worse than [the TRICARE provider] is ... [personal information omitted] ...

- I've got to say with being stationed at [personal information omitted] ... before coming to [this MTF], we were constantly referred out to [the network for] ... private care. [Personal information omitted] ... I had no issues so far between. [Personal information omitted] ... Going off base, you have the hassle of having to get a referral, going to another doctor to see them. If there is one doctor for that specialty, they need to overlap them instead of saying just don't take the care and go off base. The hassle of the referrals.

- What people keep forgetting is that referrals [outside of the MTF] cost us a lot of money. I mean they refer us all the time and every time we go [outside of the MTF] I got [hundreds of dollars] out of my pocket because the care [outside of the MTF] to see a specialist is 2 to 3 times what it is [elsewhere].

- I have only been referred off-base once [personal information omitted] ... I think for a lot of people cost is really an issue when you have to pay such an extremely large amount out-of-pocket. For some people, what I pay for [treatment out in the network] ... would break their budget.

- [Personal information omitted] ... I am actually thankful that my family and I have access to the medical care [personal information omitted] ... one of our issues is that if the one [specific specialist] on staff PCS's, we will have to forgo treatment and that will actually be a break in your treatment, which can be a huge issue and it takes months to set it up and in addition to that because there is only one doc, there is actually very limited care. They don't take into account the children that are in treatment, taking them out of school and the challenges surrounding that, so they actually limit the treatment hours to pretty much when they are in school and some of the children go off base so pulling them out of school for an hour to two hours is significant. They don't have enough technicians to provide care adequately and they start treatment only to say "by the way, you're going to pull them out of school because we don't do treatments before 8 and after 3".

Question to Audience: If you have a concern about the kind of quality you are getting here in terms of care here at [this MTF], who do you take it to? Who do you talk to about a concern?

Responses from Audience:
- I have had very poor quality experience ... I attempted to contact the patient advocate ... I tried to get past the front desk person to the person ... It took 6 months before I could walk up to a desk and ask someone I knew here "Who do I go and talk to here?" She sent me to a [leader] ... in charge of quality and complaints ... [personal information omitted] ... [it is difficult to register a complaint] about doctors I am going to have to continue to [see for treatment] ... I am not getting good quality care. The patient advocate in internal medicine is actually someone that works for the physicians that way outrank him or her and they are expected to advocate for you. They are in a position that they can't.

- [Personal information omitted] ... I actually just addressed this with the lead patient advocate of the hospital. They had not been posting the updates to the patient advocate listing and unfortunately for dependents and civilians, they probably don't have access to it on the secure side of the military network. And so when you try and use the interactive evaluation, they will end up on the same person's desk. So over the course of weeks ... by the time we have to call again a very junior NCO starts talking about "oh while I have you on the line, I also see you complained about this" and this conversation goes on. And oh yeah you used to be the [personal information omitted] ... And I told them that I don't appreciate this because you're now seeing all of my concerns ... and I don't even want to tell him about my next follow-up appointment because it's always like medical retribution, you're not going to get, you know, proper care.

Facilitator: What do you think is going to correct this issue? What needs to change in regards to how you register concerns?

Responses from Audience:
- A completely, totally independent person who is not affiliated with any of the power structure here at [this MTF] has to be an advocate. [Personal information omitted] ... I have had difficulty using the patient advocate as well. It has to be completely somebody totally new and impartial.

- I think the patient advocate has to have equal to or greater than the rank compared to the doctors providing the care. [Personal information omitted] ... I respect what NCOs are trying to do but there are limits to what they can accomplish especially if they go against the person who is their doctor and supervisor.

Questions Related to Access to Care

Question to Audience: How easy or hard is it to get an appointment at this MTF when you want to be seen?

Responses from Audience:
- I don't know about anyone else but every time I try to schedule an appointment with my PCM, it seems like he is fully booked for like the whole month and you can only get an appointment next month.

- It's usually about a month to six weeks to get an appointment. My [personal information omitted] had to wait 7 weeks to get a call-back to get a basic dental appointment.

- [Personal information omitted] ... two to three months is not unusual and I recognize military comes first so it's fine but it's still quite long.

Facilitator: So active duty takes precedence over retirees? Is that correct?

Responses from Audience:
- Everyone nods.

- I do think that the pediatrician's office ... [is] very readily available for very acute appointments which is when you are very ill and have to be seen in that day. For routine appointments, standard of care ... I just got [elsewhere] 6 months ago is 4-6 weeks. That is pretty standard for a pediatrician's office. The general practitioner or primary docs or adult dependents ... that's the appointment time that takes the longest. And specialty clinics are the worst.

Question to Audience: TRICARE standard is 24 hours for Urgent Care, 7 days for routine care, and 28 days for wellness visits and specialty care. Are they meeting those standards?

Responses from Audience:
- Internal medicine, people I deal with, I don't have any problems at all.

- [Personal information omitted] ... I have a lot of experience here with internal medicine. I've had many physicals here. [Personal information omitted] ... I've had no problems whatsoever. So, I have nothing but praise for them.

Facilitator: What do you think accounts for that huge difference in what you have experienced?

Responses from Audience:
- Depends on when you get it done. If you get it done in the summer time, two to three months because there isn't an overlap of doctors. In the wintertime, you get it sooner or more frequently.

Facilitator: So, it is staffed better in the wintertime?

Responses from Audience:
- Right, so it seems like in the summer, all the doctors leave. So as soon as school gets out, and then the other doctors don't get here until school starts.

- I think it's mostly for if you're trying to see a PCM then it's much like forever wait. But if you're trying to get into one of the other clinics like Internal Med or pain management or anything like that, usually you can get in pretty fast.

- I think a lot of it has to do with being a good patient and listening to their advice. I think it works both ways. I don't think my doctor has a magic pill.

- Your question was what is the discrepancy. I think it's the level of expectation. I think the older patients are a little bit more patient, it comes with age. But I think it's the level of expectation. My experience, the longest I've ever had to wait to see my general practitioner was about 10 days. Dermatology because of the fewer staff members may be a little bit longer but that's not critical for me. I think it's the level of expectation.

- It's important to understand that those appointments are prioritized as well in order of: it is enlisted personnel, retirees, and civilians. So ... civilians and civilian dependents ... wait quite a bit longer. If I want a dental appointment, I have to call in the morning and see if anyone military has cancelled and if they have, I can make [personal information omitted] [trip] down here to get my teeth cleaned. Otherwise, I don't get it done.

Question to Audience: Let's talk about same-day appointments. What about same-day appointments?

Responses from Audience:
- I think it's just like [other locations]. If I need them, I just have to go to the emergency room ... they do have the option to tell you that they are waiting cancellations for active

duty, they just say go online, book it online. They don't even tell me, they won't even discuss with me if they have any cancelations for the week.

- My experience has been the opposite. With family practice, we have got appointments the very same day. We have gotten them more than once.

- I had just gone to the ER with pains and they couldn't figure out why. They told me to get an appointment to see my doctor ... I got up at 7 AM to call and they couldn't get me in till [the next day] ... [Personal information omitted] ... I've had better luck with pediatricians, being able to call in and get my kids in a bit sooner on the same day. But I just had to go to the ER with a lot of pain ... I can't see my doctor until [the next day].

- If you are a civilian that does not have TRICARE, you cannot use the online booking system at all ...

- I've kind of run the whole gamut. I'm an Army brat, Army health care, prior active duty, and now dependent. I know one thing is that sick call is gone, which kind of makes it tough because if someone is sick, active duty, they have to call in to get an appointment as opposed to that little time, the 630-830 that they had to go in and see someone. So, they start filling out the slots to go to be seen so they don't have to go into work and then the other people can't come in. And I know someone else said something about expectations, well just for myself, I'm willing to wait a week. But when it's my small children, I'm not willing to wait a week when my two year old is sick because they can't tell me what's wrong. So, a lot of times, there are so many different situations, circumstances, and like others saying in the summer, same thing, I had to wait. Because even if they come in at the same time and the other ones leave, they have to be certified. That can take 30 to 60 days and therefore you have a lull in the middle of the summer because either they are not there or are not certified. So, those are the situations that I have encountered. Sometimes it's great, sometimes it stinks.

- I gotta agree with these guys here. I have not been able to get a same-day appointment. Every time I have tried to say this is happening to me, I need to see a doctor, they are like well we are booked and we can see you this many weeks out. So, I usually end up going to the ER.

Question to Audience: How often or how effectively are you booked for follow-up before you leave your appointment?

Responses from Audience:
- I just want to say [personal information omitted] ... physical therapy ... [is] ... very good about getting you in there and not messing up. You know if one person leaves, another person picks up the job and does it for you. [Personal information omitted] ... The only one bad situation where I was diagnosed with [personal information omitted] ... the doctor saw me initially and he said well, let's ... see what it does. The next time I called and had spoken to the boss. The boss walked me down and said we need to [procedure]

... this thing. It was Thursday and by Friday, they told me I had [personal information omitted] ... and I had an appointment for surgery in less than 3 weeks.

- All the variety of things are situational. [Personal information omitted] ... I would take 6 weeks on average to find an opening. And after being persistent [personal information omitted] ... I can pretty much schedule whenever and wherever I need to. And I think that is what is missing. I appreciate their willingness to want to see the same doctor but if I've got a rash, I don't need a doctor that I've been seeing for years to figure out what kind of ointment I need. I just need a physician ...

- As far as the treatment goes, there is a lack communication between the referral clinic and what the clinicians need. So, if you do get a referral, if you finally get an appointment with your doctor and they say "okay, I'll give you a referral," three or four weeks waiting for treatment, well they give you the referral, there is a lot of time pre-tests need to be done and referral management on two separate occasions has not shared that information. So by the time we show up to the appointment for the specialty clinic, they say well you don't [have] these tests done so we need to delay your treatment because we need to get more testing done so there is a lack of communication. Some of the clinics themselves like physical therapy or EMT clinic, they actually schedule very well before you leave. But I think there is a disconnect in general between practitioners, specialty clinics, and referral management.

Questions Related to Patient Safety

Question to Audience: Do you feel patient care at [this MTF] that you get is safe care? Do you get safe care?

Responses from Audience:
- [Personal information omitted] ... I cannot get anything done. So now when you say [what should I do?] ... you have an NCO on the other end of the phone saying, "I don't know what to tell you." And what has become clear to me through this process is that the NCOs are intimidated about going back to the physicians and saying this patient wants to know what your alternative plan is.

- [Personal information omitted] ... they are overly conservative in their treatment. That's why it has taken me from [fall] until [summer] to get surgery for my shoulder.

- My physician couldn't take the time to actually look at the medications that I brought him from my previous base so there would be continuity in care. He basically gave me, he said "I'm going to write you a script for what I want you to take here instead of what you've been taking" even though I've been on and off for the same medications for 15 years. The medication that he gave me, I had to take it as he thought I should, come to find out is on the list that are compounded. If you take without compound added to it, it can cause cancer. I fought with him for over a year before he would actually give me the compound.

Question to Audience: When you have issues or even when you are in for a check-up, how comfortable are you saying to your provider that I don't understand why you are giving me this? Tell me more about my condition or why you are giving me this.

Responses from Audience:
- [Personal information omitted] ... I feel comfortable asking those questions. But I get a distinct feeling that the doctors are uncomfortable answering them. The answers always come back as we just don't feel comfortable doing that or I don't give that medication. I think I asked the same question about a medication I was assigned at one time with one doctor. Went to another doctor and she didn't want to assign that medication. It took three go-arounds for her to finally explain that she wasn't comfortable with that medication. So, you know again maybe there are other people that are less comfortable asking the question but me, if they are not going to shoot me, I'm going to ask. But I don't think the doctors are comfortable with us asking and them answering the questions.

- Like you said, I can ask the question but sometimes it feels like they scurry around the question. But they don't really answer it but go around it.

- [Personal information omitted] ... I've talked to the doctor and [personal information omitted] ... I said this is the medication that I [have] used for years and years. And I know there are others, but this works. And she said, "yes I have a friend that takes it. It's 45 years old but if it works for you, use it." No complaints and I asked questions because I don't want interactions with drugs. And maybe that is a gender issue. I am a male and whether it be a female doctor or male doctor, I can ask those questions ... [personal information omitted] ... I don't know if that influences it. I don't know. I am just thinking that may be a factor.

- My experience has been that they sit down and explain it to me. If they change my medication, they value my questions and give me feedback. So, I'm very pleased with the way they sit down and explain things to me and why they have changed things on me. And I get the opportunity to ask questions.

- [Personal information omitted] ... I've received pretty good care. It's been better than what I was able to receive [in another location]. In some cases, it wasn't exactly what I wanted to hear but it worked. Well I guess what my point is I made it a point to learn about the MHS so what that means whenever I get a prescription of some sort, you know I'll ask the doc about it and I'll go in and do my own research just to make sure that I've got first-hand knowledge of it. And then at least the next time I go in, I can have an open dialogue and I find that if the doctor is not comfortable responding to your questions and you know if you have an open dialogue, he understands that you have been doing your own research and you're familiar with what ailments are and familiar with the drugs you are taking, the more apt he is to talk to you about it.

Question to Audience: I'd like you to think about if you were in charge of continuous quality improvement at [this MTF], what are some specific solutions, fixes, ideas that you have that you would like to suggest to correct, improve, the level of quality care at this MTF?

Responses from Audience:
- Ten years ago, there was a TRICARE office here at the hospital, patient would walk in there and say I just got this prescription from my doctor, can you help me? She would sit there and help you with your forms. She would call down there and check and the folks [outside of the MTF] were comfortable with it. So, get that TRICARE office back.

- We need to get sick call back so it can take care of the [Service members] so we can get same-day appointments. It will also help the emergency rooms crowding and overuse.

- One of the recent implementations has been [the secure messaging system] through RelayHealth. We have that and TRICARE and TRICARE online. And part of the issue is that doctors, the providers aren't registered with [the secure messaging system]. They won't answer your emails because someone misinterpreted the regulation that they can't respond to emails, which is not true. They are over-enforcing something about notes. So, they won't respond to your emails. And they are not registered with [the secure messaging system] to have that secure communication. And there is no provision on TRICARE online. So you have three different systems and none of them work.

Facilitator: How many of you use RelayHealth or online messaging?

Responses from Audience:
- (Show of hands) Okay, about 20 – 25% of you *(facilitator)*.

Facilitator: Is it working?

Responses from Audience:
- It is working very well for me. In fact, that's how I found out about this meeting. On the other hand, it's not logging information about me in my particular file. I am not sure if that is my responsibility or the hospital's.

- Talking about [the secure messaging system], I registered as soon as I found out about it in internal medicine. I had some lab tests so I emailed my provider and nothing came back. I checked … [and my results were in]. So I saw the provider walking down the hall and I asked "how come you didn't answer my email." [They replied] … these [results] are going to the nurse and she is going to upload it to the particular doctor so she can respond. So why can't it go to the doctor? I asked for the nurse and no nurse is available. So, anyway, it would be a good thing if it actually worked.

- I have trouble with RelayHealth. I have spent several months to get an answer as to why my medical records were not on RelayHealth. As soon as I found out about registering, I did that. But it was pointless. The only way I can do anything with it is to send an email.

At least the email part works but the rest of it doesn't. In fact, I got an email from a previous base that we were stationed there and we were there in 2010. I have had nothing to do with that base since 2010 and in the last two months, I figured out how to get my medical records on it and they did it. No one in [this MTF] has offered to help me at all.

- I think that there should be more dental appointments and optometry appointments for dependents. I understand that active duty is the reason why we are here but it shouldn't take 8 weeks to get optometry appointment. It is very frustrating.

- I have to tell you that they give a really hard time to dependents and we are given the run around. I know active duty is most important but we need help with things like [the secure messaging system] and RelayHealth.

- Ma'am can you put in your notes something about central appointments? They are trying to centralize all the appointments into one base. They need to put that back into the clinics because centralized appointments do not work. It is a bad system that makes getting appointments worse. [Personal information omitted] ... I have a tough time getting appointment through centralized appointments.

Site 7 Staff Town Hall Questions and Answers

The following text reproduces the Town Hall facilitator questions and audience responses, transcribed as close to verbatim as possible during the session. Information that could potentially identify individual participants has been omitted for privacy purposes.

Approximately 200 people attended this Town Hall meeting.

Questions Related to Quality of Care

Question to Audience: Is quality of care a priority for your facility? How do you know if it is or if it isn't?

Responses from Audience:
- I would say yes. Quality is very important here. There are several areas where we see it. Patient safety recording, everybody has an icon up on their desktops where they can report near misses and improper documentation because that can lead to something further down the road that is considered a near miss. This is briefed every week, where we discuss the number of near misses. The TeamSTEPPS® process is pushed. Communication is something that is really focused on. The safety reports that go out to everyone on a monthly basis include all of the near misses as well as the good things that have happened so that we can all continue to learn from each other.

- We also have patient advocates whose contact information can be found around the facility. Customers are welcomed to contact those patient advocates. We take their issues and address them promptly, right on the spot.

- The biggest shortsightedness issue that I have noticed is lack of continuity and it tends to show itself as people come and go. That is what I would point out as a negative issue is the lack of consistent continuity. For instance, Command oversight, one Commander comes in does something; the next Commander comes in and has a different viewpoint or leadership style which everyone has to adapt to.

- I don't know if it is a positive or a negative. I think it is what it is. We are in the military. The medical field is out there supporting different missions. For example I worked in [specific department] and we have a lot of providers that come and go who are deployed from anywhere between 8 weeks and 6 months. So for example, the continuity that was alluded to earlier, as a patient you can come into [specific department] and see a provider for the initial issue and a month later see a totally different provider for that same issue. From the patient's perspective they could go from a provider that they love, to one that they don't. Continuity of care will always be something that we struggle with.

- At times you get the sense that it is more about quantity. See this many patients, see this, see that, as opposed to simply doing the best you can for the patients that are in front of you right now. Instead it is just push them through. Doctors have to see this many patients in a given week and it is never about them taking care of the patient. It is about how many patients are they seeing. That is where there seems to be an issue about quantity.

- I think we have two success stories in [specialty clinic] ... when it comes to quality. One of those is our [specific program] ... and therefore these patients do not have to go out to the economy to get that care when before they had to do that. We have improved our quality of care by being able to provide that to our patients. Secondly, we have what we call a [second specific program] ... where we provide [this program] to our patients ... [who can see] ... one provider ... We go above and beyond in taking care of our patients. This is something that we are doing to bring more quality to our patients and our clinic.

- I definitely have a few success stories. I work in the [specific department] ... We serve a population that consists of retirees. We [perform procedures] ... [in collaboration with practitioners in the economy and elsewhere in the MHS system] ... So we have been able to do things that have never been done in the ... group before and it has been a huge success.

- In [specialty clinic]... we have a full staff of all specialties so we are able to bounce ideas off of each other and improve quality of care within the department.

- Access to care and quality in reference to that, the access to care numbers are being pushed down on us. You have a number of patients and our providers see these patients period. The quality comes in because of the level of care that we provide. Our providers routinely stay over, a normal eight hour day does not happen. They met the standards but it ends up coming out of their day. They end up working 10 hour days.

- ... when we do readiness training, they want to push patients when we are working on exercises and things like that. They have patients coming in at the same time and they are trying to take 300 people out of the hospital to do training and they are still having the same boat load of patients.

- Even though we are being told to go see a certain amount of patients, [our] providers, techs, and nurses end up staying longer than eight hours a day. We do however make sure that quality is there for the patients. For me that is the biggest success.

- The concern is the tipping point. When is it enough? We are told that these doctors, providers, [and] nurses will see these patients and we will provide good quality care but we are not staffed at the numbers where we should be. Access will still be met but at some point when the doctors and techs can't stay 10 hours every day. Quality is met but our concern is staffing.

- Since we are trying to change the world. I just wanted to make this known since it hasn't been touched on yet. The DoD in general is going through downsizing yet the policies that we have in the different services remain the same. So it may be a good idea, as they are downsizing, to adjust policies to a realistic measure. That may be asking a lot but I do think it should make its way into the report. You are hearing from several people about the manpower and workload and the extra hours that are being worked now. As we continue to reduce the force even more, the pinch that is being felt in different areas will probably increase. Policies as far as access and trying to meet that number of patients seen will remain the same.

Question to Audience: If you have a quality-related concern, what do you do?

Responses from Audience:
- ... I feel like I can take any issues or concerns that I have experienced and take it to my ... commander to ensure that the concern is pushed up the chain of command and addressed properly.

- For the most part through our incident reports, anybody can enter an incident report on anything. It doesn't necessarily mean that the patient is going to be injured. We would put in a report if a patient gets to pharmacy and their medication was not ordered yet. Little things like that go in which of course no harm has been done but it is placed. Once a report is placed and processed, someone has to respond to it. That is one of the primary ways that raise quality concerns. I think all of us are comfortable going to our ... commander as well. Overall people do not fear making a comment on an incident that they have seen.

- Definitely there is no fear to bring up anything in the hospital, I think. Whether anything gets done is another question. I don't think everything can be changed, specifically in regards to people working longer hours; we still have the access that we have to give and the numbers that we have to meet. Doing anything about it needs to be brought up higher.

- ... we can anonymously report something when we notice a near miss. We also have a way of dealing with impaired providers however those mechanisms focus on those who are impaired by the use of drugs or emotional reasons, not necessarily those who are impaired by fatigue or burnout. I think it is hard to recognize when others are impaired by fatigue or burnout when you are impaired by fatigue and burnout yourself.

Questions Related to Access to Care

Question to Audience: Do your appointment templates and schedules meet appointment demand?

Responses from Audience:
- I work in [specific department] ... and we have one of the hardest appointments to get into. Lots of times we have a lot of people who don't end up showing for their scheduled appointment but there is nothing we can do to punish them. So we have a ton of no-shows and everyone is asking for all of these appointments but there is no fix for it.

- We have got issues in terms of standards in access to care. We have patients that cancel same day. We have constant no-shows that are taking up available appointments. On top of that for instance, we have two [specialty care providers] ... that are doing the work of three.

- What it comes down to in other areas is the push between access to care where we have to get patients in as quickly as possible or it's something where the patient feels that their issue is urgent enough to be seen within 24 hours therefore they will see any provider. I believe this is where we begin to see an issue with the continuity of seeing the same provider who is seeing your case from start to finish.

- In regards to the no-shows in the [specialty clinic] ... we had 133 no-shows in May and 88 in June and there is nothing we can do about it. We cannot contact the commanders. If an active duty member does not go to their appointment we can contact their commander ... [for other no shows] I have tried everything and then when we reach out to them to see why they have not shown, they have now tied up a tech or a nurse in order to call them. It convolutes the situation.

Question to Audience: How do you fix no-shows?

Responses from Audience:
- It basically boils down to the entitlements of the MHS. If we make an appointment to an off-base provider and we no-show, we are liable for the charges for that visit. So if you charge individuals what it costs the military for missing appointments, people usually change when you affect their pocketbook.

- ... [specific procedure] are very hard to get especially for dependents. ... [yet] we have had cases where one person no-showed for four appointments in one day [when the provider was making every attempt to help that patient actually get in that same day].

- ... I never miss appointments because they are charging me. The only way to fix this is to charge somebody. Even if it is for $5, I will make my appointment to keep my $5.

- Yes it is great to charge them, but could we suspend them from receiving care? Where they would have to go to an off-base provider?

- I don't think there is anything that we can do if the command is not going to enforce it. In [specialty] ... we have ... high ... no-show rates. When we call them to investigate they tell us that the mission got in the way and we could not come. So if it is not being supported by commanders and supervisors base-wide, then there is nothing that we are going to do in this room to fix it. Something needs to be done by them to punish those that fail to show.

- Doing more with less base-wide is not the answer.

Question to Audience: When do you release appointments for booking? How often do you book each type of these appointments prior to the patient actually leaving: Follow up visits, PCM referrals to specialty clinics, outpatient procedures?

Responses from Audience:
- The access to care standard is 7 weeks out. Everyone who needs a follow up appointment typically gets booked same day.

- Our appointments are usually booked out 45 days in advance ... Most of our providers have started to book their patients' follow up appointments.

Question to the Audience: How often does your clinic respond to secure messaging from patients within the time requirements that are directed by policy and guidelines?

Responses from the Audience:
- We respond to RelayHealth messages within 3 business days which is the same time length for our telephone consults. The influx of messages is divvied out based on how each team does their [secure] messaging. People do message a lot over the weekend and holidays and they think they will get a response in three days but I'm not coming in on the weekend to answer messages.

- You cannot force everyone to use RelayHealth so some are still using the phones. Right now we are doing both and then we still have to put in the TCon (telephone consult) as well as the [secure] message. I have three people doing that every day and that turns into six. To me it is worthless unless you force everyone to use it and let our nurses off of the phones.

Question to Audience: What do you do if you are unable to meet the patient's desired appointment timeline?

Responses from Audience:
- We have no choice. We have to meet their appointments.

- Most of the time patients call our appointment line. If the clerk cannot get them an appointment then they put in a TCon (telephone consult) for ... one of the ... nurses to address the filling of the appointment. Most of the time it comes from providers taking their "call day" to see patients.

- Provider takes their lunch and free time to try to accommodate patients. I would like to see increased staffing in order to help them out because I know it is happening across all departments.

- I may be mean but I do not come from a medical background, I come from a [specific professional] background and a lot of what I am hearing is that cases cut into my personal time. I think that if you are about quality then if you can only have lunch for 10 minutes so be it. In the [specific professional] world we work 15 hour days. That is our job. We are in the military.

- I have a response to that. I don't mean any harm to anyone but I work for a ... provider... That [person] ... stays here until 1 or 2 in the morning taking care of all [their] ... TCons. I'm sorry, we give up lunch, we give up time with our families, we give up a lot just as [another profession does] ... So understand that fatigue does become an issue when you are dealing with people's lives. Quantity kills quality.

- As a dependent I have experienced only accommodations from my PCM and specialty team. My ... had an injury and they saw him after 4:30 PM. I don't know a civilian doctor who is willing to see patients after hours.

Questions Related to Patient Safety

Question to Audience: How do you report a patient safety issue or concern?

Responses from Audience:
- I think we have talked about it already but we use PSRs and PSCs to report patient safety issues or events.

- The only issue is that sometimes we take care on a local level in our clinic or within [specific department] ... here it does not get into the PSR. If we immediately identify it amongst ourselves and we address and fix the issue while putting the process improvement measures in place, therefore it may not get into PSR.

- You can find out about results if you actual identify yourself in the PSR. You will see the email track that goes along with it. If it happens from the unit, it will be something that everyone will hear about. If it is possible for anyone to make that error then there will be a conversation about it. As far as feedback it is not supposed to be punitive. Anonymous people will not get any feedback.

Question to Audience: If you were King or Queen of quality improvement here at [this MTF], what would you change?

Responses from Audience:
- Change the no-show policy

- We spend a lot of time and effort and money on advertising for sexual assault prevention. I don't think we should short [change] that but at the same time if we were to spend as much time and effort for our beneficiaries to let them know, because they seem to have this entitlement that I should get an appointment whenever I want it even if it is not acute. There should be an advertisement that goes out to let patients know what is important and needs to be seen right away and the impact of the no shows should be illustrated for them so they can see how others can't get appointments because it is blocked by individuals who fail to show up.

- We should bring back sick call

- We should not bring back sick call because it pushed back everything else. On top of the appointment that we have to see, we have to see every single person who walks in for sick call. Then we have to see all the appointments that are scheduled.

- The proportionality of what we are supposed to get to has to be adjusted. Your productivity in your section is expected to be at the 100% mark when you are being spread thin across other areas. Nobody adjusts that.

- We had a program that if you attended a class you got a sick card and you could go every month to get simple things like Tylenol and Motrin. The things that you could get over the counter but you are not wasting an appointment for.

- ... Hopefully you don't go crazy eights every week. If you are marking 10-12 hours a day, all of that stuff rolls in to DMHRSi and then [headquarters] sees it and they then try to help us out with the work load. Put in the time to describe what you do so that [headquarters] could see those numbers. We could help ourselves out with that.

- I have been involved with DMHRSi since 1996 and I was told a long time ago that it was to help me with my staffing. It is now 2014 and nothing has changed. If they are seeing, they are looking at it and turning the other cheek. I work in the [specific department] ... and I do not have the people that I need to function safely.

- I would like a military docking system that is one system not five or six. We have AHLTA, CHCS, Essentris®, etc. It would save a provider time in setting up profiles within different systems. The multiple systems do not make any sense to me.

- Just to echo what has been said in terms of manning. The mission stays the same and we have burnout which compromises safety. I believe that sufficient manning to meet demands will increase quality of work.

- Manning is one thing but at the same time the basic business model of productivity is this: if you have optimal manning you will have optimal output. As you take away manning, your productivity falls but at the same time if you cannot compromise. We need to either drop mission or find a better way to fulfill mission criteria. An example that I see in [specific department] … and that is a lot of time that I take away from my work day. If that is a mission that can be addressed by other units then it would allow me to use my time wiser for instance.

- I would like the Exceptional Family Program (EFP) to be revamped.

- If I can get a show of hands, who here works one job outside of their current job description? Two jobs? Three jobs? Four jobs? *The number of hands increases per question.* What I am trying to get at is that everyone here does more than just see patients.

Appendix 1.6
Web-based Comments

As part of the 90-day MHS Review, feedback was solicited from beneficiaries using a digital submission process. These anecdotal comments were compiled and delivered to the MHS Review Group for action. Beneficiary input received through the web portal was analyzed along with other beneficiary feedback received in site visits/town halls for inclusion in the report. There were a total of 85 web-based comments submitted.

Access comments totaled 46 (54 percent), quality comments totaled 18 (21 percent), and safety comments totaled 4 (5 percent). The remaining 17 (20 percent) were unrelated to the MHS Review. These remaining comments primarily discussed the Veterans Affairs (VA) health care delivery system or other unrelated topics.

Discussion

The primary areas of focus for the submitted comments centered on appointments and referrals, prescription services, wait times, and referral denials. The comments corresponded consistently with comments received at beneficiary town halls conducted during the MHS Review site visits.

For access, 85 percent of comments were negative (39 out of 46), 11 percent were neutral (5 out of 46), and 4 percent were positive (2 out of 46). For quality, 83 percent of comments were negative (15 out of 18), 6 percent were neutral (1 out of 18), and 12 percent were positive (2 out of 18). For safety, 75 percent of comments were negative (3 out of 4) and 25 percent were neutral (1 out of 4). As noted by one of the external subject matter experts, Dr. Brent James, input received from town hall meetings and web-based comments may be biased toward individuals dissatisfied with their access or service, and do not represent a valid sample population.

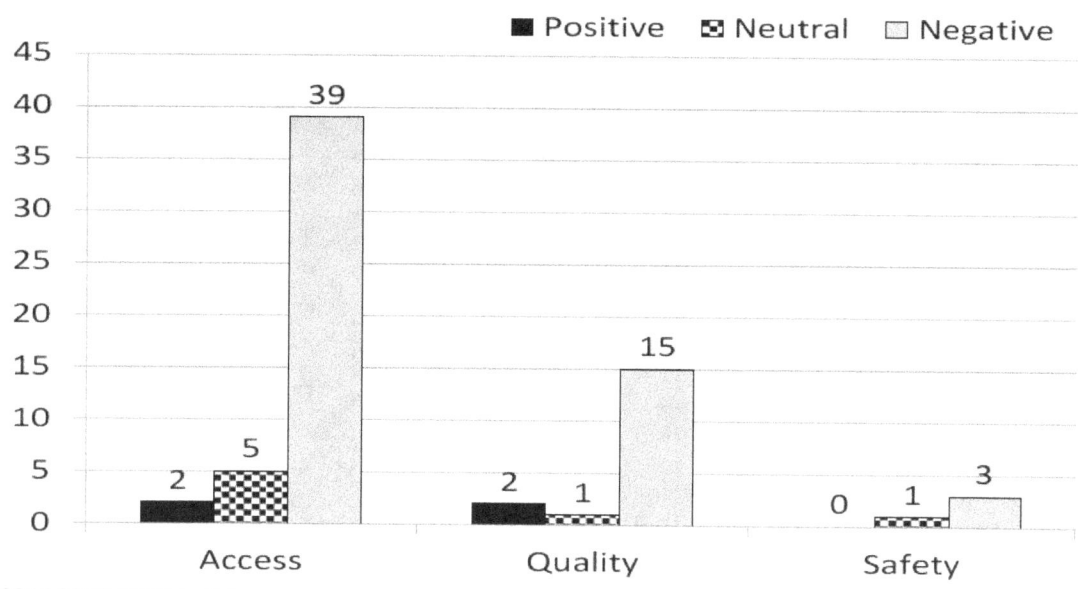

Figure 1.6-1 Breakdown of Comment Types

2014 MHS Review Group
Source: Web-based comments, June – August 2014

Appendix 1.7
The MHS Comparisons to Three Health Systems and Benchmarks

Table 1.7-1 Access to Care: Direct Care Comparison to Three Health Systems and Benchmarks

Metric Name	Direct Care	Health System 1	Health System 2	Health System 3	MHS Benchmark	California Benchmark
MTF Appointments Meeting TRICARE Access Standards	X			X	X	
% Acute Appointments	X			X	X	
% Specialty Appointments	X			X	X	
Average # of Days to Appointments	X			X	X	X
Acute Appointments	X			X	X	X
Specialty Appointments	X			X	X	X
Average # of Days to Third Next Available Appointments	X 3 Submeasures		X 3 Submeasures	X 2 Submeasures		
Acute Appointment (Primary Care)	X		X	X		
Routine Appointment (Primary Care)	X		X	X		
Available Specialty Appointment	X		X			
Satisfaction with Access to Care	X 3 Submeasures	X 2 Submeasures	X 1 Submeasure	X 1 Submeasure	X 3 Submeasures	
% Satisfaction with "Seeing Provider When Needed"	X	X			X	
% Satisfaction with Access to Care	X		X	X	X	
% Satisfaction with "Getting Care Quickly"	X	X			X	

Source: 2014 MHS Review Group, July 2014

Table 1.7-2 Quality of Care: Direct Care Comparison to Three Health Systems and Benchmarks

Metric Name	Direct Care	Health System 1	Health System 2	Health System 3	National Benchmark
Joint Commission ORYX® Core Measures Set	X 7 Submeasures	X 4 Submeasures	X 6 Submeasures	X 5 Submeasures	X 7 Submeasures
Hospital Compare Measures (Purchased Care)	X				X
Inpatient Mortality (Crude and Adjusted)	X				
Inpatient Quality Indicators: Condition Specific Mortality *	X	X		X	X
National Surgical Quality Program (NSQIP)	X			X	X
HEDIS Measures	X 16 Submeasures	X 11 Submeasures	X 11 Submeasures		
Perinatal Data					
PSI 17	X		X	X	X
PSI 18	X		X	X	X
PSI 19	X		X	X	X
Experience of Care: Health Plan					
Rate Health Care Plan	X	X	X	X	X
Rate Personal Doctor	X	X	X	X	X
Rate Health Care	X	X	X	X	X
Experience of Care: Inpatient					
% Satisfaction with Hospital	X		X	X	X
% Recommend their Hospital	X		X	X	X
30 Day Readmissions	X		X	X	

*MHS metric does not include all primary care routine appointments
Source: 2014 MHS Review Group, July 2014

Table 1.7-3 Patient Safety: Direct Care Comparison to Three Health Systems and Benchmarks

Metric Name	Direct Care	Health System 1	Health System 2	Health System 3	National Benchmark
PSI #90 Composite *	X	X	X	X	X
Sentinel Events Reporting – FY 2013 – SE Rates p 1,000 Discharges	X		X		
Patient Culture Survey	X				X
Healthcare Associated Infections					
Central Line-Associated Bloodstream Infection (DC)	X	X	X	X	X
Ventilator-Associated Pneumonia Events (DC)	X	X	X	X	X
Catheter-Associated Urinary Tract Infections (DC)	X	X	X	X	X
Root Cause Analysis **	X			X	

*Mean PSI 90 between MHS and external health systems estimated to be no different (one way analysis of variance; p<.05) **Categories of level of harm were not comparable due to systematic differences in level of harm determinations
Source: 2014 MHS Review Group

Appendix 1.8
Data Analytics Summary

Literature Review

A search for applicable comparisons to the MHS began with a review of the scientific literature to determine if access to care with regard to wait time from request to appointment has been studied or reviewed in the literature. PubMed was utilized with keyword searches performed for the following terms 'access to care', 'access standards' and 'patient appointment standards.' A scientific literature review was also performed to examine patient safety reporting systems (PSRSs) in civilian health care systems, specifically for benchmarks related to each subject. A search of PubMed was conducted using the following key words: 'Sentinel Events'; 'Patient Safety Reporting'; 'Patient Safety Culture'; and 'Root Cause Analyses.'

The Access to Care search yielded articles and reviews that were either 1) esoteric, that is, reviewing appointment with regard to a procedure type or specialty field; or 2) used the term "access" as synonym for coverage. The only global access measure identified (that is, comparable to the MHS) was that involving the Patient Experience. The CAHPS survey asks patients to evaluate their experiences with their care. No standards were ascertainable in the scientific literature relating to patient request to appoint time allowances, or clinical outcomes derived.

Results from the PSRS literature search revealed that the private sector faces equivalent patient safety challenges. The Joint Commission (TJC) publishes National Patient Safety Goals and elements of performance, but metrics are not quantified. TJC requires a root cause analysis (RCA) be performed for any sentinel event, yet a specific methodology is not prescribed.

In addition to the scientific literature search, professional organizations associated with the measurement of access, quality, and safety in the health care sector were also evaluated to determine if applicable benchmarks exist. The focus of this search was access and safety measures without readily available benchmarks and/or methodologies. This search began with an evaluation of the National Quality Forum's (NQF's) measurement clearinghouse to determine the existence of comparable measures and/or potential sources for national benchmarks. The search of NQF's clearinghouse yielded a potential State-level source for the Third-Next Available access to care measure.

TJC reports were also searched for potentially relevant information regarding the measures Sentinel Events by Type and RCA. The reporting of most sentinel events to TJC is voluntary and represents only a small proportion of actual events, but yearly counts of this reporting, as well as events identified by TJC through media outlets, are published by TJC. TJC also produces statistics on the distribution of root causes of sentinel events by year (note: TJC requires a RCA to be completed for each sentinel event within 45 days of awareness by TJC.)

Reports, publications, and tools were also evaluated for potential national benchmarks. Searches included U.S. Department of Health and Human Services (DHHS) reports, including those of the

Agency for Healthcare Research and Quality (AHRQ). A search of DHHS reports and statistics also yielded two key Office of the Inspector General reports noting the distribution and incidence of patient safety events, including degree of harm and sentinel events. This report noted inconsistencies in methods of data capture in the United States, the definitions used to define events, and the limitation of relying on self-reporting methods.

Other government statistics and reports evaluated included any potential State-level sources of comparable estimates. Many States require reporting on specific patient safety events and publish related quality and safety statistics. Some relevant State-level estimates were identified for Sentinel Event by Type distributions.

Data Analysis

Performance of the MHS direct care component is on par with other quality health care organizations in the United States. In this review, organizations demonstrate differing meaningful patterns of high-performance indicators in certain areas, all of which would be recognized as excellence by informed observers. Neither DoD nor the other institutions reviewed demonstrate distinct and consistent patterns of low performance based on numerous indicators.

Access to Care Measures

There are numerous considerations when comparing access to care measures across organizations. Access has very few nationally recognized standards or benchmarks, making direct comparisons with other health care systems difficult. Of the access measures used in this review, four were comparable with at least one of the participating health care systems. These measures include "Average number of days to appointment," "Third next available appointment," "Percent of appointments within 28 days," and "Satisfaction with Access."

Using "Average number of days to appoint" as an example, Health System 3 (HS3) reports "0" for the average number of days to acute appointments for each month in 2013 and approximately "10" or "11" days for average days to routine appointments. The comparison is difficult because the organization's definition on this measure varies on any number of points. The MHS Review Group was not able to obtain information on when the clock starts when counting the days to appointments; whether the values reported are numbers rounded up, down, or to the closest whole number; and whether "walk-ins" or phone calls are included in the measure.

A standard patient experience measure also illustrates the difficulty of comparisons. The Consumer Assessment of Health Plans and Systems (CAHPS) uses rigorous, well validated methodology and is used as the standard civilian benchmark for care in the outpatient setting. Responses regarding satisfaction are affected by multiple known factors. The factors include location within the country, age group, tenure, enrollment in a given practice or system, and others. Thus, the scores are less comparable without adjusting for the mix of patients using the CAHPS recommended methodology.

Quality of Care Measures

The quality core measures exemplify the issues associated with numeric comparisons. The direct care component measures 25 nationally recognized Quality Core Measures. None of these was available for comparison across all three civilian institutions. Top and bottom performers were variably distributed between DoD and the other institutions. On 5 of the 25 measures, DoD outperformed the national rate calculated from institutions that chose to report these measures. The ranges of scores on individual measures were less than 3 percentage points on nearly half of the measures. The three measures with lowest DoD performance had limited reporting by the comparison institutions.

HEDIS® measures provide additional perspective on cross system comparisons. At the time of this review, DoD is using 18 of the 81 existing measures. Data sources include DoD's electronic health record (AHLTA), purchased care claims, and other information systems. Health Systems 1 and 3 (HS1 and HS3) had all measures for comparison; HS2 had 11. DoD performance was comparable to HS3 with variations between individual measures, but without a dominant pattern of difference. Performance by HS1 and HS2 was generally higher, although seven scores were unavailable for HS2.

An example of the difficulty in ranking systems is seen in comparing HEDIS® scores among DoD and HS1 and HS3 (the scores were not available for HS2). For diabetes care, three glucose-related control targets and one testing goal exist. Although DoD relatively underperformed on screening, DoD performance matched for the easiest control target, and DoD relatively outperformed by increasingly greater differences on the middle and then highest treatment targets. A reasonable explanation for this might be that DoD has a larger proportion of diabetics with more easily controlled disease. Due to the extensive detail and rigorous methodology used for HEDIS®, it is often thought by many as a straightforward benchmark. In reality, for any given year, as many as six values exist for any one measure. This results from the commercial, Medicaid, and Medicare values that are then split into Health Maintenance Organization and Preferred Provider Organization groups. Additionally, the administrative and hybrid methods are two different ways of collection and reporting.

Patient Safety Measures

Patient Safety, as discussed in Chapter 5, has few nationally recognized measures. For example, numbers of sentinel events are not usually publicly available. The definition varies among potentially comparable systems. Some facilities apply sentinel event reporting to only inpatient events, per the National Committee for Quality Assurance (NCQA). The real value of sentinel event rates lies in examination of each actual event and the actions taken for system improvement.

External Comparison Data

Comparing and contrasting different health care organizations is a challenging endeavor. It requires detailed understanding and knowledge of the context and practices of the involved systems. An entire industry has evolved with many companies and organizations designing, collecting, and reporting various sets of performance measures.

Data set reviews required determinations of 1) whether the specifications of the data could be identified, 2) whether the data were sufficiently similar to the data collected from the MHS, and 3) whether the populations and timeframes would support useful comparisons. This involved knowing how data are collected, documented, reviewed, adjusted, and reported. In addition, this required knowledge of at-risk populations, demographics (such as age, gender, marital status, education level, socioeconomic status), and the health care benefits provided.

Three external health care systems graciously provided access, quality of care, and patient safety related data to support this review. Many steps were taken to access and then analyze the data from these different systems. This alone reflects the inherent complexities of health care systems throughout the United States. Comparing and improving health care systems requires sufficiently robust integrated information systems, broad ranges of professional knowledge, and supportive organizational structures. Increased standardization of data definitions and business processes throughout health care communities will make collaboration between systems more effective in increasing quality and safety.

Barriers to Data Sharing

When attempting to compare measures of safety, quality, and access, information is not always readily available. While many States have passed legislation to make some measures more available, many barriers still exist. Many health care systems limit transparency about costs, outcomes, quality improvement efforts, safety records, and leading practices in access to care. Health care organizations are caught in a balance between legal and ethical obligations to protect information and the need to move the organization forward.

Many health care systems do not have sufficient electronic health records (EHRs) to even collect the necessary types of data for comparison. Systems with EHRs are in the early stages of gathering the data collected by the MHS. Their ability to report, analyze, and improve on this data will require continued maturation of their system. These factors limited the number of external systems available for comparison. While having knowledge of one system is difficult, knowledge of multiple external health care systems presents even greater challenges. The actual selection of systems was made based on specific knowledge of the components of the candidate comparison. Being able to engage with the external comparison health care systems and quickly negotiate data sharing was critical due to unavoidable delays in authorizing, collecting, transferring, and interpreting data. The need for rapid negotiations limited potential comparison of systems to those with which MHS leaders had pre-existing professional relationships with individuals in positions of authority.

Upon selection of systems by senior leadership, the systems received a list of the measures for evaluation. These were returned with potentially matching fields and clarifying questions related to extent of data, intervals between data points, and methods. Despite extensive coordination and willing cooperation and support from the external institutions; the amount of comparable data was limited. This was due mainly to variations among institutions, their processes, data definitions, and objectives.

In addition, the MHS Review Group searched for other comparison measures. The MHS closely follows and tracks publicly available national benchmarks with the understanding that these are well defined and are validated prior to authorization for use by national organizations. If national benchmarks were not available, other sources were considered, including publicly available results, scientific literature, professional organizations, and State and Federal government statistics. Further details regarding the literature review and data sources that were identified are available in the following sections.

Data Sources

1. Healthcare Effectiveness Data and Information Set (HEDIS) Measures - National Committee for Quality Assurance (NCQA)
2. Experience of Care (Health Plan, Health Care, IP Satisfaction)
3. Prevention Quality Indicator (PQI) (Preventable Admissions) – Agency for Healthcare Research and Quality (AHRQ)
4. Readmissions (Direct Care discharges with readmission to Direct or Purchased Care) – Medicare
5. PCM Continuity – National Committee for Quality Assurance (NCQA)
6. Accreditation, Certification (including TJC, AAAHC, NCQA, URAC)
7. ORYX® Core Measures Set – The Joint Commission
8. Hospital Compare Measures (Purchased Care) – Medicare.gov
9. Inpatient Mortality (Crude and Inpatient Quality Indicators (IQI)) – AHRQ
10. National Surgical Quality Improvement Program (NSQIP) – American College of Surgeons
11. National Healthcare Safety Network (Healthcare Associated Infections (HAI)) (i.e., infection data for vents, central lines and urinary catheters) – Centers for Disease Control and Prevention (CDC)
12. Perinatal Center Data Base (PCDB) - National Perinatal Information Center (NPIC)
13. Consumer Assessment of Healthcare Providers and Systems (CAHPS) Experience of Care measures - AHRQ
14. Potential Quality Issues (i.e., Patient Safety Indicators (PSIs) for purchased care hospitals) – AHRQ

This page left intentionally blank.

APPENDIX 2. OVERVIEW

Appendix 2.1
Performance Improvement: Defense Health Agency and the Services

Military Health System Performance Improvement

Strategic Planning

Strategic Leadership offsite was held in August 2012 to identify core operating practices and processes that could be standardized. A MHS Strategic Planning Conference was held in September 2013 that resulted in leadership approving key initiatives to achieve Quadruple Aim success. Both sessions aligned quality, safety, and access processes and measures, among others, with strategic initiatives.

MHS leaders at all levels participated in the development of the MHS Strategic Imperatives Scorecard. This Scorecard starts with the Quadruple Aim, which is translated into Strategic Imperatives with Performance Measures and indicators of current state along with targets. Of the eight Strategic Imperatives, four relate to quality, safety, and access. Of the 22 measures, 11 relate to quality, safety, and access.

Governance and Performance Management

MHS Review and Analysis (R&A) is conducted quarterly to evaluate MHS Strategic Imperatives Scorecard performance targets against actual results and documents needed adjustments to strategy. Strategic Initiatives are identified and implemented to close noted strategic gaps and drive improvement.

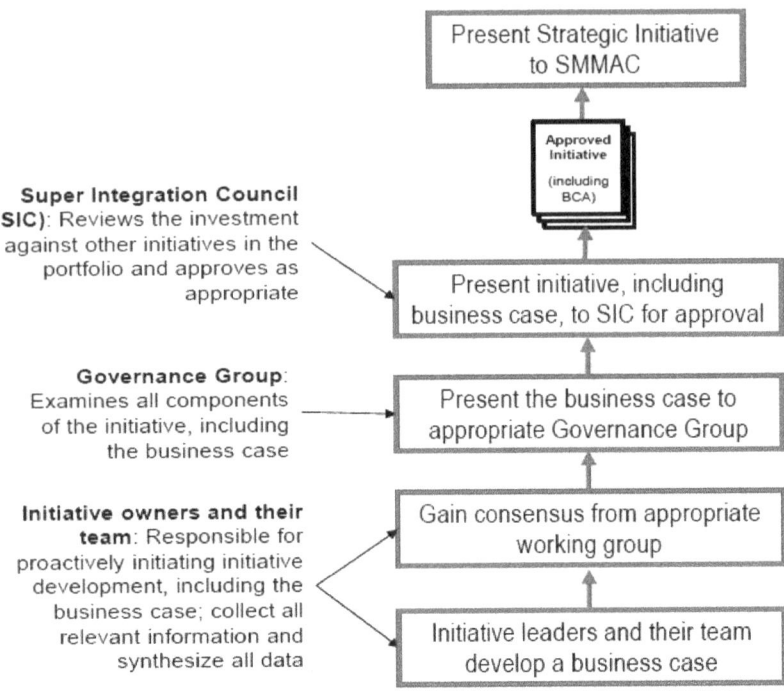

Figure 2.1-1 Strategic Initiatives Process

Purchased Care Performance Management:

1. Monthly contract assessments are reviewed for common cause and special cause variation and events against the standard of care
2. Each contractor has its own compliance office to manage corrective action
3. Contractors identify areas of non-conformance
4. Contractors implements corrective action plan
5. Contractors provide Monthly, Quarterly, and Annual Quality Status Reporting (includes Safety and Access)

Performance Management Tools and Methodology

MHS Conference content is focused on strategy, education, and communication. The MHS Strategic Plan, Quadruple Aim, and Strategic Initiatives are all themes that provide the enterprise perspective for performance improvement activities throughout the MHS. As part of establishing the enhanced Multi-Service Markets (eMSM), incentives have been linked to achieving specific targets. Targets include quality, safety and access measures.

Current Capabilities

The DHA has standardized Business Case Analysis (BCA) and Business Process Reengineering (BPR) methods (below) to evaluate the ten shared services' processes and to deliver efficiencies that are estimated to save $3.7 billion over 5 years. This approach is now part of the MHS standard work for evaluating MHS initiatives.

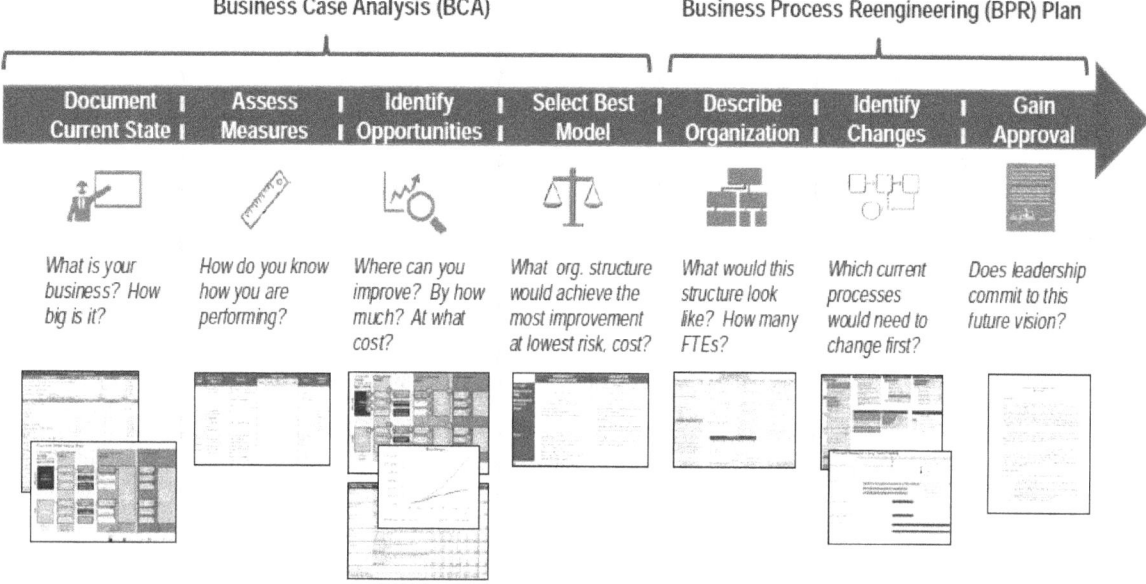

Figure 2.1-2 Standard BCA and BPR Process

Any DHA assets with Lean or Six Sigma training are engaged in supporting BCA and BPR efforts outlined in the Report to Congress. Thus far, 10 of the 87 projects identified to produce desired results are complete and another 17 are underway.

Knowledge Management and Replication

MHS Conferences have provided valuable knowledge and sharing opportunities within and among Services and from leading health care industry experts. An example is the Safety Bundles initiative first highlighted by the Institute for Healthcare Improvement.

National Capital Region Medical Directorate (NCR MD) Performance Improvement

Strategic Planning

The Business Performance Plan for the eMSM is the primary document that directs the integration and focus of strategic initiatives within the NCR MD. This plan outlines specific market initiatives under which project teams are formed to address process and performance initiatives that will positively impact the goals of the eMSM to operate efficiently, increase fiscal responsibility, and ensure the highest quality and safety in the delivery of care to the NCR MD population. Current data analysis is provided by a Market Analysis and Evaluation (MAE) directorate organic to the eMSM and will be further augmented by a Market Board Decision Support Committee (future state) consisting of key market health care and business operations analysts/leaders.

Governance and Performance Management

Under the governance construct of the eMSM, project team analyses and recommendations for process improvements are vetted via the Medical Executive Committee (MEC) and the Market Board, both consisting of leadership representatives of the eMSM MTFs. This ensures that decisions are made collaboratively and allows for execution of initiatives with full standardization, uniformity, and integration throughout the NCR MD market. Monitoring and sustainment is conducted via the MAE, but is limited due to staffing constraints and lack of organic project management tools and dynamic dashboard capability (static scorecards are currently present).

Performance Management Tools and Methodology

Currently up to 200 annual labor hours are available for Black Belt Lean Six Sigma (LSS) capability via an onboard contractor to NCR MD. LSS capabilities to include Black Belts are at both Joint facilities; however, coordination of field capabilities is not yet mature within the MAE. Application of Business Case Analysis tools is centralized within the MAE division of NCR MD. Each Joint facility has basic analytic capability through their Healthcare/Business Operations Directorates and root cause analysis (RCA) capability via their Quality Management Programs. Training to include Clinic Managers Training assists with basic analysis and assessment techniques at the MTF clinical level and TeamSTEPPS® training and implementation is underway throughout the NCR MD.

Knowledge Management and Replication

The Market Executive Council and Market Board facilitate communications at the leadership level among eMSM MTF Leadership. Bi-weekly meetings of NCR MD Market Business Operation allows for communications with market MTF analysts and action officers.

Areas for Future Analysis

Future analytical areas desired are focus areas in support of NCR MD Initiatives that assist in promoting efficient, quality, safe, and fiscally responsible care delivered within an integrated system of the NCR. This requires significant focus on standardizing business and clinical processes based on informed decision support data. This may also include analysis that helps inform optimal courses of action to meet foci within the Quadruple Aim and MHS Core Measures. Some topics include operating room utilization, referral management, patient centered medical home enrollment optimization, outpatient market demand and capacity analysis, general and product line analysis, inpatient bed market demand projections, and graduate medical education demand analysis.

Army Medicine

Army Medicine Strategy Shapes Performance Improvement

Army Medicine 2020 Campaign Plan (AM2020CP) is the strategy to achieve mission by guiding, tracking, and focusing actions to improve operational and fiscal effectiveness to increase value to Soldiers, retirees, their family members, and commanders. AM2020CP has 4 Lines of Effort with 10 Campaign Objectives cascading to 34 Programs and Service Lines. Through alignment of strategic planning with measureable objectives, ongoing performance management, and financial incentives, U.S. Army Medical Command (MEDCOM) accelerates performance excellence. To further focus efforts, The MEDCOM Commander/The Surgeon General (TSG) directs four priorities: Combat Casualty Care, Readiness and Health of the Force, Ready and Deployable Medical Force, and Health of Families and Retirees. MEDCOM continually aligns strategy with both the Army and MHS strategies.

In each strategic objective, program and service line, MEDCOM measures performance and sets stretch targets using national health care benchmarks, DoD or HQDA mandates, or self-determined targets based on analysis. The difference between measured current performance and those targets creates "performance gaps." Gaps are addressed by resourcing and executing initiatives using transparent data and performance improvement tools.

Governance and Performance Management

AM2020CP defines the strategic governance characterized by routine performance management venues during which leaders continually assess objective performance through transparent measures and performance gaps. Leadership discusses initiatives to sustain or improve and directs supportive action leveraging command resources, knowledge management at actionable points across the organization (see Table 2.1-1).

Table 2.1-1 Army Performance Management

Weekly	Monthly	Quarterly	Annually	Other
Command Update Brief (CUB)	Chief of Staff Update	Command Team Leader Development Training Session (CTLDTS)	MTF Performance Planning	Fiscal Accountability & Recovery Mission (FARM) (4-6 sites per year)
Campaign Synchronization Working Group (CSWG)	Regional Analytic Data Review (RADR)	Campaign Assessment Board to CofS (CAB)	Strategy Review & Refining	Organizational Inspection Program (OIP)
MHS Synchronization Work Group	PCMH Monthly Review & Analysis	Command Management Review	Human Capital Distribution Plan (HCDP) (2yr)	
MHS Governance Boards x 4		Campaign Assessment & Performance Board (CAPB) to TSG	PB Development	
		Integrated Resourcing & Incentive System (IRIS) Reconciliation	POM	
		ACP Performance Reviews		

KEY: Strategy Governance: AM2020CP & ACP
Focused Performance Management
Synchronization/Knowledge Management
Resourcing Strategy
Compliance and Staff Assistance

In a command with a Tier 1 Headquarters Staff in two locations, 10 Tier 2 Major Subordinate Commands (MSC) spread worldwide, and 71 Tier 3 organizations, multi-tiered performance reviews are key to driving strategic change. Each enables data-driven decision making and leverages an Operating Company Model to best optimize and accelerate value creation, improve health outcomes, and standardization, thus providing a consistent patient experience.

For example:

- Weekly, MEDCOM's G-3/5/7 conducts *Campaign Synchronization Work Groups* where each strategic program cycles through to report their metrics and execution.
- Monthly, the Deputy Commanding General for Operations conducts *Regional Analytic Data Reviews* focusing on the six highest expense Service Lines analyzing access, quality, safety, satisfaction, productivity, and shared leading practices.
- Quarterly/Semi-Annually, the Chief of Staff conducts *Campaign Assessment Boards* and TSG conducts *Campaign Assessment and Performance Boards;* each performance review with inputs from the preceding venues for decisions which written governance specifies for each of their roles.
- Quarterly, selected key Army Medicine performance measures cascade to *Army Campaign Plan (ACP)-level Performance Reviews* to Army senior leaders.
- Annually, Tier 3 hospitals participate in the *MHS Performance Planning* process forecasting beneficiary health care to maximize value and achieve clinical and business outcomes. Performance is assessed against their plan through the year.

A Variety of Tools Ensures Performance Management and Progress

Transparent Data and Dashboards: Data transparency through enterprise web-based performance dashboards is critical to change management. Enterprise transparency clarifies data identity, measure calculation, and comparative performance, and creates competitive tension inciting innovation, which can then be leveraged through knowledge management. Leaders and employees use tools such as Army's Strategic Management System (SMS), MEDCOM's Command Management System (CMS), and the Performance Planning Dashboard to monitor performance. For example, individual health care providers see their provider-level workload and value analysis using the MEDCOM's Practice Management Revenue Model (PMRM) tool to evaluate where they spend their time, how much they "earn," how their performance changes over time, and how they compare to peers. This enables individual improvement at provider level.

Financial Incentives: MEDCOM began using performance based budgeting in 2006 to align funding with strategic targets to accelerate performance. Then called the Performance Based Budget Model (PBAM), near continuous performance improvement was demonstrated in all areas incentivized under PBAM. Using PBAM's lessons-learned, MEDCOM transitioned to the *Integrated Resource and Incentive System (IRIS)* in 2014 funding primary care through capitation based on planned enrollment, behavioral health linked to performance, and expanded incentives to 27 performance factors in access, quality, safety, capacity, care utilization, cost, and administrative efficiency. Headquarters distributes IRIS incentives quarterly to subordinate organizations to fund performance and enable incremental learning during the year. IRIS execution is likewise captured and transparently displayed in a web-based Financial Management Information System.

Targeted Performance Assistance, Education, and Knowledge Management: MEDCOM assembles teams of functional subject matter experts (SME) who travel to subordinate organizations to strengthen local capabilities to be self-sustaining and performance-focused with correct use of tools. MEDCOM's Deputy Chief of Staff for Resources, Infrastructure & Strategy leads the *Fiscal Accountability and Recovery Mission (FARM)* engagements: a 120-day preparation, execution, and follow-up process involving Headquarters, Regional Medical Command, and local hospital SMEs centered around a one-week on-site assessment and knowledge sharing visit. MEDCOM's *Organizational Inspection Program (OIP)* sends SMEs on a recurring basis to subordinate organizations to assess and teach. Similarly, TSG's *Command Team Leader Development Training Sessions (CTLDTS)* provide subordinate organizations' command teams with training by SMEs for collective leader development and knowledge sharing against strategic issues and performance.

Lean Six Sigma Tools and Methods Enable Robust Process Improvement

MEDCOM uses myriad performance improvement initiatives and tools appropriate to each challenge (e.g., root cause analysis, TeamSTEPPS®, "plan-do-check-act" [PDCA], risk management analysis).

Building Necessary Infrastructure to Enable LSS Success: MEDCOM designs and resources each MSC headquarters with necessary infrastructure, including a Directorate of Strategy and Innovation (DSI) or equivalent office. The DSI directors and their staff serve as advisors, responsible for LSS Program governance, strategic planning and management, and knowledge management in accordance with Army and MEDCOM guidance. This office is uniquely suited to integrate analytics, strategic management, and process improvement to support decision-making and achievement of sustainable results.

MEDCOM Standardizes LSS Processes Yielding Improved Capabilities: MEDCOM's LSS program is an enterprise-wide formal program designed to drive organizational change through continuous process improvement. The map below outlines the program's current high-level process from Project Selection to Replication.

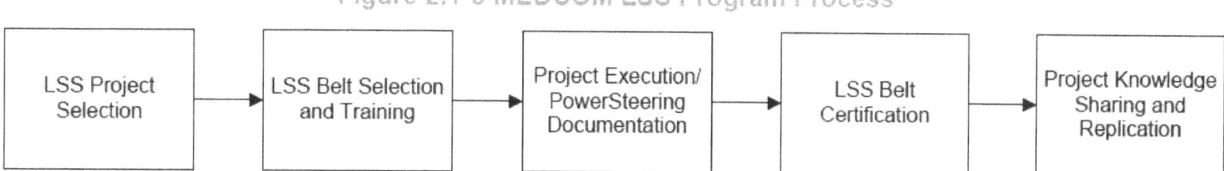

Figure 2.1-3 MEDCOM LSS Program Process

Recognizing that successful LSS programs are leader-driven and responsive to organizational strategic priorities, the 6 Dec 13-published *Office of the Surgeon General/ US Army Medical*

Command Lean Six Sigma Program Guide documents processes to standardize LSS execution and drive improvement within the command's LSS program.

The Program Guide calls for each LSS project to be aligned to strategic priorities and documented performance gaps from the Army Medicine 2020 Campaign Plan, organizational Balanced Scorecards, Project Identification Selection Workshops, or directives from senior Army Medicine leaders. Local command teams or executive committees must approve project charters. Projects must be aligned with strategic goals, but also be important to the customer, have Project Sponsor support, senior leader commitment, a sense of urgency, projected financial and/or operational benefit, a high benefit to risk ratio, and be feasible in scope and resources.

Local command teams or executive committees select LSS belt candidates based on demonstrated leadership and problem-solving abilities; the Program Guide publishes the full list of candidate selection criteria. During and after training, belt candidates execute projects in accord with the LSS standardized methodology. Project work is documented in the Army's web-based project portfolio management software system, PowerSteering (PS). PS provides senior leaders, LSS deployment directors, process owners, and belt project managers real-time visibility, strategy alignment, and the ability to make more effective project investment decisions, reduce costs, and prioritize projects. Once completing training, executing a project in accordance with standardized LSS methodology and documenting the project in PS, the belt is submitted for Army LSS certification and the project is evaluated for replication opportunities.

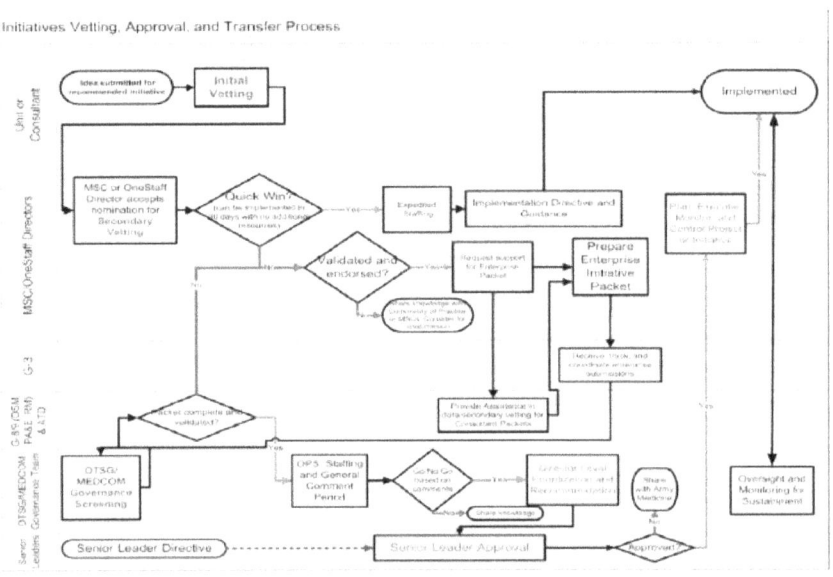

Figure 2.1-4 MEDCOM Initiatives Vetting, Approval, and Transfer Process

Knowledge Management and Replication Advances Enterprise Improvement
MEDCOM acknowledges that enterprise-wide performance improvement, data driven decision-making, and shared knowledge within an Operating Company Model will drive accelerated change. MEDCOM's methodology for identifying replication opportunities, vetting them, and actively transferring them across the command is a tiered process involving multiple levels of the organization. The *Initiative Transfer Process* map shown here is published in the AM2020CP as an important component of the effort to standardize key processes throughout the command. The process is intended to formalize an approach MEDCOM piloted to identify, validate, and replicate not only LSS Project successes, but all leading practices or initiatives with the potential to benefit the command.

In April 2014, MEDCOM launched a new initiative communicating the results of successful LSS Projects through an Executive Summary (EXSUM) and one-slide quad chart to HQs Process Owners and Consultants for visibility and potential replication opportunities. Project EXSUMs are then shared with TSG and all Army Medicine senior leaders.

Further Analysis and Process Improvement Will Continue Positive Change

MEDCOM's LSS Program Guide publishes program performance measures which are built into the SMS tool with drill down capabilities to all Tier 3 organizations. These have targets and are routinely monitored, and action is taken to improve through the command's LSS Community of Practice.

As of 1 Jul 2014, MEDCOM trained 634 Green Belts (GB)/certified 165 GB; trained 558 Black Belts (BB)/certified 178 BB; and trained 34 Master Black Belts (MBB)/certified 17 MBB. Of those trained, the current MEDCOM certification rate is 26 percent for GB and 32 percent for BB. Of 360 certified belts, 73 (20 percent) have completed more than one project. FY 2014 targets increase belt certification rates and certified belts completing more than one project, with a focus on non-gated projects such as Rapid Improvement Events.

Finally, MEDCOM's LSS Program self-assessment is based on the Army's LSS Maturity Model as published in the Army Lean Six Sigma Deployment Guidebook. This self-assessment identifies MEDCOM's LSS program strengths such as Training and Organization, but more importantly identifies future improvement opportunities.

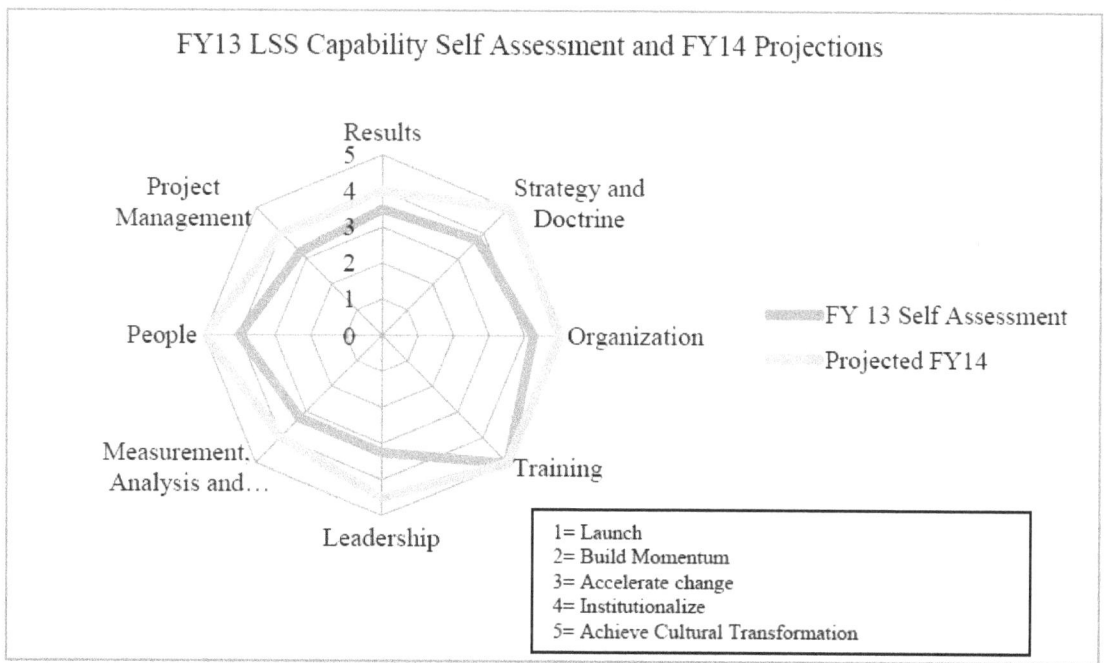

Figure 2.1-5 MEDCOM FY 2103 LSS Capability Self-Assessment and FY 2014 Projections

Navy Medicine Performance Improvement

Strategic Planning

Navy Medicine has three overarching strategic priorities: Readiness, Value and Jointness. These strategic priorities combine with six strategic objectives and three enabling objectives as depicted in Figure 2.1-6. Each priority and objective is aligned with MHS strategy and each is underpinned by patient safety, quality, and access.

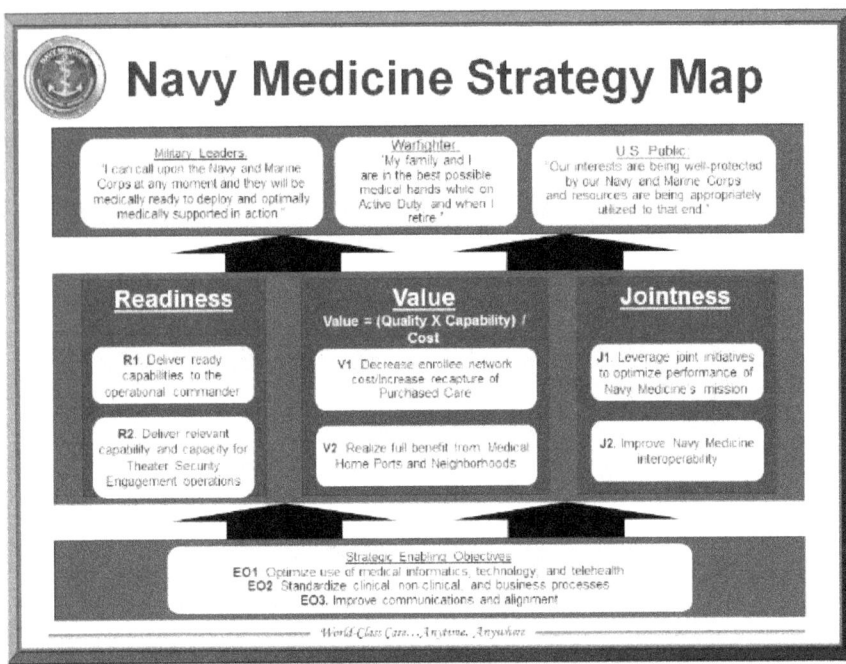

Figure 2.1-6 Navy Medicine Strategy Map

Specific strategic objectives in patient safety, quality, and access include:

V2 - Realize full benefit from Medical Home Ports (MHP) and Neighborhoods - Our objective is to attain better health for patients, and when they do need care, to provide the best care possible in a patient-centered care environment.

EO1 - Optimize use of medical informatics, technology, and telehealth - Leverage informatics, technology, and telehealth with standardized interoperable tools and processes throughout the enterprise. Quality metrics and data are then used to optimize clinical and business decision making, workflows, and outcomes within the Operational, Joint, and Interagency environment.

EO2 - Standardize clinical, non-clinical, and business processes - Through appropriate standardization of processes, improve delivery of Navy Medicine capabilities and services, clinical outcomes, quality of care, and overall efficiency while reducing costs and resource utilization.

EO3 - Improve Communications and Alignment - Navy Medicine drives strategic alignment using communication capabilities and clear governance structure while holding each level of Navy Medicine accountable for execution. Alignment and communication ensures that Navy Medicine's intent and strategic plan is understood by all stakeholders and provides two-way communication.

These goals are articulated to the lower echelons of the organization through communication from the Surgeon General and other Senior Navy Medicine Officials. An annual Navy Surgeon

General Symposium, with attendance by all senior leaders throughout Navy Medicine, is conducted to promulgate and emphasize the organization's strategic goals. Additionally, biannual Regional Command and MTF performance reviews, quarterly Senior Strategy Board reviews and monthly Value Objective reviews are conducted to ensure improvement strategies are aligned with strategic and enabling objectives and are promulgated throughout Navy Medicine.

Governance and Performance Management

Navy Medicine's Strategic Plan drives tactical governance which includes biannual, quarterly, and monthly recurring performance reviews of strategic objectives. These performance reviews facilitate implementation and sustainment of improvement activities and hold each level of Navy Medicine accountable for strategic execution.

Specific programs dedicated to continuous Performance Improvement within Navy Medicine include the Lean Six Sigma (LSS) and Industrial Engineering (IE) programs. Both programs report through the interim Quality Improvement Officer and each has an extensive portfolio of ongoing projects that target improving patient safety, quality of care, clinical efficiency, access to care and standardization throughout Navy Medicine.

The portfolio of performance improvement initiatives for both programs is managed through a series of governance committees and meetings between Headquarters, the Regions, and the MTFs. Project requests are driven through a variety of channels, including MTF, Specialty Leader, or leadership. Project requests are routed through the Quality Committee (QC) which approves and prioritizes these efforts. All projects are managed centrally by the Regional LSS offices or the Bureau of Medicine and Surgery (BUMED) IE program staff. On a monthly basis, IE, LSS, and each Regional Command (Navy Medicine East and Navy Medicine West) staff meet and review recently completed, ongoing, or upcoming projects. This coordination ensures all major stakeholders are involved in management and oversight of each effort.

Performance Management Tools and Methodology

Performance Dashboards and Summary Reports: Consistent with our strategic priorities, enterprise-wide clinical, non-clinical and business data dashboards and summary reports are used to measure, trend, and manage key strategic performance metrics. These provide standardized, transparent, concise and relevant performance measurement to facilitate data driven decision making at all levels of Navy Medicine. Each performance metric includes enterprise, Regional, MTF, and peer-level views and comparisons. Leadership at all levels uses these tools to monitor and manage performance.

Lean Six Sigma: A foundational modality of Performance Improvement, Navy Medicine uses LSS methodology, a robust process improvement methodology that targets elimination of waste, defects, and unnecessary processes, redirecting human effort toward value added operations. LSS tools include value stream mapping of current and future state, risk prioritization, continuous process flow, Failure Mode Effects Analysis (FMEA), data analysis, statistical process control, mistake proofing, visual cuing, and process standardization. Navy Medicine's

LSS program was launched in 2006 pursuant directives from the Deputy Secretary of Defense, Secretary of the Navy, and Secretary of Defense.

This enterprise-wide formal process drives continuous process improvement and organizational change. Each enterprise project launched in Fiscal Year 2014 aligns with one of Navy Medicine's strategic priorities of Readiness, Value, and Jointness. LSS projects are managed by MTF Green or Black Belts, with mentoring from Regional Black Belts or Master Black Belts.

Industrial Engineering: The Industrial Engineering (IE) program supplements Navy Medicine's LSS toolset with additional capabilities in process engineering, data analytics, and software development. IE projects are typically large scale and involve several process aspects including facilities, information technology, staffing, and both administrative and clinical operations. Dedicated process improvement resources work on projects over a typical six-month project length, using LSS, simulation modeling, and project management tools. At a high level, the project approach involves describing the current state and defining the ideal future state (Diagnostic Phase), implementing the future state (Implementation Phase), and continued monitoring of performance (Sustainment). Extensive collaboration and stakeholder involvement is used to gain buy in and support for project analysis and recommendations. Examples of implemented recommendations include standardized workflows, checklists, software tools, including monitoring dashboards, and facility modifications.

Incentives: The Strategic Health Incentivization Program (SHIP) was introduced in Fiscal Year 2014 and includes 26 strategic metrics. Metrics are generally classified as belonging to one of three groups including Readiness, Health, and Value. SHIP metrics are intended to challenge the status quo and encourage a reexamination of perspectives and of system processes. During Fiscal Year 2015, monthly webinars will be hosted which will focus on the health care system dynamics of the individual metrics.

Current Capabilities

Projects: 340 LSS projects have been completed to-date with an additional 45 active projects in progress that target improving patient safety, quality, clinical efficiency, and standardization. Additionally, there are 11 ongoing IE projects in Navy Medicine East (NME) and eight ongoing projects in Navy Medicine West (NMW). Since 2009, 28 projects have been completed across Navy Medicine. Initiatives span clinical and administrative areas, including primary care enrollment and access to care, operating rooms, obstetrics, medical boards processing, supply chain, and ancillary services.

Assets: Navy Medicine has a total of 11 staff members who provide full-time support to the LSS program; BUMED-5 total; NME-3 total; NMW-3 total. These individuals serve as Regional Black Belts, Master Black Belts, Black Belts, and administrative support staff for training, software management, program communication and logistics.

The LSS governing structure includes senior military members that serve as the Regional Black Belts, providing oversight and direction of LSS activities at the respective region; and Master

Black Belts that serve as process experts and technical advisors on project management, tool selection, and statistical analysis.

IE resources include seven full time civilian industrial engineers and additional contract project leads, industrial engineers, data analysts, programmers, and subject matter experts. Current contracts for performance improvement include a contract with Johns Hopkins University Applied Physics Laboratory, a University Affiliated Research Center, and also an Indefinite Delivery, Indefinite Quantity (IDIQ) contract with prime contractors Altarum, Booz Allen Hamilton, Deloitte, and Improvement Path Systems. Additionally, a contract with the Center for Naval Analyses, a Federally Funded Research and Development Center (FFRDC), provides analytical support and research on topics related to policy.

Knowledge Management and Replication

Knowledge Sharing: All Navy Medicine LSS projects are recorded into, and managed through, the Power Steering Continuous Process Improvement Management System (CPIMS). This is a web-accessed tool utilized by other Navy entities, including Marine Corps, to capture all project activity. This tool is visible across Navy Medicine and is used to share information across the service.

Knowledge gained from IE projects is shared within the organization through the project reporting structure, which includes briefings to a Steering Committee consisting of MTF leadership and an Oversight Committee including MTF leadership and flag-level leadership at BUMED. On an ongoing basis, IE staff members participate in established BUMED Working Groups, including the Emergency Management Working Group and the Operating Room Optimization Working Group. Additionally, IE project information is being integrated into the CPIMS site for sharing.

The process for sharing LSS and IE information between services is informal and evolving. For example, Navy performance improvement teams presented to the Extremity Trauma and Amputation Center of Excellence and the Veterans Administration on subject matter related to wounded warrior care. Further, sharing of project work with the other services has begun to take place since the migration of headquarters functions to the Defense Health Headquarters (DHHQ). For example, the Army has recently requested to implement an operating room (OR) dashboard at their hospitals that was developed as part of previous Navy performance improvement projects. Moreover, improvement information and best practices are shared with the other services as part of the MHS governance structure which includes Advisory Boards and Work Groups such as the Patient Centered Medical Home Advisory Board and the MHS Access Improvement Work Group. With the recent development of the enhanced Multi-Service Market structure, projects have expanded to include other services where relevant, such as laboratory services that could be coordinated across various MTFs.

Sustainment: Sustainment of both implemented improvements and ongoing performance improvement capabilities is ensured through the current program structure.

To keep visibility on the results of performance improvement projects, key performance indicators are assigned and tracked for each project. As part of every IE project, the team helps develop and implement automated dashboards which monitor these metrics. These tools are used in sustainment to help stakeholders track improvements or identify when a process is slipping back to the original state.

The training curriculum provided by the LSS program ensures ongoing capability in performance improvement techniques. The curriculum provides participants advanced knowledge on LSS Methodology. A total of 2,815 Navy Medicine staff has been trained, including 1,140 Champions, 185 Black Belts and 1,490 Green Belts. Additionally, 30,969 CEUs and 3,677 CMEs have been awarded. The goal of the training program has been to infuse a culture of continuous improvement throughout the Navy Medicine enterprise. Additionally, as of July 2014, seven organic staff have been certified as LSS instructors.

In the effort to ingrain the LSS methodology within Navy Medicine culture, a Department of the Navy (DON) Additional Qualification Designator (AQD) was approved for Green Belts and Black Belts for officers, and a Navy Enlisted Classification (NEC) code for Green Belt was approved for enlisted staff. BUMED also established a certification process to recognize Black Belts and Green Belts for training and project work to improve the enterprise processes.

Areas for Future Analysis

Navy Medicine is in the initial stages of integrating its IE component with its LSS program. It is hoped this initiative will prove highly successful in streamlining the Performance Improvement Process throughout Navy Medicine. It should have the added benefits of facilitating communications between the two entities and also inspire a synergistic effect in the approach to Performance Improvement in Navy Medicine.

One of the initiatives of this recent effort is the establishment of the Performance Improvement Board of Directors. Its initial monthly meeting took place on 24 Jun 2014. The Board consists of the Navy Medicine Chief Performance Improvement Officer and Deputy Chief Performance Improvement Officer, the Heads of the Performance Improvement Offices at Navy Medicine East and Navy Medicine West, the Senior Master Black Belt at BUMED; others in attendance are from both the IE staff and the LSS staff. The basic agenda of this meeting is to facilitate the dissemination of information, standardization of methods and processes among the Regions, BUMED, and any other relevant stakeholders.

Air Force Medical Service Performance Improvement

Strategic Planning

The overarching goals of the Air Force Medical Service (AFMS) Strategy – Readiness, Better Care, Better Health, and Best Value – are depicted in Figure 2.1-7. Patient safety, quality and access are foundational elements in each of these goals.

Figure 2.1-7 Air Force Medical Service Strategy Map

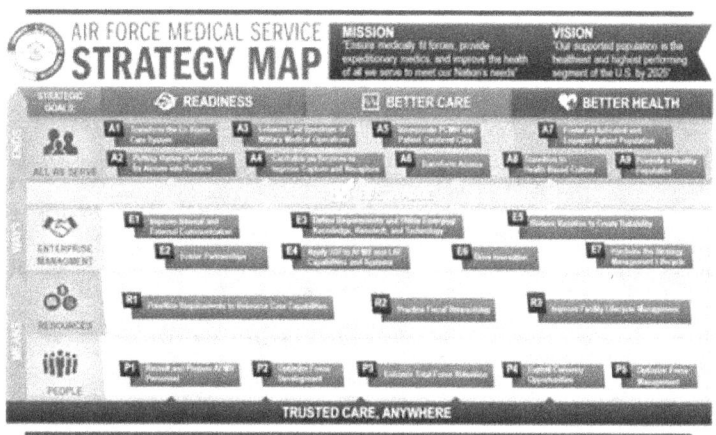

Several Strategic Objectives aligned under these overarching goals are more specific to patient safety, quality and access, and drive us toward higher reliability in these areas. These objectives are:

E5 - Reduce Variation to Create Reliability
A4 - Capitalize on Services to Improve Capture and Recapture
A5 - Incorporate PCMH into Patient-Centered Care
A6 - Transform Access
A7 - Foster an Active and Engaged Population
E1 - Improve Internal and External Communication
E6 - Drive Innovation
E7 - Hardwire Strategy
P4 - Exploit Currency Opportunities

As the operational entity overseeing home station care for the AFMS, the Air Force Medical Operations Agency (AFMOA) developed cross-organizational cells directly aligned to the AFMS Strategic Objectives listed above. The cells are responsible for execution of these objectives through partnering and coaching the MTFs to achieve designated performance. (See Table 2.1-2).

Table 2.1-2 Alignment of Cells to AFMS Strategic Objectives

Cross Functional Cell	Objective
Patient Centered Medical Home (PCMH); **Hospital, Specialty Care and Ambulatory Procedures (HAS)**	E5 Reduce Variation to Create Reliability
Medical Enterprise Resource Information Tool (MERIT); **Enhanced Multi-Service Market (eMSM);** **HSA**	A4 Capitalize on Services to Improve Capture and Recapture
	P4 Exploit Currency Opportunities
PCMH **HSA**	A6 Transform Access
	A5 Incorporate PCMH into Patient Centered Care
	A7 Foster an Active and Engaged Population
Performance Management	E7 Hardwire Strategy
Enterprise Level	E1 Improve Internal and External Communication
	E6 Drive Innovation

As objectives are operationalized and performance measures and targets identified, performance toward targets is analyzed by AFMOA. If not making progress toward targets, performance improvement initiatives are undertaken. This "Operational Management of Strategy Execution" is depicted below in Figure 2.1-8, adapted from the VA graphic of Department-wide strategic management process.

Figure 2.1-8 Operational Management of Strategy Execution

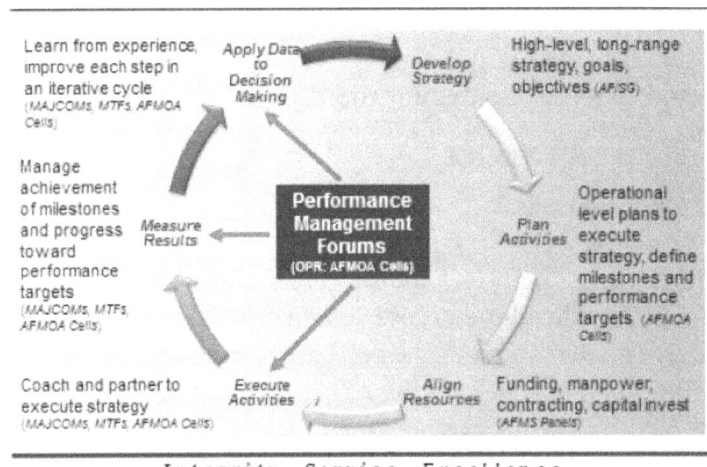

Integrity - Service - Excellence

Governance and Performance Management

As noted in the Operational Management of Strategy Execution in Figure 2.1-8, AFMOA, and more specifically the AFMOA cells, are responsible for four of the six key elements: Plan Activities, Execute Activities, Measure Results, and Apply Data to Decision Making. The other two elements of Develop Strategy and Align Resources are the responsibility of the Office of the Air Force Surgeon General and AFMS Panels.

Operational level plans to execute strategy are developed by the cells with milestones, meaningful and actionable operational performance measures, and performance targets defined. AFMOA partners with the Major Commands (MAJCOMs) and MTFs through the Performance Management Forums to implement in the MTFs, measure results, and use the data for informed decision making on improvement initiatives.

The Performance Management Forums were started in 2011 as a method to communicate with the Air Force specialty hospitals on key issues surrounding access, capture/recapture, currency, and a multitude of other key performance indicators. They are held quarterly and executed by three MTF peer groups: specialty hospitals, small hospitals, and clinics. The overarching Performance Management Cell standardizes the structure and processes of the forums.

These forums continue to evolve and drive improved performance by sharing aggregated and MTF specific strategic and operational measure performance. They consist of invaluable peer-to-peer discussions on successes and challenges to achieving milestones and progress in meeting performance targets. The enterprise gains group consensus on key items, issues, and improvement solutions, as well as leading practices to be replicated across the AFMS. Actions and process improvement activities from the forums and performance at both the MTF and enterprise-level are tracked by AFMOA.

Current Capabilities

Continuous process improvement within the Air Force focuses on growing Airmen into effective and efficient thinkers and problem solvers, primarily through the use of Lean. It is about moving the organization to the point where everyone is committed to asking themselves "What have I improved today?" It is about leadership owning the responsibility to make the best use of Airmen's time; thereby, improving efficiency and effectiveness of operational capabilities.

The AFMS went one step further and adopted Lean Healthcare and the teachings of the University of Tennessee. The underpinning of Lean Healthcare is the application of management prescriptions, concepts, and tools aimed at furthering the organizational mission by strengthening operating processes. Management prescriptions are focusing on the process and value from the customer's (patient's) perspective, and constantly seeking to eliminate waste. Primary concepts are work is accomplished through a series of processes (not functions) and improving process lead and cycle times is beneficial to everyone. There are a multitude of lean tools, to include problem solving, process mapping, workplace organization, pull systems, standard work, and flow and variation reduction. Identifying which tools to use in problem solving for improvement depends on the problem and the best approach to identifying root causes and solutions.

The Air Force prescribed systematic method for problem solving is the Observe-Orient-Decide-Act Loop, which is further broken down into the eight-step process: 1) Clarify and validate the problem; 2) Break down the problem/identify performance gaps; 3) Set improvement targets; 4) Determine root causes; 5) Develop countermeasures; 6) See countermeasures through; 7) Confirm results; and, 8) Standardize successful processes. This method is applied across the gamut of small, local activities (such as decreasing no-show rates in a clinic) to large, enterprise-wide projects (such as Surgical Services Analysis and Process Improvement Project).

Improvement initiatives may be generated through the formalized process of identifying improvements that move an organization along strategic lines of effort to those generated through risk management, patient safety, and inspection findings. Use of the eight-step process is highly encouraged. However, some MTFs fall back to the prescribed method of external agencies, such as the 10-step method of the Accreditation Association from Ambulatory Health Care.

Training within the AFMS follows the AF standardized curriculum. Training includes the following courses: Basic Awareness, Senior Leader, Executive Leader, 8-Step, Green Belt, and Black Belt. The AFMS contracted with the University of Tennessee over the last several years to deliver the UT Lean for Healthcare Course, and is now investigating the ability to offer the course with internal resources.

Green and black belt courses are the didactics required for green and black belt certification. The Air Force and AFMS do not prescribe the required numbers of green and black belt certified facilitators within organizations and across the enterprise. In addition, designated billets for Wing and Headquarters black belts were recently significantly decreased due to resource realignments. Green and black belt resources are now interspersed and inconsistent, leaving some MTFs with no designated on-site certified green or black belt facilitators.

The Air Force uses the Continuous Process Improvement Management Tool (CPI-MT) as its central repository for process improvement activities. This is the same system used by the Army and Navy, but called by different names. The CPI-MT is not consistently used across the Air Force, and is concerning in respect to housing quality protected medical activities. Activities with quality protected information are either redacted or not put in CPI-MT. There is no other central repository for process improvement activities across the AFMS. However, AFMOA is the repository for enterprise-wide activities, such as Emergency Services Analysis and Process Improvement Project, Surgical Analysis and Process Improvement Project, and Implementation of Real Time Demand Capacity.

Process improvement activities occur every day across the AFMS, but may not be captured as a formalized process improvement activity. These activities may or may not be shared with higher headquarters. With the goal of the Air Force being to grow Airmen into the most effective and efficient thinkers and problem solvers, the emphasis is on doing and not on reporting. The most important aspect of AFMS continuous process improvement is improving efficiency and effectiveness of operational capabilities. This improvement will cascade up into improving performance in those most important aspects aligned to strategy, as described in the previous section.

Knowledge Management and Replication

Information sharing on improvements and leading practices is described above in the Performance Management Governance/Process Venues section. There is no formal process for sharing improvement information and leading practices with other services. However, AFMS personnel frequently share information with their counterparts in other services through their function specific venues and other forums: for example, the MHS PCMH Advisory Board and the Tri-Service Workflow forum.

Areas for Future Analysis

Many opportunities exist to improve the application and management of continuous process improvement in the MHS). Variation exists across the Services in the method prescribed for process improvement, the training provided, requirements for certified facilitators, and instilling a daily environment of continual improvement. This needs to become more standardized as the MHS works jointly and in e-MSMs in order to target outcomes and move with more agility in the future. Further analysis could also be done on how to best share information within and among Services, to include a sensible solution for a shared and interactive repository. Joint Information Management Information Technology (IMIT) solutions need to be agreed upon and built quickly to reach these goals. Specific topics for consideration as improvement projects across the enterprise include the use of Healthcare Artifact and Image Management Solution (HAIMS) and standardized metrics and technology that supports timely data available at all levels.

This page left intentionally blank.

APPENDIX 3. ACCESS TO CARE

Appendix 3.1
Code of Federal Regulations 32 CFR 199.17 (p)(5)

Access standards. Preferred provider networks will have attributes of size, composition, mix of providers, and geographical distribution so that the networks, coupled with the MTF capabilities, can adequately address the health care needs of the enrollees. Before offering enrollment in Prime to a beneficiary group, the MTF Commander (or other authorized person) will assure that the capabilities of the MTF plus preferred provider network will meet the following access standards with respect to the needs of the expected number of enrollees from the beneficiary group being offered enrollment:

(i) Under normal circumstances, enrollee travel time may not exceed 30 minutes from home to primary care delivery site unless a longer time is necessary because of the absence of providers (including providers not part of the network) in the area.

(ii) The wait time for an appointment for a well-patient visit or a specialty care referral shall not exceed four weeks; for a routine visit, the wait time for an appointment shall not exceed one week; and for an urgent care visit the wait time for an appointment shall generally not exceed 24 hours.

(iii) Emergency services shall be available and accessible to handle emergencies (and urgent care visits if not available from other primary care providers pursuant to paragraph (p)(5)(ii) of this section), within the service area 24 hours a day, seven days a week.

(iv) The network shall include a sufficient number and mix of board certified specialists to meet reasonably the anticipated needs of enrollees. Travel time for specialty care shall not exceed one hour under normal circumstances, unless a longer time is necessary because of the absence of providers (including providers not part of the network) in the area. This requirement does not apply under the Specialized Treatment Services Program.

(v) Office waiting times in non-emergency circumstances shall not exceed 30 minutes, except when emergency care is being provided to patients, and the normal schedule is disrupted.

Appendix 3.2
Access Improvement Working Group Charter

Table 3.2-1 The Military Health Systems (MHS) Access Improvement Working Group (AIWG)

Military Health Systems (MHS) Access Improvement Working Group (AIWG)

Sponsor(s): Tri-Service Patient-Centered Care Advisory Board

Scope:
The mission of the MHS Access Improvement Working Group, a working group of the Tri-Service Patient-Centered Care Advisory Board, is to develop and sustain comprehensive and standardized Department of Defense ATC guidance to improve and sustain the following ATC processes: appointment/scheduling/templating operations, ATC performance measures, appointing information systems management, empanelment, and related training opportunities. Where relevant, the Advisory Board should make recommendations to the Tri-Service PCMH Advisory and Tri-Service Specialty Care Advisory Boards for implementation approval.

Chairperson(s): USAF, then rotating among services annually

Stakeholders/Names:
Army Representative-
Navy Representative-
Air Force Representative-
Coast Guard Representative-
DHA Representatives-
Referral Management Representatives-
Medical Management Representatives-
Service Medical Home Representatives-
Specialty Representatives from Orthopedics, OR Specialties, OB/GYN, Mental Health and Ambulatory Specialties-

Business Case/Opportunity Statement:
With the adoption of the Quadruple Aim and Patient Centered Medical Home (PCMH) as MH strategic goals, there is a significant need to update, execute and sustain a standardized set of guidance on access management in order to meet 32 CFR 199.17 access standards and the tenets of PCMH, the Quadruple Aim and the access imperatives of the uniformed services. The MHS guide to Access Success, last updated in 2008, will be replaced with this policy guidance to support current MHS strategy.
Additionally, in order to support fully integrated delivery system, the MHS is implementing the Medical Neighborhood with oversight by the Tri-Service Patient-Centered Care Advisory Board. The MHS AIWG will report directly to the Tri-Service Patient-Centered Care Advisory Board to facilitate coordination.

Goal Statement:
The goal for this working group is to meeting at least monthly to discuss and develop processes to implement and sustain standard access improvement business practice across the MHS. One of the first projects will be to write a MHS Access to Care Operations Manual. This document will be used to provide updated guidance currently contained in the MHS Guide for Access Success.
Due to the closely related nature of ATC business practices to a number of related process improvement efforts, the AIWG will coordinate closely with the Tri-Service PCMH Advisory Board, Tri-Service Specialty Care Advisory Board, the Medical Management Advisory Board and the Referral Management Working Group. Representation from these groups will be both ADHOC and permanent on the AIWG.

Deliverables:
1. MHS Access to Care Operations Manual reflecting standardized ATC business rules across the Services.
   a. MHS Core Access to Care Guidance to include development of standardized clinic management and appointing practices.
   b. Drafting of MHS Access to Care Operations Manual appendices providing in depth how-to guidance in various areas of access management to include warriors in transition access management, information systems operations, use of technology, online appointing, use of secure messaging, access performance measurement, patient communications/customer services, operations checklist and more.
2. Development of marketing and education plan for users and stakeholders.
3. Integration of ATC guidance into functional requirements of MHS information systems.
4. Monthly meetings to continue to discuss and develop ATC guidance for the MHS.

Tasks/Milestones:	Target Date	Date Achieved
Charter drafted and approved	February 2014	
MHS AIWG chair selected	February 2014	
Develop/distribute CHCS problem resolution worksheet	March 2014	
Standardize provider specialty code sorting process to delineate extenders (PharmD, BHOP, etc) working in PCMH clinics	March 2014	
Develop "Simplified Appointing" Model, creating a two or three appointment type Primary Care appointing system	April 2014	
MHS Access Ops Manual Core guidance completed/approved	August 2014	
All appendices drafted and approved	June 2015	

Tasks/Milestones:	Target Date	Date Achieved
Development and approval of a marketing and educational plan to include identification of faculty and course	December 2015	
Continuing development of policies and guidance	Ongoing	
Is there a Regulatory Requirement for this IWC/Workgroup/Committee:	NO	
Approved by the Chair of the Medical Operations Group:		

Source: 2014 MHS Review Group

Appendix 3.3
Summary of Access to Care Policies and Orders

DoD Policies

10 U.S. Code, Chapter 55, *Medical and Dental Care.* The U.S. Code is a consolidation and codification by subject matter of the general and permanent laws of the United States; it is currently divided into 51 titles. Title 10 contains laws relating to the Armed Forces. The provisions of law that affect military health care are codified in chapter 55 of title 10. Section 1072 defines the term "TRICARE Program" as the managed health program established by the DoD, principally by Section 1097. Section 1073 tasks the Secretary of Defense with responsibility for administering the medical and dental benefits provided in chapter 55 of title 10, including broad authority to implement and administer the TRICARE program.

Code of Federal Regulations (32 CFR), Part 199.17 *TRICARE Program.* Pursuant to the above statutory authority, the Secretary of Defense has promulgated rules and regulations at 32 CFR 199.17 governing the TRICARE Program for the purpose of implementing a comprehensive managed health care program for the delivery and financing of health care services in the Military Health System. Section 199.17(p)(5) addresses access standards, including specific wait and travel time standards, for TRICARE Prime enrollees.

The Military Health System's (MHS) *Guide to Access Success,* **15 December 2008.** The guide establishes roles, responsibilities, definitions, and guidance for implementing, sustaining, and managing MTF ATC in the MHS that meets or exceeds the access standards stated in 32 Code of Federal Regulations (CFR) 199.17. This very detailed and comprehensive guide provides MTFs with direction on appointing and schedule management, appointing in the electronic scheduling system known as the Composite Health Care System (CHCS), the Open Access model, patient eligibility and enrollment, TRICARE On Line, referrals, and specialty and mental health access. The guide provides step-by-step CHCS operations related to access to care and data quality. Templates for an access improvement plan, access manager job description, measures, and optimization strategies are included in the appendices.

Health Affairs Policy 11-005, *TRICARE Policy for Access to Care,* **23 February 2011.** HA Policy 11-005 rescinded and replaced eight previous policies. It provides guidance for access standards for health care benefits under the TRICARE Program consistent with 32 CFR, Part 199.17(p)(5). The wait and travel times, priority of access to MTF care by beneficiary status, TRICARE Prime Service Area, and beneficiary waiver of travel standards are all described in detail. The standards apply to all MTFs (to the extent practicable in overseas locations).

Health Affairs Policy 09-15, *Policy Memorandum Implementation of the Patient Centered Medical Home [PCMH], Model of Priority Care in MTFs.* The policy is an established model of primary care associated with better outcomes, reduced mortality, fewer hospitalizations for patients with chronic diseases, lower utilization, improved patient compliance with recommended care, and reduced medical spending.

Health Affairs Policy 01-015, *Policy Memorandum to Refine Policy for Access to Care in Medical Treatment Facilities and Establish the TRICARE Plus Program,* **22 June 2001.** HA Policy 01-015 establishes the TRICARE Plus program, an MTF primary care enrollment program available to beneficiaries not enrolled in TRICARE Prime and limited to available MTF capacity.

Army Policies

The Army Medical Department policies provide specific guidance on how to improve ATC in areas such as schedule and template management, enrollment, and referral management. In the last five years, the Army Medical Department (AMEDD) implemented an Access to Care Campaign to facilitate the transition to the PCMH model with evidence of improved access, continuity of care, and higher levels of staff and patient satisfaction. The Army monitors and reviews access-related metrics in multiple venues from the tactical level of the MTF to Health Affairs requirements. Access metrics are incorporated into the Army Medicine Campaign Plan, Annual Performance Planning Guidance, and Organizational Inspection Program. All commands have access to the TRICARE Operations Center (TOC) as the premier health care information web portal for the MHS, providing decision makers at all levels of the organization with meaningful, easy-to-use, web-based operational reports. The Army continually works with regional medical commands and MTF managed care and clinical operations to improve access principles and processes that impact Title 10 health care entitlements and the TRICARE Prime health plan.

The Office of the Surgeon General (OTSG)/ Medical Command (MEDCOM) Policy 12-006, *MEDCOM MTF Enrollment, Access and Appointment Standards for all Uniformed Service Members, with Special Emphasis on Enhanced Access to Care for Specified Populations,*[1] **13 January 2012.** This policy implements many of the requirements outlined in HA Policy 11-005 and the *MHS Guide to Access Success*.

OTSG/MEDCOM Policy 11-089, *Improving MTF Practices for Provider Template and Schedule Management,* **25 October 2011** is designed to increase command and control, efficiency, and effectiveness by minimizing redundancies while also increasing access, including additional requirements for TOL and AudioCare.

OTSG/MEDCOM Policy 12-085, 18 January 2011, 21 December 2012 enhances access to care and primary care continuity through standardized appointing services.

OTSG/MEDCOM Policy 13-061, *MEDCOM MTF Referral Management Office - Overarching Core Business*. **1 November 2013.** This policy formalizes MEDCOM-wide objectives, business design plans, and MHS tools for Referral Management Operations.

---

[1] "Specified Populations" include Wounded Warriors, Special Operating Forces, and Deploying and Re-Deploying Forces.

OTSG/MEDCOM Policy 13-065, *AMEDD Enrollment Policy,* **17 December 2013** formalizes MEDCOM-wide objectives, business designs, and tools for consistent, maximum enrollment of TRICARE Prime/Plus beneficiaries within MEDCOM.

OTSG/MEDCOM Policy 14-007, *No-Show Policy,* **7 February 2014** formalizes MEDCOM-wide objectives, business designs, and tools for MTF no-show management to improve patient access to care by limiting the number of missed appointments. Limiting no-shows improves access compliance, provider schedule management, and beneficiary expectations.

Operations Order 09-36, *Access to Care Campaign,* **30 March 2009,** and subsequent fragmentary orders were launched to refocus MTF commanders on their mission-essential task of providing timely access to care. Eleven key focus areas included patient appointing and access, TOL, schedule and template management, referral management, patient satisfaction measures that provide more specific access compliance targets, and reporting requirements beyond previously issued policy guidance.

Operations Order 11-05, *Community Based Primary Care Clinics* [CBPCCs], **4 November 2010** initiated the opening of CBPCCs in off-post leased facilities closer to where our Army families live in order to improve access to quality health care. Operations Order 11-05 was subsequently renamed, *Community-Based Medical Home*.

Operations Order 11-20, *Army Patient Centered Medical Home,* **25 January 2011,** and subsequent fragmentary orders standardize health care delivery by transitioning 100 percent of direct-care enrollees to the PCMH model not later than FY 2015 in order to improve access to care, outcomes, wellness, prevention, and satisfaction while ensuring a uniform patient care experience for all beneficiaries.

Operations Order 12-50, *Soldier-Centered Medical Home* [SCMH] **4 February 2013,** and subsequent fragmentary orders implement the SCMH model at installations across the Army beginning not later than 01 March 2013 and to be completed not later than 1 October 2014 in order to improve medical readiness and ensure consistently superior health care.

Army PCMH Operations Manual Leaders Guide to Army Patient Centered Medical Home Transformation, **19 January 2013** describes the methods and processes for operating an Army PCMH, defines the essential tasks and standards, and details metrics at the PCMH, MTF, regional, and Army Medical Command levels. This operations manual fully supports execution of previously issued policy and operations orders and fragmentary orders.

Navy Policies

Navy's access policies are heavily focused on the PCMH model of care and the patient experience. The policies require MTF leadership to build and sustain a culture of patient-centric care within the MTF that is continuously improved upon. To ensure compliance with the access standards, Navy policy requires the frequent monitoring of access to care through measures/metrics. These are reviewed by MTF and regional and higher-level headquarters' leadership to identify problems or deficiencies that can then be addressed quickly with operational and process changes. Navy access policy references both the *MHS Guide to Access Success* and PCMH policy as the primary drivers of access management at the Navy MTF. Both external and internal inspection agencies validate the MTFs' ability to meet access standards and adherence to policies, with onsite inspections and face-to-face patient interviews and MTF metrics briefs.

BUMEDINST 6300, *Primary Care Services in Navy Medicine,* **5 April 2010** is the primary policy for Navy medicine with regard to access to care. This policy was created to implement a new delivery model of patient- and family-centered care from an individual patient and individual provider to a team-based model for primary care services. This new design would be comprehensive to fully meet primary care health and wellness needs of patients. The primary goal is the health and wellness of Sailors, Marines, and their families, as well as acute care needs when they become ill. By providing comprehensive support in primary care, they operationalize force health protection. By utilizing the team approach, they mitigate challenges such as operational tempo, staffing shortfalls, and personnel turnover. They also increase access to care, standardize primary care services, and improve the partnership between the patient, provider(s), and the primary care team. Ultimately, this will align with civilian models of PCMH. In Navy Medicine, this is referred to as "Medical Home Port." This instruction outlines the transition from current practices to implementation of the new model, defines terms and standards of the primary care team, clarifies roles and responsibilities, applies appointment standards, outlines facility standards, sets forth business rules in which to operate, documents information management/information technology guidance, standardizes metrics for performance, and approves BUMED provider administrative discounts.

NAVMED Policy 09-004, *Access to Care Management Policy for Navy Medicine Military Treatment Facilities,* **(12 March 2009)** is the secondary policy that identifies how Navy Medicine executes the access standards. The policy provides a framework for MTFs to implement and sustain a systematic Access plan to ensure that the access standards as specified in 32 CRF 199.17 are carried out. The policy refers the user back to the *MHS Guide to Access Success* of 2008 as a reference in standardizing roles, responsibilities, definitions, and guidance for implementing, sustaining, and managing access to care across Navy medicine. Primary care guidance within this policy is now superseded by later instruction related to the PCMH and the establishment of the Medical Home Port Program within Navy Medicine, BUMEDINST 6300.19.

Air Force Policies

Relevant Air Force policies focus on the timely access to appropriate care and patient safety. The goal is to build and sustain a culture of continuous process improvement within the MTF, with frequently monitoring to identify issues and resolve them quickly. Policy implementation requires a robust training for both new and existing staff. In addition, as with the other Services, external and internal inspection agencies conduct onsite inspections and patient interviews to validate the MTFs' ability to meet access standards.

Air Force Instruction (AFI) 44-176, *Access to Care Continuum*, **12 September 2011,** is the leading Air Force ATC policy, and the culmination of several previously published access policy memoranda from 28 March 2001, *Improving Appointing and Access Business Practices*, through 22 Feb 11, *AFMS Access to Care Functions Guidance*. AFI Policy 44-176 defines the roles and responsibilities of headquarters, MTF commanders, and MTF staff in ensuring that 32 CFR, Section 199.17 ATC standards and the DHA ATC policy 11-005, *TRICARE Policy for Access to Care* are met. The AFI also incorporates the guidance from the Military Health System's *Guide to Access Success,* (December 2008). AFI directives and recommended guidance documents the following topics: appointing and schedule execution and management; enrollment empanelment levels; telephony metrics; maximizing use of TOL and AudioCare Appointment Reminder applications; specialty care and mental health access; nurse-run clinics; open/enhanced access strategies; appointing agent and group practice manager training; referral management; reserve component access to care; non-enrolled patient access to care; and actions when demand exceeds available appointments. The AFI requires MTFs to have processes in place to perform ongoing reviews of booked and unused appointments and effectiveness of the MTF's ATC program. Specific access, referral management, and telephony metrics are measured and reported to MTF leadership and higher headquarters. The AFI references and is consistent with AFI 44-171, PCMH, Family Health Operations, and other relevant Air Force policies. The Air Force Inspection Agency's inspection criteria include elements to ensure compliance with AFI 44-176.

Air Force Instruction (AFI) 44-171, *Patient Centered Medical Home and Family Health Operations*, **18 January 2011** defines and implements standards for Air Force Family Health Clinic business practices and supports to meet the PCMH goals of optimal patient-centered care for enrolled patients using evidence-based clinical practice grounded in established population health principles, patient and staff satisfaction, and continuous process improvement. AFI Policy 44-171 is consistent and aligns with DHA policy 09-015, *Policy Memorandum Implementation of the Patient-Centered Medical Home Model of Primary Care in MTFs*. The AFI consolidates published policy memoranda on optimizing primary care and PCMH from 2004 to 2010. AFI Policy 44-171 defines specific roles and responsibilities of policy execution/accountability from AF/SG, intermediary commands, through the individual PCMH team members. The AFI outlines directives and recommended guidance on clinical, business, and deployment operations and identifies the following measures to be reported monthly: continuity of care with PCM; technician availability; available appointments/week; HEDIS measures; RVU productivity; patient satisfaction; use of purchased care emergency room/urgent primary care clinics; and the case mix index. The AFI recommends that the measures be reviewed with the clinic staff on a monthly basis and states that the AF Inspection Agency will inspect MTF compliance with policy criteria.

AFMS Referral Management Guide (1 May 2014). To increase patient satisfaction, meet specialty care access standards, and assist providers with obtaining specialty care referral results, the Air Force Medical Service (AFMS) published the first *AFMS Referral Management Guide* in 2003, establishing a Referral Management Center (RMC) at each MTF and standardized referral operations across the enterprise. To continuously improve the referral process, the business rules are reviewed and updated approximately every two years by multi-disciplinary stakeholders. The guide is an inclusive reference for 32 C.F.R. § 199.17, MHS, and AFMS policies, TRICARE contractor roles and responsibilities in the referral process, and civilian accreditation requirements for care coordination and referral management. The guide includes standardized business rules, outlining the referral process from the time the referral is written to the time the referring provider is notified of the referral results scanned into the electronic health record. The RMC is charged with educating the patient about the referral process, booking the patient's MTF specialty care appointment before leaving the MTF, providing the referring provider/PCM with the initial and follow-up referral results, thus alleviating the provider and clinical team from the administrative burden of referral tracking, and facilitating recapture of MTF direct care capabilities in support of readiness, currency, and decreasing purchased care costs. The referral management business rules were added to the 2014 revision of AFI 44-176, *The Access to Care Continuum*, currently in formal coordination.

Defense Health Agency, National Capital Region Medical Directorate (NCR MD) Policies

The Joint Task Force for the National Capital Region (JTF CAPMED) was a transitional organization put in place to oversee the consolidation of the medical assets of the area. Policy for the operation of the NCR MD facilities was established as JTF CAPMED Policy. In 2013, JTF CAPMED was disestablished and replaced by the NCR MD as a directorate of the DHA. JTF CAPMED policies remain in effect until NCR MD generates newer policies. JTF CAPMED INST 6015.01 links directly to the 32 C.F.R. § 199.17 and establishes the referral management process, delineates responsibility for template management, and a number of other operational aspects of access to care. In addition, it utilizes the 2008 *MHS Guide to Access Success* as a core reference for best practices regarding access to care. NCR MD is currently revising this instruction under TASKORD 140612 01 NCR MD.

JTF CAPMED 6015.1, Appointing, Template, Demand and Referral Management, 03 January 2013. This policy establishes the Integrated Referral Management Appointing Center (IRMAC) as the authority to optimize appointing and Referral Management services for TRICARE beneficiaries in the NCR MD. It provides consolidated guidance to meet access standards, as well as instructions to maximize access through defined referral management processes, and the efficient use of patient appointing and template management at MTFs within the NCR MD. The instruction also delineates responsibilities for execution of the integrated referral and appointment management procedures at the JTF CAPMED Commander, IRMAC Director and Template Coordinator, Joint MTF Commander, and Center Directors levels respectively.

NCR MD Standard Operating Procedure For Appointing, Template, Demand, and Referral Management (Draft) establishes standard operating procedures within the Enhanced Multi Service Market, NCR.

Purchased Care Policies

This section outlines the policies for the purchased care component within the 50 United States and District of Columbia (US) and outside the United States (Overseas) (also called the TRICARE Overseas Program (TOP)).

TRICARE Policy Manual. The policy manual is written and maintained by the DHA. The manual provides a description of program benefits, adjudication guidance, policy interpretations, and decisions implementing the TRICARE Program.

TRICARE Operations Manual (TOM) Chapter 5, Section 1. Paragraphs 1.0 – 2.0. The TOM is written and maintained by the DHA. Chapter 5 directs the contractor to establish provider networks based on specific requirements and standards included in the chapter. Paragraph 2.2 notes that the access standards specified in reference 32 C.F.R. § 199.17 shall apply in each network area and that the contractor is responsible for developing and implementing a system for continuously monitoring and evaluating network adequacy.

TOM Chapter 6. This chapter of the TOM provides the contractor with specific instructions concerning enrollment of eligible beneficiaries in the TRICARE Prime program. Paragraph 9.0 details the access standards and provides guidance as to how travel times are to be calculated. Contractual access requirements for the Provider Network include the following:

- The Contractor shall ensure that the standards for access, in terms of beneficiary travel time, appointment wait time, and office wait time for various categories of services are met for beneficiaries residing in TRICARE Prime Service Areas (PSAs). These standards shall be met in a manner that achieves beneficiary satisfaction with access to network providers and services as set forth in the contract. The Contractor shall define metrics, and collect data about them, that give insight to the degree to which the access standards are being met.

- TOM 6010.56M, February 1, 2008, Chapter 5, Section 1, Paragraph 2.2: Each PSA is considered to be a separate service area to which access standards apply. The contractor shall develop and implement a system for continuously monitoring and evaluating network adequacy.

    The contractor shall establish provider networks for the delivery of Prime and Extra services to ensure that all access standards are met at the start of health care delivery and continuously maintained in all PSAs in the Region.

    The contractor shall adjust provider networks and services as necessary to compensate for changes in MTF capabilities and capacities, when and where they occur over the life of the contract, including those resulting from short-notice unanticipated facility expansion, MTF provider deployment, downsizing and/or closures. Changes in MTF capabilities and capacities may occur frequently over the life of the contract without prior notice. The Contractor shall ensure that all eligible beneficiaries who live in PSAs have the opportunity to enroll, add additional family members, or remain enrolled in the Prime program regardless of such changes. The Contractor shall ensure that MTF enrollees residing outside PSAs have the opportunity to add additional family members or remain enrolled in the Prime program regardless of such changes.

Each TRICARE Regional Contractors is required to have a credentialed provider network. The West is accredited by the National Credentialing Quality Association; the North and South networks are accredited by URAC (formerly known as the Utilization Review Accreditation Commission). To receive this status, the TRICARE Regional Contractors must demonstrate access to the full range of providers and services, provider credentialing, and quality oversight as prescribed by these organizations. If certain government requirements are more stringent, the contractor is required to abide by the more stringent requirements.

The TRICARE Regional Contractors provide each TRO with region-specific Network Adequacy Reports monthly, comparing total unique providers contracted to the projected number of contracts required. When the report shows areas where there may be a shortage of contracted physicians, the TRICARE Regional Contractors examines network performance in the area to identify the precise effect of the shortage and work to identify and recruit additional providers as necessary.

The TRICARE Regional Contractors also submit monthly Network Inadequacy Reports, defined in the contract as any occurrence of a TRICARE Prime beneficiary being referred to a network provider outside of the time and/or distance standards (except when the beneficiary waives the access standard), or any beneficiary being referred to a non-network provider. The TRICARE Regional Contractors report "significant" network inadequacies to the Contracting Officer and/or designee within 48 hours of identification of the significant network inadequacy.

The TROs work with the TRICARE Regional Contractors to monitor and improve access to care through their Performance Management Review (PMR) meetings. They routinely monitor the 96 percent referrals to network, drive time, referrals to non-network providers, and satisfaction data for access to care. In the PMR, the TROs and TRICARE Regional Contractors routinely review appointment wait times, referral volume, and referral utilization, and take action as needed.

TRICARE policy requires beneficiaries to obtain a referral for urgent care clinic visits when their primary care manager (PCM) is unavailable.

Appendix 3.4
Summary of External Reviews Related to Access to Care

External Reviews

A 10-year retrospective review of DoD Inspector General (IG) and Government Accountability Office (GAO) reports identified 34 reports with potential relevance to access to care. Seven GAO reports issued between 2007 and 2014 were determined to be relevant, and all but one focused on access to purchased care primary care. None of the reports addressed the access standards required by 32CFR 199.17, and only one included recommendations for executive action.

The reports focused primarily on access to civilian providers for non-enrolled TRICARE Standard and Extra beneficiaries, a population for whom access standards are not defined by federal law. Each report is described below, with slightly more detail on the only one (GAO 14-384) that included recommendations.

GAO-07-941R TRICARE: Changes to Access Policies and Payment Rates for Services Provided by Civilian Obstetricians.

FINDINGS: Our finding that more than three-fourths of Prime Service Areas (PSAs) met their physician supply targets for all reported periods is an indicator that access was not likely a problem for most TRICARE beneficiaries seeking obstetric care. However, we could not be conclusive about access from the contractors' data alone because of other factors that can influence access. (No recommendations.)

GAO-13-205 DoD HEALTH CARE: Domestic Health Care for Female Service Members.

FINDINGS: This report describes 1) the extent that DoD's policies for assessing individual medical readiness including unique health care issues of female service members; 2) the availability of health care services to meet the unique needs of female service members at domestic Army installations; and 3) the extent to which DoD's research organizations have identified a need for research on the specific health care needs of female service members who have served in combat. (No recommendations.)

GAO-14-384 DEFENSE HEALTH CARE: More-Specific Guidance Needed for Assessing Non-enrolled TRICARE Beneficiaries' Access to Care.

FINDING: GAO found that the TROs' efforts to implement the action memo's recommendations have resulted in limited and inconsistent methods for identifying and addressing areas with potential access problems, which in some instances have included the use of judgment in place of clear criteria for making these determinations.

RECOMMENDATION: Secretary of Defense requires the Director of DHA to enhance existing guidance for the TROs to include more specificity on assessing non-enrolled beneficiaries' access to care. Specifically, the guidance should contain criteria for analyzing and interpreting the non-enrolled beneficiary and civilian provider surveys' results and the beneficiary population sizing model to facilitate a more rigorous and consistent approach across regions for identifying locations with potential access problems and determining whether actions should be taken.

GAO-13-364 TRICARE Multilayer Surveys Indicate Problems with Access to Care for Non-enrolled Beneficiaries.

FINDINGS: Overall, during 2008-2011, an estimated one in three non-enrolled beneficiaries experienced problems finding any type of civilian provider—primary, specialty, or mental health care provider—who would accept TRICARE. Non-enrolled beneficiaries' satisfaction did not differ across types of areas, but was generally lower than that of Medicare fee-for-service beneficiaries. Civilian providers' acceptance of new TRICARE patients has decreased over time; mental health providers report lower awareness and acceptance than other provider types. Collective results of TMA's beneficiary and civilian provider surveys indicate specific geographic areas where non-enrolled beneficiaries have experienced access problems.

GAO-11-500 DEFENSE HEALTH Access to Civilian Providers under TRICARE Standard and Extra.

FINDINGS: Reimbursement rates have been cited as the primary impediment that hinders beneficiaries' access to civilian health care and mental health care providers under TRICARE Standard and Extra. Another main impediment to TRICARE beneficiaries' access to civilian providers is a shortage of certain provider specialties, both at the national and local levels. However, TMA is limited in its ability to address provider shortages because this impediment affects the entire health care delivery system and is not specific to the TRICARE program. Access to mental health care is a concern for all TRICARE beneficiaries, and it has been affected by provider shortages and other issues, including providers' lack of knowledge about combat-related issues, providers' concerns about reimbursement rates, and providers' lack of awareness about TRICARE. TMA and its contractors have used various feedback mechanisms, such as surveys, to gauge beneficiaries' access to care under TRICARE Standard and Extra. More recently, TMA officials have taken steps to develop a model to help identify geographic areas where beneficiaries that use TRICARE Standard and Extra may experience access problems. However, because this initiative is still evolving, it is too early to determine its effectiveness.

GAO-10-402 DEFENSE HEALTH CARE 2008 Access to Care Surveys Indicate Some Problems, but Beneficiary Satisfaction Is Similar to Other Health Plans.

FINDINGS: DoD's implementation of beneficiary and provider surveys for 2008 followed the Office of Management and Budget survey standards and generally addressed the survey requirements outlined in the NDAA. In general beneficiaries rated their satisfaction similarly to users of other health plans. Survey results from 2008 indicate that a higher percentage of non-enrolled beneficiaries in PSAs experienced problems accessing care from primary care physicians or nurses than those in non-PSAs. Non-enrolled beneficiaries in PSAs and non-PSAs surveyed in 2008 rated satisfaction with their health care similarly to each other and to beneficiaries of commercial health care plans. These provider survey results are not representative of all providers in surveyed areas but provide limited information that indicates differences among providers' awareness and acceptance of TRICARE.

GAO-07-48 Access to Care for Beneficiaries who have not enrolled in TRICARE's Managed Care Option.

FINDING: TMA's surveys to network and non-network civilian providers on their willingness to accept non-enrolled TRICARE patients and beneficiary satisfaction with access to care met the NDAA directive. GAO stated that DoD did not designate a senior official to have oversight responsibility as required in the NDAA. TMA disagreed with meeting the directive to designate a senior official to oversee non-enrolled TRICARE beneficiaries' access to care.

Appendix 3.5
Access to Care Education Courses

Access improvement seminars provide training to managers on the most up-to-date information on access policy, access data analysis, PCMH operations, secure messaging, performance measurements, demand management, population/empanelment management, appointing and schedule management, appointing information systems and telephony management, customer service management, referral management, and general process improvement techniques. The courses include:

CHCS Managed Care Program Course: Appointment Booking Fundamentals (2 hours). This course trains all CHCS users who book appointments on the booking process for primary care clinics and referrals in specialty clinics. Emphasis is given to the proper use of access to care standards linked to appropriate appointment types.

CHCS Patient Appointing Services (PAS): Schedule Creation and Maintenance (2 hours). This VC course trains lead clerks and super-users to create provider schedules for later use in patient appointment booking. Students learn on how to create, open, replicate, and print provider schedules. The course also focuses on steps used to maintain/modify provider schedules. Students learn how to change providers in a schedule, freeze and release schedules, add appointments to the wait list, cancel appointments by facility, and modify, add, and delete appointments in a schedule.

CHCS PAS: Template Creation (2 hours). This VC course trains designated PAS users to create, replicate, print, and delete daily and weekly provider templates for later use in developing clinic schedules.

CHCS PAS/Monthly Capitation Payment: Front Desk Functions (2 hours). This course instructs front desk clerks to complete specified clinic functions through both AHLTA and legacy CHCS. Students learn to process unscheduled visits (walk-in, sick-call, and telephone consultations), and how to check-in individual and multiple patients, cancel and display patient appointments, and perform end-of-day (EOD) processing.

CHCS PAS/MCP: Advanced Front Desk Functions (1.5 hours). This VC course ensures that PAS/MCP clerks, clerk supervisors, and super users are able to effectively join/split appointment slots, log non-MTF appointments, cancel/reschedule appointments, enter an appointment refusal, and locate, and print PAS/MCP reports.

CHCS PAS/MCP: Consult Tracking Process (1.5 hours). This course follows the flow of consult tracking when using both AHLTA and CHCS, and includes ordering, reviewing and booking a consult, patient check-in, resulting and closing a consult. Students learn how to view consults in progress in both AHLTA and CHCS, and review T-cons as entered from AHLTA. This course is intended for multiple types of users consults: providers who enter consult orders in AHLTA, referral management department staff who use CHCS) to review and book consult orders, medical personnel who check in consult order appointments in AHLTA, and specialty providers who enter the patient encounter results in AHLTA.

CHCS PAS/MCP: Notify Patients Menu (1 hour). This course addresses three clinic lists that are associated with changes/issues regarding a patient's clinic appointment: cancellation list, no-show list, and the wait list. Site personnel who notify patients of changes/issues related to their clinic appointments learn to notify patients by telephone or mailer when an appointment is cancelled (by facility, division, or clinic), rescheduled, or when an appointment was not kept. Notification of the patient prior to booking an appointment from the clinic's wait list is also covered.

Army Basic Healthcare Administration Course (Phase 1&2) (60 hours). This course prepares clinic management professionals on the basic concepts, principles, and applications of health administration in MTFs. Training includes information on PCMH, data quality management control, CHCS, Armed Forces Health Longitudinal Technology Application (AHLTA), Medical Expense and Performance Reporting System, Defense Medical Human Resources System internet, Performance-Based Adjustment Mode, Army Provider-Level Satisfaction Survey, leadership, teamwork, change management, customer service, health care continuing education, and strategic and performance (business) planning. Implemented in March 2011, 4 instructors trained 1,359 individuals (U.S. Army Medical Department (AMEDD) active Army officers, non-commissioned officers, and Department of the Army civilians) between FY 2011 and FY 2013. Trainees' job roles included: Health System Administrator, Health System Specialist, Medical Records Administrator, Medical Records Technician, Medical Support Assistant, Miscellaneous Administration and Program (Medical), and Miscellaneous Clerk and Assistant (Medical).

Navy Clinic Management Course (32 hours). This 4-day course targets primary and specialty clinic teams to advance their expertise in the skills, knowledge, and tools necessary to successfully integrate the MHS and the Navy's Bureau of Medicine and Surgery' strategic goals into their daily practices as an accountable care organization in a variety of health care settings. Teams of 3-4 members are nominated to represent clinic teams for each class. Parent commands identify the clinics of focus for improvement efforts and identify members of that clinic team to attend the course. Updated in 2010, 3 traveling staff trained 823 individuals (O, E, GS, and contract) between FY 2011 and FY 2013.

Air Force Medical Service (AFMS) Appointing Information Systems Hands-on Training Course (23.4 hours). The course provides students with the detailed know-how on various appointing functions, operations, and management utilizing the Composite Health Care Systems (CHCS). Comprehensive training is provided combining MHS/AFMS policy and correct CHCS templates, schedules, and file and table building. Taught over a 4-day period, the course provides hands-on training, lectures, and practical exercises arming students with knowledge to make improvements in MTF appointing operations and to improve access at their MTF. Instruction on data analysis and report review teaches the most efficient approaches to finding, extracting, printing, and analyzing provider schedules/patient appointment data within CHCS, AFMS, and MHS data. Implemented in 2006, the course's three instructors trained 141 individuals (officer (O), enlisted (E), general schedule (GS), and contract) between FY 2011 and FY 2013.

AFMS Access Improvement Seminar (18.4 hours). This course provides access managers with instruction on the most up-to-date information in the areas of access policy, access data analysis, PCMH operations, secure messaging, access performance measurements, demand management, population/empanelment management, appointing and schedule management, appointing information systems and telephony management, customer service management, referral management, and general process improvement techniques. Implemented in 2003, the course's 12 instructors trained 795 individuals (O, E, GS, and contract) between FY 2011 and FY 2013. Trainees had the following job roles: group practice managers (GPM), assistant GPMs, selected enlisted, chief of the medical staff, medical operations and support squadron commanders, clinic nurses, PCMH physicians/providers, template managers, appointment center supervisors, family health/primary care element leaders & non-commissioned officers in charge, and any other clinic staff involved in appointing management.

AFMS Group Practice Management Course (40 hours). This course provides training for those personnel being assigned to group practice manager (GPM) positions. Emphasis is placed on the skills required to prepare the health services administrator to effectively manage and support the assigned clinics to ensure that beneficiaries receive access to medical care within standards. The curriculum consists of practice management concepts, including and responsibilities, population health overview, data management, templating/scheduling skills in MHS appointing information systems, and training for electronic hands-on web-based tools. Implemented in 2011, 1 instructor trained 161 individuals (O, E, and GS) between FY 2011 and FY 2013. Trainees' job roles included: officers and GS-equivalents currently assigned or pending assignment to a GPM position, enlisted members filling the role of GPM, assistant, office manager, or similar role requiring knowledge of GPM practices.

Appendix 3.6
Access to Care Standards

A review of the access to care literature revealed no national benchmarks or scientific evidence to support appointment scheduling standards for three general appointment types: urgent (acute) care, routine care, and specialty care referrals, although some private providers have established standards based on patient perception of reasonable access.[2] Table 3.6-1 compares MHS with 16 health care providers in terms of acute, routine, and specialty care standards.

Table 3.6-1 Comparison of MHS Access Standards with those of Other Health Care Providers

PLAN	Urgent/ Acute Care (Within X Hours)	Routine Care (Within X Days)	Specialty Care Referrals (Within X Days)
MHS (Military Health System)	24	7 calendar	28 calendar
Aetna Plans	24	7 (assume calendar)	(open access)
Anthem Blue Cross (CA)	24	10 business (12 calendar)	15 business (21 calendar)
Blue Cross-Blue Shield (MI)	48	4 calendar	n/a
Blue Cross-Blue Shield (NC)	24	3 calendar	14 calendar
Boston HealthNet Plan (MA)	48	10 (assume calendar)	30 (assume calendar)
Care1st Health Plan (CA)	48	10 business (12 calendar)	15 calendar
Community Health Plan (WA)	24	7 calendar	n/a
Coventry Health Care (WV)	48	3 calendar	n/a
Dept. of Managed Care (CA)	48	10 business (14 calendar)	15 business (21 calendar)
Emblem Health (NY)	24	28 (assume calendar)	28 calendar
Humana ChoiceCare PPO	24	7-14 calendar	21 business (26 calendar)
Independence Blue Cross (PA)	24	14 (assume calendar)	28 calendar
Managed Health Services (WI)	24	7 calendar	60 calendar
MVP Health Care (NY)	24	3 calendar	28 – 42 calendar
Preferred IPA (CA)	24	7 calendar	14 calendar
UnitedHealthcare	24	14 (assume calendar)	n/a

2014 MHS Review Group
Source: Multiple Sources

---

[2] Health plan members' experiences: percentage of adult health plan members who reported how often it was easy to get needed care. 2013 September. National Quality Measures Clearinghouse: 009073 National Committee for Quality Assurance - Health Care Accreditation Organization. Available at: http://www.qualitymeasures.ahrq.gov/browse/by-topic-detail.aspx?id=40307&ct=3&term=access.

Appendix 3.7 MTF-Level Access Data

Table 3.7-1 All Measure Results, by Facility

DMIS ID	Facility Name	Service	Facility Type	MTFs	Enrolled	% Meeting Standard		Time to Appointment		Days to Third Next Appointment			TOL	Getting Needed Care		Satisfaction	HCSDB	
						A	S	A	S	PriCare		S	% TOL enrolled	Svc	TROSS	ATC (mos)	Get Care Quickly	Get Needed Care
										A	P							
0001	FOX ARMY HEALTH CENTER	Army	Clinic	1	11,561	98%	93%	0.36	11.35	1.0	4.6	18.6	82%	82%	76%	65%	75.9	87.6
0003	LYSTER AHC	Army	Clinic	1	17,469	98%	93%	0.24	12.90	0.7	5.0	10.4	88%	90%	76%	64%	80.1	83.8
0004	42ND MEDICAL GROUP	Air Force	Clinic	1	15,832	97%	97%	0.47	9.86	3.1	6.1	9.1	66%	94%	58%	54%	74.7	74.7
0005	BASSETT ACH	Army	Hospital	5	24,439	96%	95%	0.39	11.48	2.0	5.4	11.5	62%	84%	68%	56%	n/a	n/a
0006	673rd MEDICAL GROUP	Air Force	Hospital	2	36,887	92%	92%	0.62	13.43	1.3	6.8	13.4	66%	97%	74%	58%	75.1	75.2
0008	R W BLISS ARMY HEALTH CENTER	Army	Clinic	1	12,503	94%	97%	0.91	9.26	2.9	7.6	9.8	83%	83%	81%	61%	75.6	74.2

Appendix 3. Access to Care

August 29, 2014

	Facility Information					% Meeting Standard		Time to Appointment — Days to Appointment		Days to Third Next Appointment — PriCare		TOL	Getting needed care		Satisfaction — ATC (mean)	HCSDB	
DMIS ID	Facility Name	Service	Facility Type	MTFs	Enrolled	A¹	S²	A¹	S²	A¹	S²	% TOL enabled	Svc	TROSS		Get Care Quickly	Get Needed Care
0009	56th MEDICAL GROUP	Air Force	Clinic	1	26,650	98%	96%	0.25	12.38	0.9	5.0	14.1	76%	98%	82%	66%	73.9	84.4
0010	355th MEDICAL GROUP	Air Force	Clinic	1	21,244	87%	95%	0.79	12.12	2.9	9.1	10.8	76%	96%	81%	58%	84.1	80.6
0013	19th MEDICAL GROUP-LITTLE ROCK	Air Force	Clinic	1	14,168	97%	96%	0.39	10.64	1.2	5.8	15.7	82%	96%	62%	51%	67.1	76.6
0014	60th MEDICAL GROUP	Air Force	Medical Center	3	38,832	89%	94%	1.08	12.76	5.6	9.6	14.5	64%	95%	67%	54%	64.5	76.9
0015	9th MEDICAL GROUP	Air Force	Clinic	1	9,918	95%	99%	0.42	7.90	1.9	5.0	10.5	65%	94%	64%	45%	n/a	n/a
0018	30th MEDICAL GROUP	Air Force	Clinic	1	7,796	95%	97%	0.49	9.37	1.4	5.3	14.6	68%	96%	75%	62%	75	78.6
0019	412th MEDICAL GROUP	Air Force	Clinic	1	7,193	97%	98%	0.34	8.47	1.3	4.2	11.4	77%	95%	79%	64%	63.7	78.9

Military Health System Review – Final Report
August 29, 2014

DMIS ID	Facility Name	Facility Information			Enrolled	Time to Appointment							TOL	Getting needed care		Satisfaction	HCSDB	
		Service	Facility Type	MTFs		% Meeting Standard		Days to Appointment		Days to Next Appointment		Days to Third		% TOL enrolled	Svc	TROSS	ATC (TROSS)	Get Care Quickly	Get Needed Care
						A	S	A	S	A	S	A	S						
0024	NH CAMP PENDLETON	Navy	Hospital	12	57,873	94%	96%	0.72	12.36	0.8	4.4		10.8	56%	93%	65%	58%	74.8	79.6
0028	NH LEMOORE	Navy	Hospital	2	13,782	93%	97%	0.66	12.50	0.9	2.9		10.9	51%	96%	68%	64%	83.1	n/a
0029	NMC SAN DIEGO	Navy	Medical Center	12	95,047	93%	91%	0.79	13.16	1.2	6.4		15.5	28%	94%	71%	55%	76	84.3
0030	NH TWENTYNINE PALMS	Navy	Hospital	3	13,864	98%	96%	0.32	12.04	1.0	3.1		8.7	31%	96%	72%	65%	n/a	84.9
0032	EVANS ACH	Army	Hospital	14	70,934	97%	96%	0.28	11.72	1.5	3.7		12.8	55%	80%	70%	62%	78.4	80.8
0033	10TH MEDICAL GROUP	Air Force	Clinic	1	28,556	96%	96%	0.47	13.34	1.3	4.1		11.1	65%	99%	78%	65%	70.1	85.9
0036	436th MEDICAL GROUP	Air Force	Clinic	1	11,597	97%	95%	0.42	13.38	1.5	7.1		12.8	81%	95%	66%	56%	n/a	n/a
0038	NH PENSACOLA	Navy	Hospital	11	52,304	96%	96%	0.49	9.36	0.7	3.2		9.0	69%	96%	80%	70%	78.3	86.3

Appendix 3. Access to Care

	Facility Information					Time to Appointment						TOL	Satisfaction			HCSDB	
						% Meeting Standard		Days to Appointment		Days to Third Next Appointment			Getting needed care				
DMIS ID	Facility Name	Service	Facility Type	MTFs	enrolled	A†	S‡	A†	S‡	PreCare		% TOL enrolled	Svc	TROSS	ATC (TROSS)	Get Care Quickly	Get Needed Care
										A†	R†	S‡					
0039	NH JACKSONVILLE	Navy	Hospital	6	59,539	94%	96%	0.81	10.09	0.9	3.9	11.9	68%	93%	69%	60%	80.2	76.9
0042	96th MEDICAL GROUP	Air Force	Hospital	2	36,861	93%	92%	0.67	14.14	1.7	9.1	14.6	75%	95%	69%	58%	59.1	70.3
0043	325th MEDICAL GROUP	Air Force	Clinic	1	13,200	99%	87%	0.30	16.90	1.0	9.7	11.4	74%	93%	78%	66%	72.9	78.4
0045	6th MEDICAL GROUP	Air Force	Clinic	2	38,007	95%	93%	0.55	13.63	2.7	5.3	12.8	66%	98%	75%	66%	72.2	79.9
0046	45th MEDICAL GROUP	Air Force	Clinic	1	14,592	95%	96%	0.44	9.67	1.4	11.9	10.5	82%	96%	78%	72%	79.3	74.1
0047	EISENHOWER AMC	Army	Medical Center	6	44,883	98%	95%	0.32	10.41	0.8	3.3	10.9	73%	83%	72%	62%	82.6	75.9
0048	MARTIN ACH	Army	Hospital	11	53,856	92%	95%	0.79	9.79	1.4	7.5	7.4	72%	81%	66%	54%	n/a	n/a
0049	WINN ACH	Army	Hospital	5	60,846	95%	93%	0.68	12.78	1.5	8.0	12.7	64%	78%	61%	59%	n/a	n/a

Military Health System Review – Final Report
August 29, 2014

	Facility Information				Time to Appointment					TOL		Satisfaction		HCSDB	
DMIS ID	Facility Name	Service	Facility Type	MTFs	Enrolled	Meeting Standard		Days to Appointment	Days to Third Next Appointment		% TOL enrolled	Getting needed care		ATC (TRISS)	Get Care Quickly	Get Needed Care
						Ac	Sp	Ac	Sp	PrCare	Sp		Sp	TRISS			
0050	23rd MEDICAL GROUP	Air Force	Clinic	1	10,398	96%	95%	0.28	9.56	1.1	6.5	9.2	91%	98%	72%	56%	n/a	n/a
0051	78th MEDICAL GROUP	Air Force	Clinic	1	15,318	97%	96%	0.31	8.47	2.0	4.6	6.6	53%	95%	76%	71%	75.7	88.2
0052	TRIPLER AMC	Army	Medical Center	4	67,200	92%	94%	0.90	12.28	2.0	4.8	11.8	55%	83%	68%	61%	85.3	82.9
0053	366th MEDICAL GROUP	Air Force	Hospital	1	10,134	97%	97%	0.32	12.19	2.2	6.5	15.3	84%	93%	73%	62%	79.5	88.8
0055	375th MEDICAL GROUP	Air Force	Clinic	2	24,141	97%	96%	0.45	12.92	1.5	5.0	15.6	71%	97%	75%	59%	81.8	80.6
0057	IRWIN ACH	Army	Hospital	8	41,779	82%	96%	2.31	11.06	2.6	5.3	10.5	81%	82%	68%	65%	88.9	77.7
0058	MUNSON ARMY HEALTH CENTER	Army	Clinic	3	16,963	99%	96%	0.21	11.96	0.7	3.0	12.8	82%	91%	81%	72%	81.6	79.9
0059	22nd MEDICAL GROUP	Air Force	Clinic	1	11,622	96%	93%	0.48	10.20	2.1	5.2	11.5	89%	96%	81%	65%	n/a	n/a

195

Appendix 3. Access to Care

		Facility Information				% Meeting Standard		Time to Appointment — Days to Appointment		Time to Appointment — Days to Next Appointment PriCare				TOL	Satisfaction — Getting needed care		Satisfaction — ATC mross	Satisfaction — HCSDB	
DMIS ID	Facility Name	Service	Facility Type	MTFs	Enrolled	A¹	S²	A¹	S²	A¹	S²			% TOL enabled	Svc	TROSS		Get Care Quickly	Get Needed Care
0060	BLANCHFIELD ACH	Army	Hospital	11	72,709	97%	93%	0.31	12.60	1.9	5.3		10.7	43%	82%	68%	59%	57.9	78.4
0061	IRELAND ACH	Army	Hospital	6	31,436	96%	92%	0.37	14.66	0.9	7.4		13.4	72%	81%	71%	62%	76.3	67.3
0062	2nd MEDICAL GROUP	Air Force	Clinic	1	16,899	96%	96%	0.46	11.58	1.6	4.5		14.7	85%	94%	73%	60%	71.9	77.9
0064	BAYNE-JONES ACH	Army	Hospital	6	23,225	98%	97%	0.32	11.49	1.3	5.4		12.3	72%	86%	70%	63%	80.2	73.3
0066	779th MEDICAL GROUP	Air Force	Clinic	3	28,672	93%	87%	0.70	15.25	2.3	6.6		19.9	68%	92%	74%	61%	71.4	72
0067	WALTER REED NATIONAL MILITARY MEDICAL CNTR	NCR	Medical Center	4	40,211	73%	87%	2.53	14.53	3.1	9.7		16.0	44%	88%	69%	61%	67	64.7
0068	NHC PATUXENT RIVER	Navy	Clinic	4	14,898	92%	92%	0.59	11.48	1.0	9.5		11.2	0%	96%	70%	59%	71.3	72.4

Military Health System Review – Final Report
August 29, 2014

	Facility Information					Time to Appointment						TOL	Getting needed care		Satisfaction		HCSDB	
Digits ID	Facility Name	Service	Facility Type	MTFs	Enrolled	% Meeting Standard		Days to Appointment		Days to Next Appointment								
						A	S*	A*	S*	PriCare	A*	S*	% TOL enrolled	Sec TRDSS	Sec TRDSS	ATC (mins)	Get Care Quickly	Get Needed Care
0069	KIMBROUGH AMBULATORY CARE CENTER	Army	Clinic	10	59,676	89%	90%	0.63	13.06	1.9	5.5	15.1	77%	86%	69%	60%	75.7	71.1
0073	81st MEDICAL GROUP	Air Force	Medical Center	1	25,880	95%	93%	0.61	14.58	5.5	7.1	14.8	56%	97%	75%	59%	72.2	79.7
0074	14th MEDICAL GROUP	Air Force	Clinic	1	3,944	91%	99%	1.09	9.38	0.7	6.4	11.1	66%	96%	77%	64%	77.7	87.3
0075	L. WOOD ACH	Army	Hospital	3	23,148	82%	96%	2.20	10.73	1.6	4.4	9.9	66%	85%	69%	60%	74.5	74.6
0076	509th MEDICAL GROUP	Air Force	Clinic	1	12,107	98%	95%	0.22	11.41	1.1	10.8	16.7	76%	92%	74%	58%	66.9	76.6
0077	341st MEDICAL GROUP	Air Force	Clinic	1	9,829	97%	96%	0.54	10.91	2.7	9.6	9.6	84%	97%	66%	63%	67.6	73
0078	55th MEDICAL GROUP	Air Force	Clinic	1	27,115	97%	95%	0.39	11.75	1.7	5.3	11.3	91%	97%	70%	58%	77.1	75.3

Appendix 3. Access to Care

	Facility Information					Time to Appointment							TOL	Getting needed care		Satisfaction	HCSDB	
DMIS ID	Facility Name	Service	Facility Type	MTFs	Enrolled	% Meeting Standard		Days to Appointment		Days to Next Appointment			% TOL enrolled	Svc	TROSS	ATC (TROSS)	Get Care Quickly	Get Needed Care
						A*	S*	A*	S*	PreCare A*	R*	S*						
0079	MIKE O'CALLAGHAN FEDERAL HOSPITAL	Air Force	Medical Center	2	48,894	88%	91%	1.20	14.42	4.5	12.5	15.9	52%	98%	67%	55%	69.7	73.6
0083	377th MEDICAL GROUP	Air Force	Clinic	1	12,342	97%	94%	0.30	12.24	1.2	3.5	7.5	72%	93%	83%	63%	72.1	76.8
0084	49th MEDICAL GROUP	Air Force	Clinic	1	10,168	97%	97%	0.27	10.74	1.6	7.2	4.1	72%	97%	64%	50%	n/a	n/a
0085	27th SPECIAL OPERATIONS MEDICAL GROUP	Air Force	Clinic	1	11,104	94%	91%	0.38	15.24	2.0	9.5	27.2	76%	97%	66%	53%	n/a	n/a
0086	KELLER ACH	Army	Hospital	7	13,033	93%	94%	0.72	12.30	2.0	5.5	12.3	64%	89%	76%	75%	n/a	n/a
0089	WOMACK AMC	Army	Medical Center	13	124,077	94%	93%	0.81	11.68	1.1	4.7	15.4	78%	76%	63%	59%	67.9	72.8
0090	4th MEDICAL GROUP	Air Force	Clinic	1	10,521	97%	94%	0.14	10.02	2.1	4.6	6.3	66%	95%	72%	60%	n/a	n/a

Military Health System Review – Final Report
August 29, 2014

MHS ID	Facility Name	Service	Facility Type	MTFs	Enrolled	Meeting standard		Time to Appointment			Days to 3rd Next Available			TOC		Getting needed care		Satisfaction		HCSDB	
						A*	S*	A*	S*		A*	S*		% TOC enabled	Svc	TRICARE	ATC Access	Get Care Quickly	Get Needed Care
0091	NH CAMP LEJEUNE	Navy	Hospital	8	36,615	91%	93%	0.64	10.67		1.3	7.3	14.4	43%	92%	72%	67%	73	62.5
0092	NHC CHERRY POINT	Navy	Clinic	1	21,669	99%	96%	0.24	9.81		0.8	2.8	8.6	64%	93%	73%	64%	70.9	74
0093	319th MEDICAL GROUP	Air Force	Clinic	1	5,053	93%	96%	0.44	9.12		2.6	6.5	19.3	16%	97%	80%	75%	n/a	n/a
0094	5th MEDICAL GROUP	Air Force	Clinic	1	12,813	92%	96%	0.60	12.23		1.6	6.6	17.0	94%	98%	81%	69%	68.3	89.2
0095	88th MEDICAL GROUP	Air Force	Medical Center	1	37,403	95%	90%	0.55	14.52		3.3	9.7	16.9	86%	97%	76%	65%	76.3	73
0096	72nd MEDICAL GROUP	Air Force	Clinic	1	18,523	85%	96%	1.05	10.86		3.2	11.5	13.4	39%	96%	73%	39%	63.9	75.3
0097	97th MEDICAL GROUP	Air Force	Clinic	1	4,598	88%	89%	0.62	12.00		1.2	4.8	11.2	80%	99%	87%	74%	n/a	n/a
0098	REYNOLDS ACH	Army	Hospital	4	30,414	93%	95%	0.61	11.31		2.3	5.9	11.7	87%	84%	68%	58%	75.5	86.3

Appendix 3. Access to Care

	Facility Information					% Meeting Standard		Time to Appointment — Days to Appointment		Days to Third Next Appointment — PriCare			TOL	Getting needed care		Satisfaction	HCSDB	
DMIS ID	Facility Name	Service	Facility Type	MTFs	Enrolled	A¹	S²	A¹	S²	A¹	R²	S²	% TOL enabled	Svc	TROSS	ATC (mcss)	Get Care Quickly	Get Needed Care
0100	NAVAL HLTH CLINIC NEW ENGLAND	Navy	Clinic	4	26,545	96%	96%	0.38	8.21	0.7	4.9	6.5	45%	95%	73%	61%	84.1	78.1
0101	20th MEDICAL GROUP	Air Force	Clinic	1	13,682	94%	97%	0.50	9.80	2.1	6.2	13.1	69%	91%	76%	63%	71.1	71
0103	NAVAL HEALTH CLINIC CHARLESTON	Navy	Clinic	1	15,669	97%	95%	0.37	9.95	0.9	1.7	13.7	52%	94%	78%	66%	75.1	84.7
0104	NH BEAUFORT	Navy	Hospital	3	10,960	97%	98%	0.44	6.95	1.1	2.8	7.3	42%	96%	85%	72%	69.2	89.2
0105	MONCRIEF ACH	Army	Hospital	4	25,058	92%	96%	0.80	11.19	1.7	4.7	14.5	79%	84%	71%	69%	75	87.2
0106	28th MEDICAL GROUP	Air Force	Clinic	1	10,985	99%	98%	0.18	10.22	0.8	2.5	9.8	76%	95%	83%	76%	n/a	n/a
0108	WILLIAM BEAUMONT AMC	Army	Medical Center	8	73,245	94%	94%	0.65	12.47	4.1	3.4	12.0	74%	82%	67%	65%	61.1	59.8

Military Health System Review – Final Report
August 29, 2014

| DMIS ID | Facility Information | | | | | Time to Appointment | | | | | | TOL | Satisfaction | | | | |
| | Facility Name | Service | Facility Type | MTFs | Enrolled | % Meeting Standard | | Days to Appointment | | PCMs | | | Getting needed care | | ATC (TRISS) | HCSDB | |
						A	S	A	S	A	S	Days to Third Next Appointment	>3 TOL enabled	Svc	TRISS		Get Care Quickly	Get Needed Care
0109	BROOKE AMC-SAN ANTONIO MMC JBSA FSH	Army	Medical Center	6	56,862	96%	92%	0.45	14.08	2.0	7.5	10.8	83%	85%	69%	60%	76.7	88.5
0110	DARNALL AMC	Army	Medical Center	14	100,277	55%	94%	5.83	12.27	4.1	8.7	13.7	87%	77%	61%	60%	55.7	64
0112	7th MEDICAL GROUP	Air Force	Clinic	1	10,419	96%	98%	0.29	7.41	3.2	5.5	9.4	58%	95%	64%	50%	75.1	79.6
0113	82nd MEDICAL GROUP	Air Force	Clinic	1	9,675	92%	96%	1.04	10.06	2.5	4.5	7.6	54%	99%	66%	50%	75.4	75.9
0114	47th MEDICAL GROUP	Air Force	Clinic	1	3,643	96%	91%	0.37	10.35	1.0	3.7	16.1	51%	98%	79%	62%	n/a	75.8
0117	59th MEDICAL WING	Air Force	Medical Center	3	55,339	96%	93%	0.39	13.60	1.6	5.3	14.6	80%	98%	69%	60%	68.6	80.1
0118	NHC CORPUS CHRISTI	Navy	Clinic	3	12,956	86%	94%	0.67	9.57	1.0	4.8	10.5	27%	92%	77%	60%	66.8	67

Appendix 3. Access to Care

August 29, 2014

	Facility Information				% Meeting Standard		Time to Appointment		Days to Third Next Appointment			TOL	Getting needed care		Satisfaction	HCSDB	
DMIS ID	Facility Name	Service	Facility Type	MTFs	Enrolled	A¹	S²	A¹	S²	Pri-Care A¹	R²	S²	% TOL availed	Svc	TROSS	ATC (TROSS)	Get Care Quickly	Get Needed Care
0119	75th MEDICAL GROUP	Air Force	Clinic	1	17,292	98%	97%	0.38	8.50	1.6	5.3	10.1	81%	97%	74%	66%	74.2	69.8
0120	633rd MEDICAL GROUP	Air Force	Hospital	1	37,735	86%	90%	1.37	15.44	5.5	9.2	17.3	82%	96%	60%	51%	59.7	87
0121	MCDONALD ARMY HEALTH CENTER	Army	Clinic	4	26,151	95%	92%	0.49	14.26	1.1	3.3	16.8	76%	86%	73%	61%	63.1	67
0122	KENNER AHC	Army	Clinic	4	21,058	94%	95%	0.60	12.53	1.0	7.2	8.5	72%	80%	66%	61%	71.2	78.5
0123	FORT BELVOIR COMMUNITY HOSPITAL	NCR	Hospital	3	78,983	87%	89%	1.40	14.92	2.0	8.5	17.5	59%	80%	64%	58%	58.6	58.2
0124	NMC PORTSMOUTH	Navy	Medical Center	10	104,151	93%	91%	1.32	14.46	1.0	9.2	15.9	42%	92%	68%	64%	70.9	66.7
0125	MADIGAN AMC	Army	Medical Center	15	118,070	94%	92%	0.70	13.72	2.1	6.0	16.1	63%	81%	68%	53%	71.4	56.6

Military Health System Review – Final Report
August 29, 2014

	Facility Information				Time to Appointment						TOL			Satisfaction		HCSDB	
DMIS ID	Facility Name	Service	Facility Type	MTFs	Enrolled	% Meeting Standard		Days to Appointment		Days to Third Next Appointment				Getting needed care		Get Care Quickly	Get Needed Care
						A*	S*	A*	S*	A*	S*	% TOL enrolled	Svc	TRO$$	ATC (TRO$$)		
0126	NH BREMERTON	Navy	Hospital	4	34,272	96%	95%	0.77	12.43	0.7	4.1	11.8	67%	94%	72%	61%	82.4	78.9
0127	NH OAK HARBOR	Navy	Hospital	1	14,481	97%	93%	0.32	11.80	0.4	3.6	10.8	63%	96%	78%	72%	77.7	72.7
0128	92nd MEDICAL GROUP	Air Force	Clinic	1	10,912	99%	98%	0.44	9.12	1.4	4.5	6.9	57%	97%	78%	73%	85.6	74
0129	90th MEDICAL GROUP	Air Force	Clinic	1	8,755	95%	96%	0.35	13.59	1.4	8.3	15.6	60%	93%	75%	68%	73.1	n/a
0131	WEED ACH	Army	Hospital	6	10,413	98%	95%	0.46	13.72	1.2	2.5	11.0	86%	77%	65%	58%	66.8	72
0203	354th MEDICAL GROUP	Air Force	Clinic	1	5,575	96%	98%	0.29	11.64	2.3	5.6	8.7	68%	94%	76%	63%	n/a	n/a
0248	61st MEDICAL GROUP	Air Force	Clinic	2	7,695	99%	97%	0.21	11.97	0.8	4.1	17.2	88%	97%	65%	44%	71.8	64.6
0252	21st MEDICAL GROUP	Air Force	Clinic	2	26,632	97%	98%	0.41	10.76	1.6	8.4	13.7	53%	97%	72%	65%	70.1	70

203

Appendix 3. Access to Care

		Facility Information				% Meeting Standard		Days to Appointment		Days to Third Next Appointment				TOL	Getting needed care		Satisfaction	HCSDB	
DMIS ID	Facility Name	Service	Facility Type	MTFs	Enrolled	A*	S*	A*	S*	PriCare		S*		% TOL enabled	Svc	TROSS	ATC (TROSS)	Got Care Quickly	Got Needed Care
										A*	R*								
0280	NHC HAWAII	Navy	Clinic	5	29,857	63%	98%	8.16	9.00	0.8	3.3		12.4	38%	94%	75%	67%	79	81.4
0287	15th MEDICAL GROUP	Air Force	Clinic	1	14,394	95%	94%	0.52	13.53	1.3	7.5		10.6	68%	93%	76%	57%	n/a	n/a
0306	NHC ANNAPOLIS	Navy	Clinic	6	12,593	95%	98%	0.44	6.49	1.0	3.8		5.8	35%	95%	79%	76%	74.5	86.9
0310	66th MEDICAL GROUP	Air Force	Clinic	1	5,808	96%	87%	0.26	9.32	2.1	5.1		8.3	88%	96%	69%	61%	74.7	78
0326	87th MEDICAL GROUP	Air Force	Clinic	1	17,453	96%	95%	0.44	11.87	1.4	9.3		14.4	84%	95%	64%	44%	n/a	n/a
0330	GUTHRIE AHC	Army	Clinic	7	32,569	98%	93%	0.31	14.39	1.6	4.8		10.4	79%	81%	67%	61%	n/a	n/a
0338	71st MEDICAL GROUP	Air Force	Clinic	1	4,042	91%	94%	0.44	12.40	3.8	2.9		13.6	78%	96%	81%	67%	n/a	n/a
0356	628th MEDICAL GROUP	Air Force	Clinic	1	12,242	97%	96%	0.42	10.29	2.0	4.4		7.8	77%	97%	76%	51%	n/a	n/a

Military Health System Review – Final Report
August 29, 2014

	Facility Information						% Meeting Standard		Time to Appointment						TOL	Getting needed care		Satisfaction		HCSDB	
DMIS ID	Facility Name	Service	Facility Type	MTFs	Enrolled		A*	S*	Days to Appointment			Days to Next Appointment PriCare		S*	% TOL enrolled	Svc	TRICSS	ATC (TRICSS)	Get Care Quality	Get Needed Care
									A*	S*	A*	R*								
0364	17th MEDICAL GROUP	Air Force	Clinic	1	8,959		98%	92%	0.37	13.51	1.9	6.5	10.2	84%	98%	80%	56%	82.1	82.4
0366	359th MEDICAL GROUP	Air Force	Clinic	1	24,365		95%	97%	0.62	11.64	1.6	6.0	7.4	90%	93%	81%	63%	69.9	72.4
0385	NHC QUANTICO	Navy	Clinic	5	19,973		83%	90%	1.00	10.13	0.9	3.3	11.0	0%	95%	65%	49%	65.6	59.7
0395	62nd MEDICAL SQUADRON	Air Force	Clinic	1	3,925		98%	97%	0.29	10.28	1.2	4.1	12.6	21%	87%	54%	40%	n/a	n/a
0413	579TH MEDICAL GROUP	Air Force	Clinic	1	8,646		90%	94%	0.61	8.57	2.2	6.5	10.0	79%	96%	63%	49%	n/a	n/a
0607	LANDSTUHL REGIONAL MEDCEN	Army	Medical Center	12	50,495		95%	93%	0.46	12.11	1.2	7.6	11.4	84%	80%	70%	73%	73	69.1
0609	BAVARIA MEDDAC	Army	Clinic	8	29,164		97%	96%	0.25	7.68	1.3	4.6	9.8	87%	88%	77%	73%	61.9	67.3

205

Appendix 3. Access to Care

	Facility Information				Time to Appointment							TOL	Satisfaction			HCSDB	
DMIS ID	Facility Name	Service	Facility Type	MTFs	Enrolled	% Meeting Standard		Days to Appointment		Days to Third Next Appointment			% TOL enabled	Getting needed care		ATC (mross)	Get Care Quickly	Get Needed Care
						A[1]	S[2]	A[1]	S[2]	PriCare A[1]	R[2]	S[2]		Svc	TROSS			
0610	BG CRAWFORD F. SAMS USAHC-CAMP ZAMA	Army	Clinic	1	2,064	99%	96%	0.21	11.14	0.7	4.4	10.4	97%	92%	83%	78%	n/a	n/a
0612	BRIAN ALLGOOD ACH	Army	Hospital	8	32,920	96%	95%	0.38	13.50	1.4	6.0	14.4	69%	77%	77%	57%	n/a	n/a
0615	NH GUANTANAMO BAY	Navy	Hospital	1	2,800	64%	97%	4.27	8.56	0.6	7.9	6.9	0%	93%	72%	85%	n/a	n/a
0617	NH NAPLES	Navy	Hospital	2	5,221	93%	96%	0.96	9.91	0.6	3.5	10.8	67%	95%	78%	72%	n/a	n/a
0618	NH ROTA	Navy	Hospital	1	2,606	92%	98%	1.08	8.81	0.7	0.7	6.2	70%	95%	88%	79%	n/a	n/a
0620	NH GUAM	Navy	Hospital	2	13,547	96%	96%	0.47	12.64	0.9	5.3	10.2	58%	95%	78%	73%	79.7	74.9
0621	NH OKINAWA	Navy	Hospital	9	32,075	95%	95%	0.43	11.55	0.8	4.4	10.3	53%	92%	71%	56%	80.5	71.6
0622	NH YOKOSUKA	Navy	Hospital	9	30,696	98%	97%	0.31	11.07	0.8	2.8	9.6	58%	95%	76%	69%	79.9	71.7
0624	NH SIGONELLA	Navy	Hospital	3	8,760	97%	98%	0.29	8.60	0.8	2.0	7.9	40%	95%	84%	71%	n/a	n/a

Military Health System Review – Final Report
August 29, 2014

OHS ID	Facility Name	Facility Information					Time to Appointment							TDI		Getting needed care			Satisfaction		HCSDB	
		Service	Facility Type	MTF	Enrolled	% Meeting Standard		Days to Appointment		Days of Time Until Appointment			% TDI enabled	Svc	TRO3S	ATC (mean)	Get Care Quality	Get Needed Care
						A*	S*	A*	S*	A*	P*	S*							
0629	65th MEDICAL GROUP	Air Force	Clinic	1	1,217	95%	97%	0.37	7.33	0.9	4.3	6.8	91%	99%	74%	80%	n/a	n/a
0633	48th MEDICAL GROUP	Air Force	Hospital	1	18,141	91%	94%	0.69	14.47	2.1	6.6	17.7	81%	95%	73%	66%	71.5	76.6
0635	39th MEDICAL GROUP	Air Force	Clinic	1	2,279	87%	94%	1.01	9.82	1.4	6.5	7.9	52%	97%	84%	72%	n/a	n/a
0637	8th MEDICAL GROUP	Air Force	Clinic	1	2,327	98%	97%	0.32	8.96	3.6	4.5	7.5	26%	No Data	70%	63%	n/a	n/a
0638	51st MEDICAL GROUP	Air Force	Hospital	1	7,639	97%	96%	0.47	11.06	1.7	7.2	14.2	88%	92%	67%	56%	71.6	n/a
0639	35th MEDICAL GROUP	Air Force	Hospital	1	7,171	60%	93%	6.82	12.46	2.5	5.2	10.5	65%	93%	69%	65%	n/a	n/a
0640	374th MEDICAL GROUP	Air Force	Hospital	1	7,017	90%	94%	0.60	13.24	3.0	9.1	13.1	82%	94%	76%	67%	83.3	n/a

207

Appendix 3. Access to Care

August 29, 2014

Facility Information					% Meeting Standard		Time to Appointment Days to Appointment		Days to Third Next Appointment PriCare			TOL	Getting needed care		Satisfaction	HCSDB	
DMIS ID	Facility Name	Service	Facility Type	MTFs*	Enrolled	A¹	B²	A¹	B²	A¹	B²	% TOL enabled	Svc	TROSS	ATC (mean)	Get Care Quickly	Get Needed Care
0653	422 ABS MEDICAL FLIGHT	Air Force	Limited Scope MTF	1	1,017	97%	98%	0.43	10.79	3.0	6.0	21.2	96%	93%	80%	73%	n/a	n/a
0799	470 MEDICAL FLIGHT	Air Force	Limited Scope MTF	1	2,291	97%	94%	0.31	12.39	1.0	4.3	ND	87%	97%	89%	66%	n/a	n/a
0802	36th MEDICAL GROUP	Air Force	Clinic	1	5,975	94%	96%	0.52	12.38	2.3	7.7	13.6	87%	93%	77%	53%	n/a	n/a
0804	18th MEDICAL GROUP	Air Force	Clinic	1	16,081	98%	97%	0.20	13.42	2.2	6.8	14.7	69%	94%	64%	63%	58.4	70.7
0805	52nd MEDICAL GROUP	Air Force	Clinic	1	7,584	97%	82%	0.37	18.01	1.0	4.4	14.4	76%	93%	81%	63%	77.3	86
0806	86th MEDICAL GROUP	Air Force	Clinic	1	19,878	96%	95%	0.46	12.86	1.9	6.2	17.0	66%	95%	78%	61%	78.6	77.1
0808	31st MEDICAL GROUP	Air Force	Hospital	1	7,262	97%	95%	0.42	11.90	1.0	5.5	16.7	76%	95%	78%	72%	n/a	n/a

Military Health System Review – Final Report
August 29, 2014

		Facility Information			Time to Appointment							TOL	Satisfaction			HCSDB	
					% Meeting Standard		Days to Appointment		Days to Third Next Appointment				Getting needed care				
DMIS ID	Facility Name	Service	Facility Type	MTFs	Enrolled	A¹	S²	A¹	S²	PriCare	R³	S²	% TOL enabled	Svc	TROSS	ATC (TROSS)	Get Care Quickly	Get Needed Care
0814	423 MDS-RAF ALCONBURY	Air Force	Limited Scope MTF	1	2,294	96%	89%	0.37	11.62	1.2	2.7	37.1	84%	98%	78%	52%	n/a	n/a
7139	1st SPECIAL OPERATIONS MEDICAL GROUP	Air Force	Clinic	1	15,825	96%	89%	0.30	12.92	3.1	5.8	13.5	41%	96%	73%	56%	59.7	74
7200	460th MED GRP-BUCKLEY AFB	Air Force	Clinic	1	8,570	97%	83%	0.37	17.16	1.0	5.7	14.1	84%	95%	79%	66%	n/a	n/a
7234	MENWITH HILL MEDICAL CENTER	Air Force	Limited Scope MTF	1	658	97%	91%	0.26	10.23	0.7	3.7	19.7	99%	97%	82%	85%	n/a	n/a
	MHS Average for FY14				3,380,654	92%	93%	0.97	12.4	1.86	6.2	12.9	70%	82%	71%	60%	75%	73%

1 Acute
2 Specialty
3 Routine

2014 MHS Review Group
Source: TRICARE Operations Center (TOC); TRICARE Outpatient Satisfaction Survey (TROSS); Air Force Services Delivery Assessment (SDA); Army Provider Level Satisfaction Survey (APLSS); Patient Satisfaction Survey (PSS), Healthcare Survey of DoD Beneficiaries (HCSDB): June 2014

Appendix 3.8
Percent of Appointments Met Analysis – Direct Component

Percent of Acute Appointments Meeting the TRICARE Access Standard

The total number of routine appointments booked in primary and specialty care is measured against the MHS access standard of 24 hours. The MHS goal is for 90 percent of acute appointments booked to be within the acute access standard. This measure evaluates appointments coded in CHCS as acute and open access.

Overall: In FY 2014 to date, 92 percent of acute appointments booked in CHCS are meeting the MHS access standard of 24 hours, which is better than the MHS goal of 90 percent (see Figure 3.8-1).

Figure 3.8-1 Acute Appointments Meeting Access Standard - Direct Care Component Overall: MHS Goal >90%

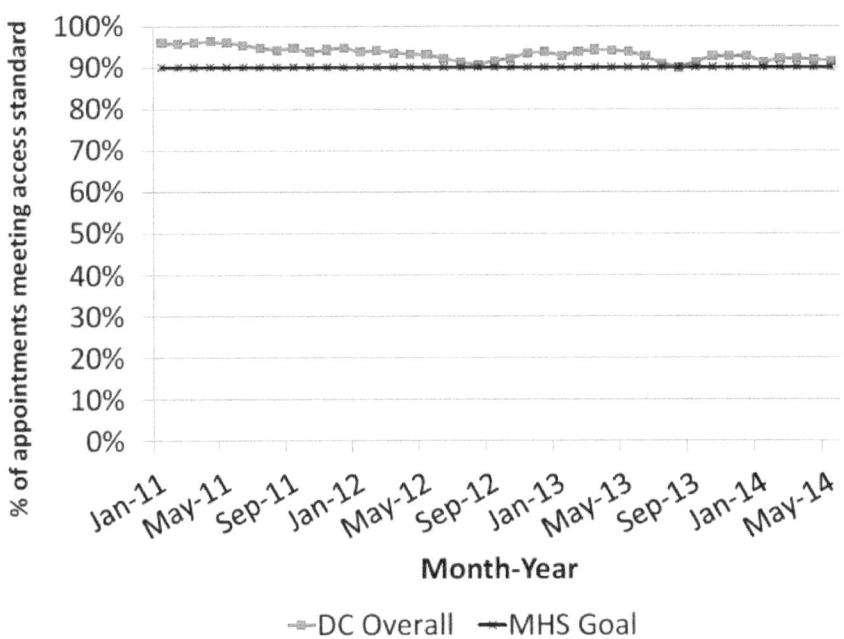

2014 MHS Review Group
Source: TRICARE Operations Center (TOC), June 2014

Civilian Comparison: The average percent of acute appointments meeting the MHS access standard is 92 percent, which is higher than Health System 3, which reports 86 percent of all appointments are within 28 days.

Service-Level: All Services except NCR MD are meeting the MHS goal of 90 percent or more acute appointments meeting the MHS access standard for acute care. The Air Force, Navy, and Army are all performing better than the MHS goal of 90 percent, at 95 percent, 92 percent and 91 percent, respectively. NCR MD is performing below the MHS goal at 84 percent.

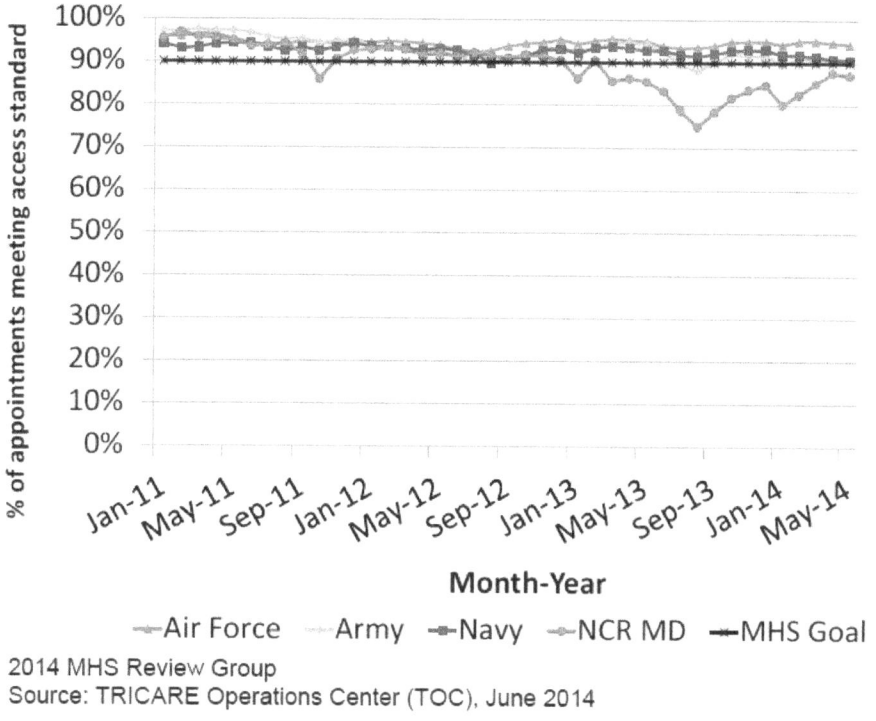

Figure 3.8-2 Acute Appointments Meeting Access Standard, by Service – MHS Goal: >90%

2014 MHS Review Group
Source: TRICARE Operations Center (TOC), June 2014

Facility Type: Clinics and hospitals did better than the MHS goal of 90 percent, averaging 93 percent and 92 percent, respectively. The medical center FY 2014 average of 89 percent did not meet the MHS goal of 90 percent of acute appointments meeting the MHS access standard.

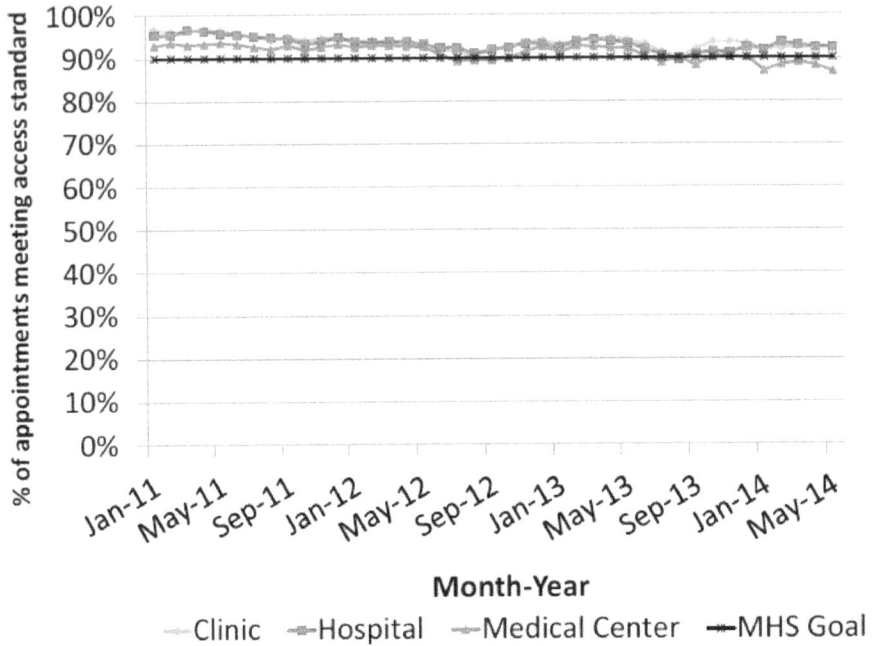

Figure 3.8-3 Acute Appointments Meeting Access Standard, by Facility Type – MHS Goal: >90%

2014 MHS Review Group
Source: TRICARE Operations Center (TOC), June 2014

Location: Facilities located overseas had better performance compared to facilities located in the United States. The percent of acute appointments meeting the MHS access standard was 94 percent overseas, compared to 92 percent in the United States, with both groups meeting the MHS goal.

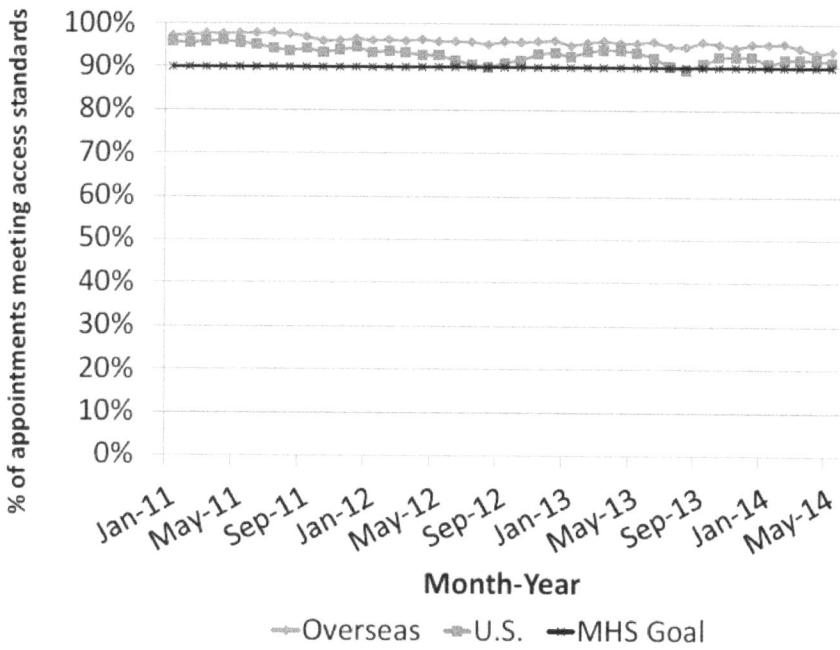

Figure 3.8-4 Acute Appointments Meeting Access Standard, by Location – MHS Goal: >90%

2014 MHS Review Group
Source: TRICARE Operations Center (TOC), June 2014

Percent of Specialty Appointments Meeting the Tricare Access Standard

The total number of specialty appointments booked is measured against the MHS access standard of 28 days. The MHS goal is for 90 percent of specialty appointments booked to be within the MHS specialty access standard. This measure evaluates specialty appointments.

MHS Overall: In FY 2014 to date, 93 percent of specialty appointments booked in CHCS are meeting the MHS standard of 28 days, which meets the MHS goal of 90 percent or more.

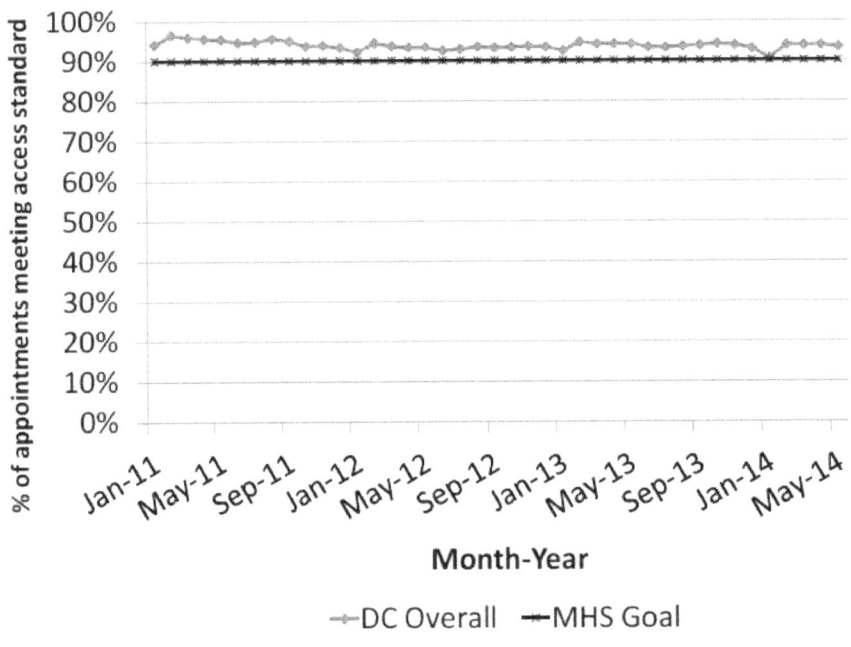

Figure 3.8-5 Specialty Appointments Meeting Access Standard – Overall: MHS Goal >90%

2014 MHS Review Group
Source: TRICARE Operations Center (TOC), June 2014

Civilian Comparison: The average percent of specialty appointments meeting the MHS access standard is 93 percent, which is higher than Health System 3, which reports 86 percent of all appointments are within 28 days.

Service-Level: All Services except NCR MD are meeting the MHS goal of 90 percent or more specialty appointments meeting the MHS access standard. The Air Force, Navy, and Army are all performing better than the MHS goal of 90 percent, at 93 percent, 94 percent and 94 percent, respectively. NCR MD is performing below the MHS goal at 88 percent.

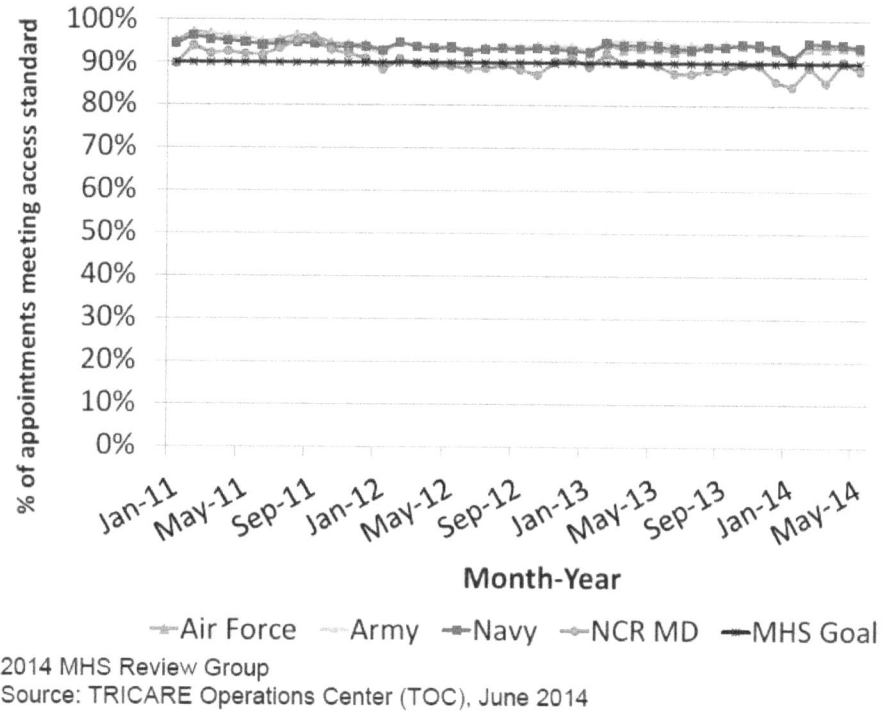

Figure 3.8-6 Specialty Appointments Meeting Access Standard, by Service – MHS Goal: >90%

2014 MHS Review Group
Source: TRICARE Operations Center (TOC), June 2014

Facility Type: Clinics, hospitals and medical centers outperformed the MHS goal of 90 percent, averaging 95 percent, 94 percent and 92 percent, respectively. All MTF type groups meet the MHS access standard.

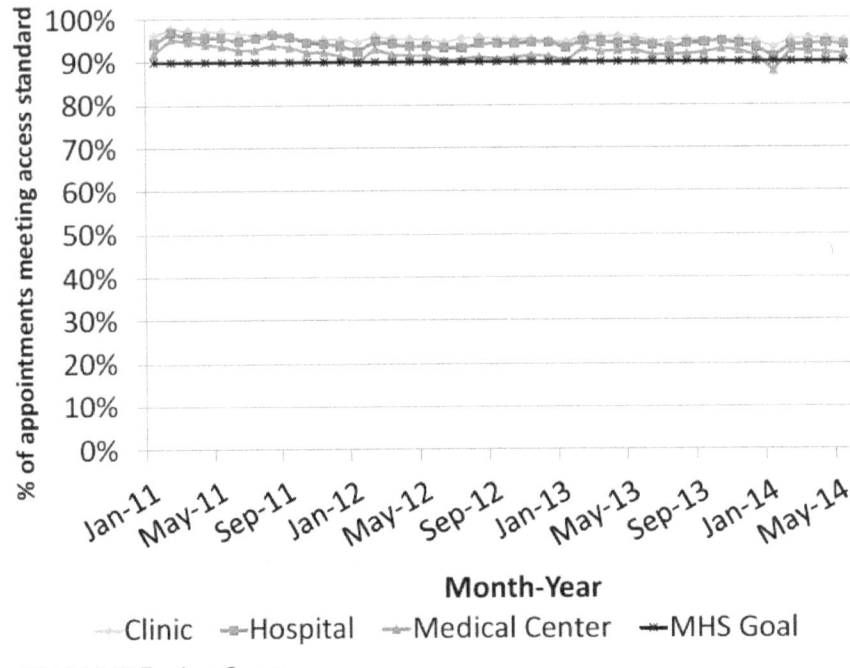

Figure 3.8-7 Specialty Appointments Meeting Access Standard, by Facility Type – Goal: >90%

2014 MHS Review Group
Source: TRICARE Operations Center (TOC), June 2014

Location: Facilities located overseas had better performance compared to facilities located in the United States. The percent of specialty appointments meeting the MHS access standard was 94 percent overseas, compared to 93 percent in the United States, with both groups meeting the MHS goal.

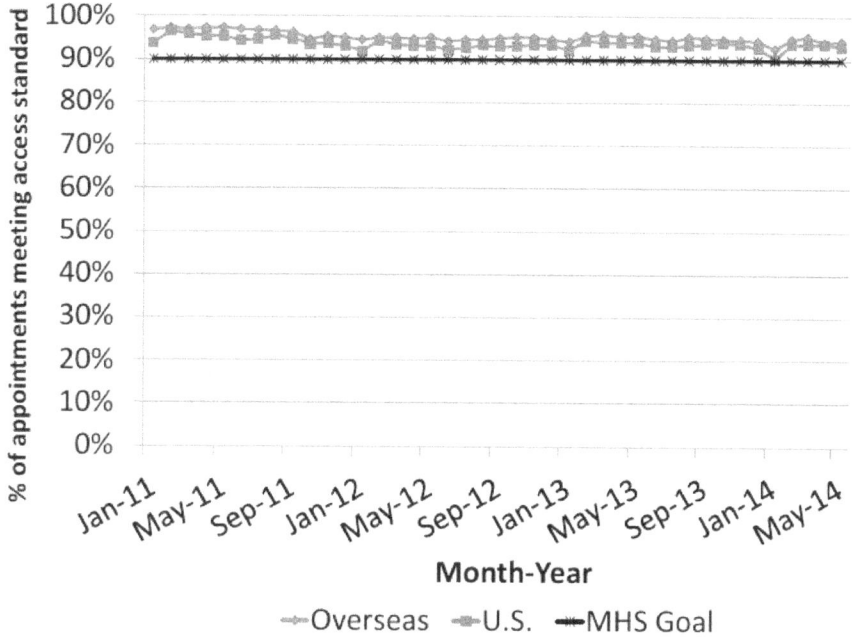

Figure 3.8-8 Specialty Appointments Meeting Access Standard, by Location – Goal: >90%

2014 MHS Review Group
Source: TRICARE Operations Center (TOC), June 2014

Appendix 3.9
Overseas and United States Access Measures – Direct Care Component

Acute Appointments

Number of Days to Acute Appointment

Facilities located overseas had better performance compared to facilities located in the United States. The average days to acute appointments overseas is 0.61 days in FY 2014 compared to 1.03 days for facilities located in the United States. Both groups performed better than the CA acute access standard.

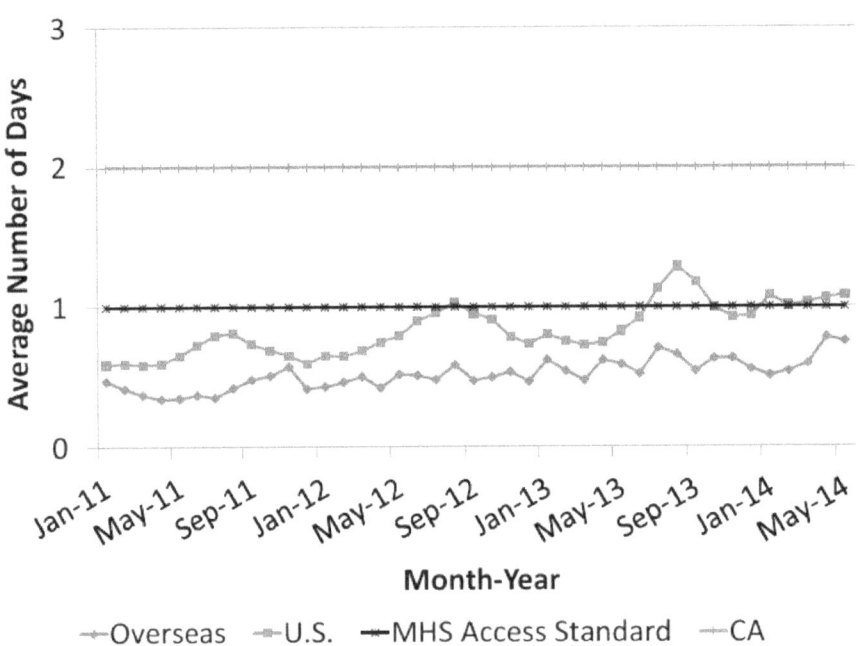

Figure 3.9-1 Average Number of Days to an Acute Appointment, by Location – Direct Care Component: MHS Access Standard ≤ 1 day

2014 MHS Review Group
Source: TRICARE Operations Center (TOC), June 2014

Third next available acute appointment

Facilities located overseas had better performance compared to facilities located in the United States. The average days to acute appointments overseas is 0.80 days in FY 2014 compared to 1.9 days for facilities located in the United States. Both groups performed better than the CA acute access standard.

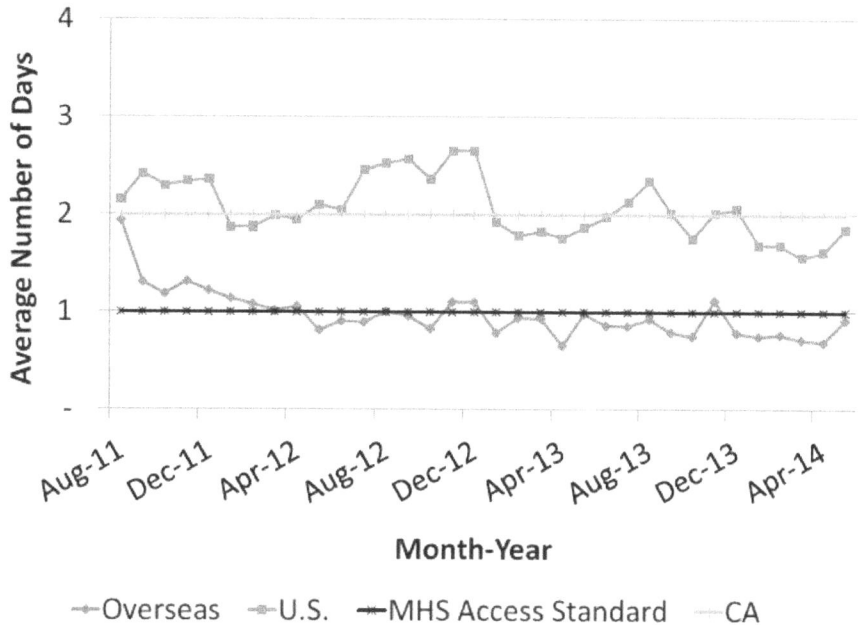

Figure 3.9-2 Average Number of Days to Third Next Acute Appointment, by Location – Direct Care Component: MHS Access Standard ≤ 1 day

2014 MHS Review Group
Source: TRICARE Operations Center (TOC), June 2014

Routine Appointments

Number of days to third next routine appointment in primary care

Facilities located overseas had better performance compared to facilities located in the United States. The average days to routine appointments overseas is 5.2 days in FY 2014 compared to 6.3 days for facilities located in the United States. Both groups performed better than the MHS standard of 7 days and the CA standard of 10 business days (14 calendar days).

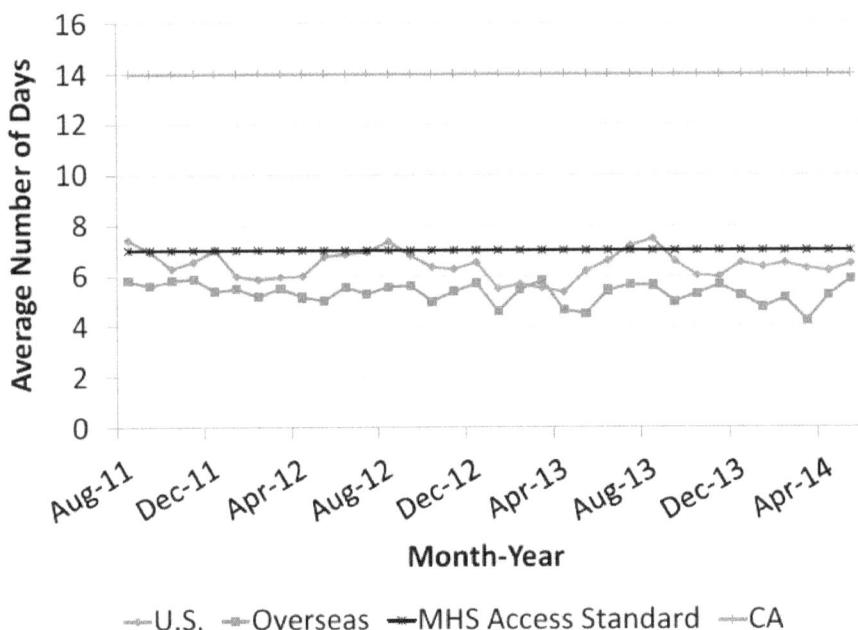

Figure 3.9-3 Average Number of Days Third Next Routine Appointment, by Location – Direct Care Component: MHS Access Standard ≤ 1 day

2014 MHS Review Group
Source: TRICARE Operations Center (TOC), June 2014

Military Health System Review – Final Report
August 29, 2014

Specialty

Number of Days to Specialty Appointment

Facilities located overseas had slightly better performance compared to facilities located in the United States. The FY 2014 average number of days to specialty appointments overseas is 11.5 days compared to 12.5 days in facilities located in the United States. Both groups performed better than the MHS standard of 28 days and the CA standard of 15 business days (21 calendar days).

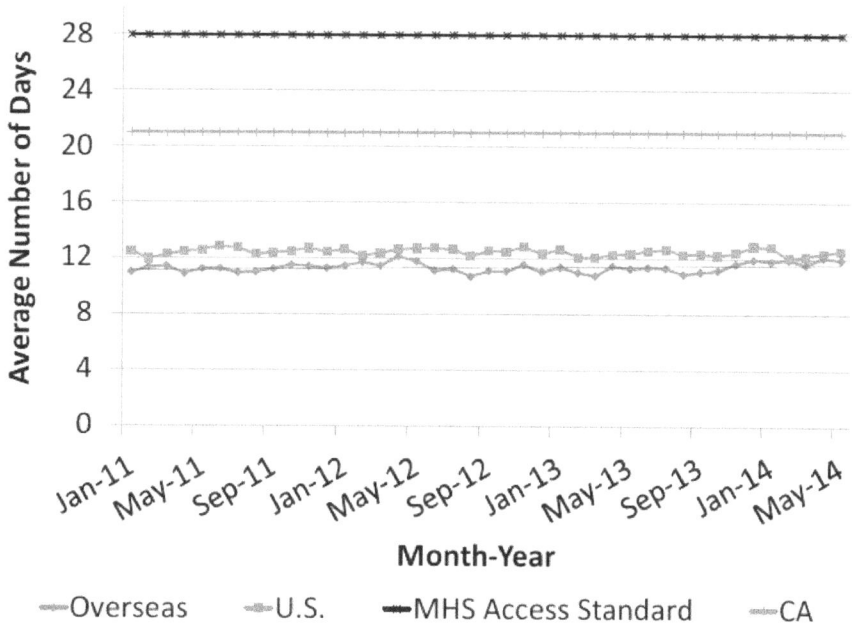

Figure 3.9-4 Average Number of Days to Specialty Appointment, by Location – MHS Access Standard

2014 MHS Review Group
Source: TRICARE Operations Center (TOC), June 2014

Number of Days to Third Next Specialty Appointment

Facilities located overseas had slightly better performance compared to facilities located in the United States. The FY 2014 average number of days to specialty appointments overseas is 11.8 days compared to 13.2 days in facilities located in the United States. Both groups performed better than the MHS access standard of 28 days and the CA specialty access standard of 15 business days (21 calendar days).

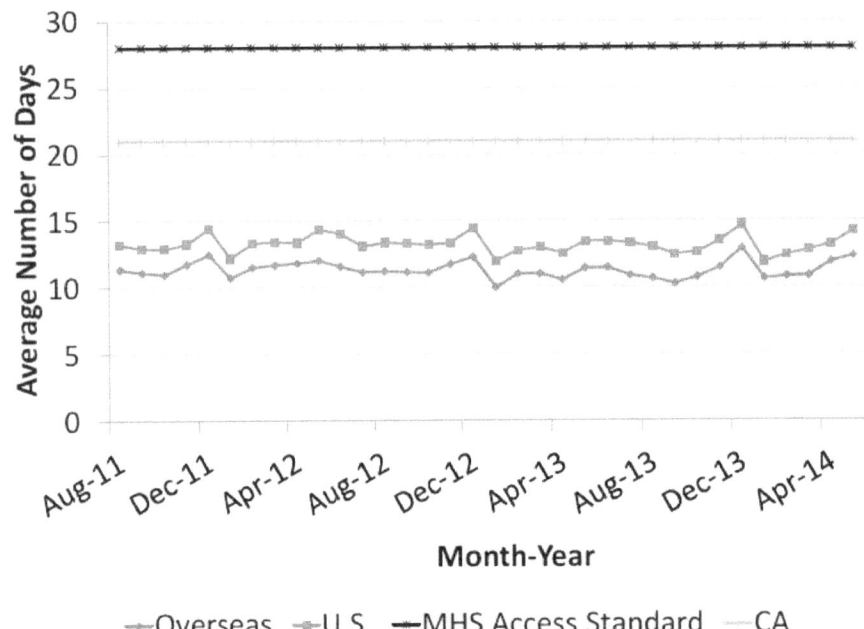

Figure 3.9-5 Average Number of Days to Third Next Specialty Appointment, by Location – MHS Access Standard

2014 MHS Review Group
Source: TRICARE Operations Center (TOC), June 2014

Appendix 3.10
Outlier Analysis

Average Number of Days to an Acute Appointment

The FY 2014 mean was 0.97 days and the median was .45 days; 87 percent of MTFs have a lower average number of days to acute appointments than the mean. There are four high outliers and seven extreme outliers (see Table 3.10-1 and Figure 3.10-1).

Table 3.10-1 Average Number of Days to an Acute Appointment Summary, FY 2014 to Date

Min	Max	Median	25 perc	75 perc	IQR	IQR* 1.5	IQR* 3	Low outlier	Low extreme	High outlier	High extreme
0.14	8.16	0.45	0.33	0.67	0.34	0.51	1.02	(0.18)	(0.69)	1.18	1.69

2014 MHS Review Group
Source: TRICARE Operations Center (TOC), June 2014

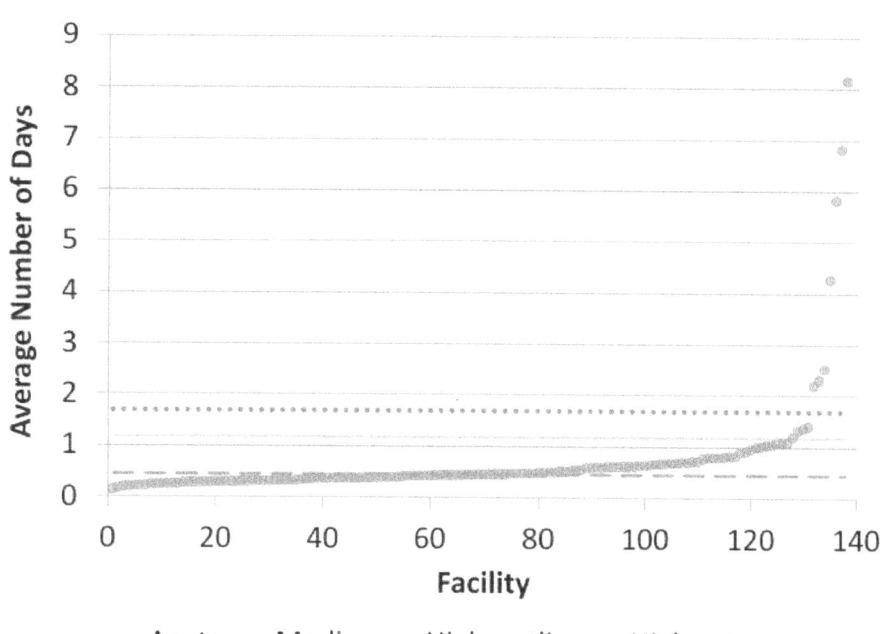

Figure 3.10-1 Average Number of Days to an Acute Appointment – by Facility, FY 2014 to Date

2014 MHS Review Group
Source: TRICARE Operations Center (TOC), June 2014

Average Number of Days to Third Next Acute Appointment in Primary Care

The FY 2014 mean was 1.86 days and the median was 1.4 days; 64 percent of MTFs have a lower average number of days to third next appointment than the mean. There are six high outliers and one extreme outlier (see Table 3.10-2 and Figure 3.10-2).

Table 3.10-2 Average Number of Days to Third Next Acute Appointment – Summary FY 2014 to Date

Min	Max	Median	25 perc	75 perc	IQR	IQR* 1.5	IQR* 3	Low outlier	Low extreme	High outlier	High extreme
0.4	5.6	1.4	0.99	2.14	1.14	1.72	3.44	(0.73)	(2.45)	3.86	5.58

2014 MHS Review Group
Source: TRICARE Operations Center (TOC), June 2014

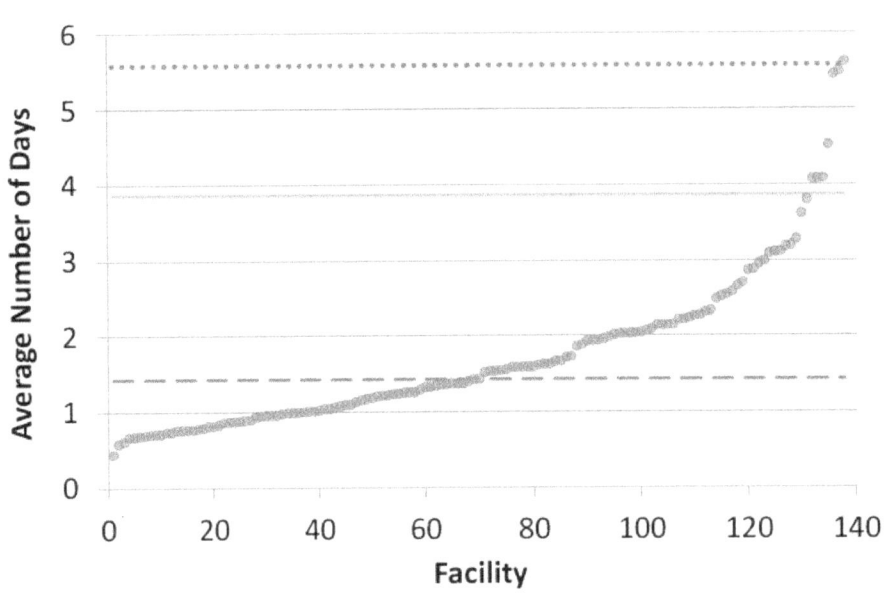

Figure 3.10-2 Average Number of Days to Third Next Acute Appointment – by Facility, FY 2014 to Date

2014 MHS Review Group
Source: TRICARE Operations Center (TOC), June 2014

Average Number of Days to Third Next Routine Appointment in Primary Care

The FY 2014 mean was 6.2 days and the median was 5.3 days; 64 percent of MTFs have a lower average number of days to third next appointment than the mean. There are three high outliers and no extreme outliers (see Table 3.10-3 and Figure 3.10-3).

Table 3.10-3 Average Number of Days to Third Next Routine Appointment – Summary FY 2014 to Date

Min	Max	Median	25 perc	75 perc	IQR	IQR* 1.5	IQR *3	Low outlier	Low extreme	High outlier	High extreme
0.70	12.5	5.30	4.36	7.14	2.78	4.17	8.33	0.19	(3.98)	11.30	15.47

2014 MHS Review Group
Source: TRICARE Operations Center (TOC), June 2014

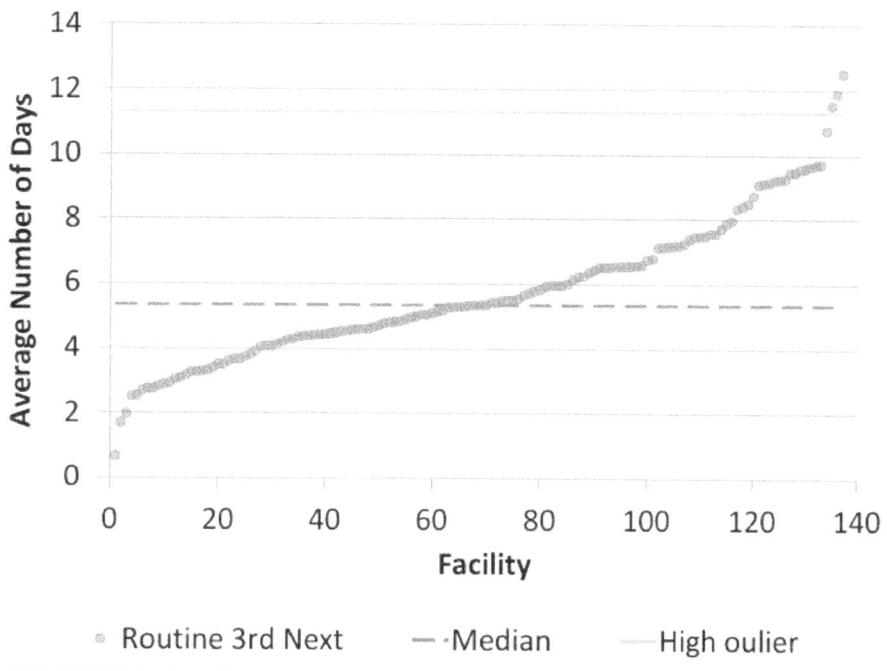

Figure 3.10-3 Average Days to Third Next Routine Appointment – by Facility, FY2014 to Date

2014 MHS Review Group
Source: TRICARE Operations Center (TOC), June 2014

Average Number of Days to Specialty Appointment

The FY 2014 mean was 12.4 days and the median was 11.6 days; 67 percent of MTFs have a lower average number of days to third next appointment than the mean. There is one high outlier, which is still within the MHS access standard and no extreme outliers (see Table 3.10-4 and Figure 3.10-4).

Table 3.10-4 Average Number of Days to Specialty Appointment – Summary FY 2014 to Date

Min	Max	Median	25 perc	75 perc	IQR	IQR *1.5	IQR *3	Low outlier	Low extreme	High outlier	High extreme
6.49	18.01	11.64	10.04	12.91	2.87	4.30	8.60	5.74	1.44	17.21	21.51

2014 MHS Review Group
Source: TRICARE Operations Center (TOC), June 2014

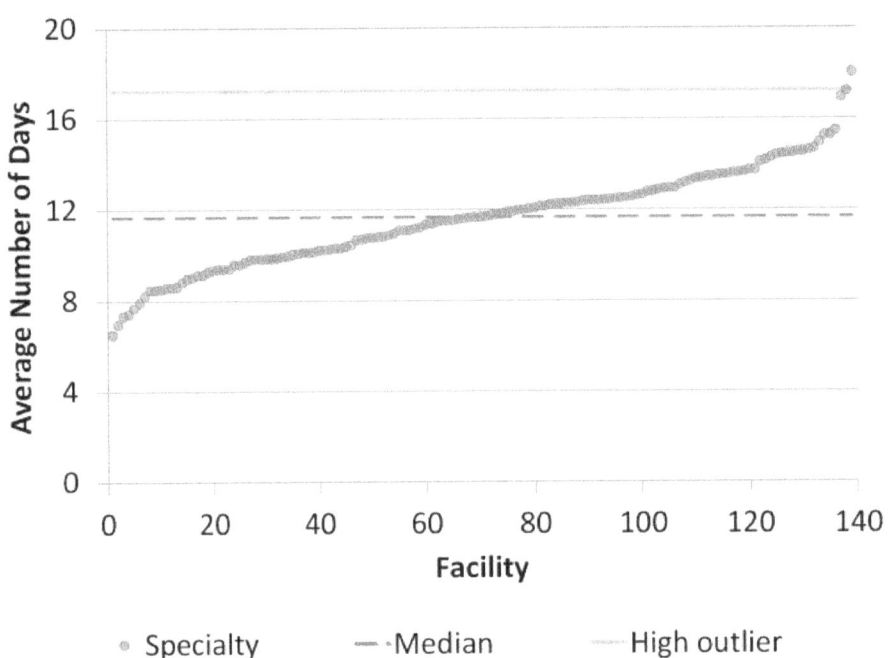

Figure 3.10-4 Average Number of Days to Specialty Appointment – by Facility, FY 2014 to Date

2014 MHS Review Group
Source: TRICARE Operations Center (TOC), June 2014

Average Days to Third Next Specialty Care Appointment

The FY 2014 mean was 6.2 days and the median was 5.3 days; 64 percent of MTFs have a lower average number of days to third next appointment than the mean. There is one high outlier, although it is still within the MHS access standard for specialty care and one extreme outlier (see Table 3.10-5 and Figures 3.10-5).

Table 3.10-5 Average Number of Days to Third Next Specialty Appointment – Summary FY 2014 to Date

Min	Max	Median	25 perc	75 perc	IQR	IQR* 1.5	IQR* 3	Low outlier	Low extreme	High outlier	High extreme
3.1	37.1	11.5	9.9	14.5	4.7	7.0	14.0	2.8	(4.2)	21.5	28.5

2014 MHS Review Group
Source: TRICARE Operations Center (TOC), June 2014

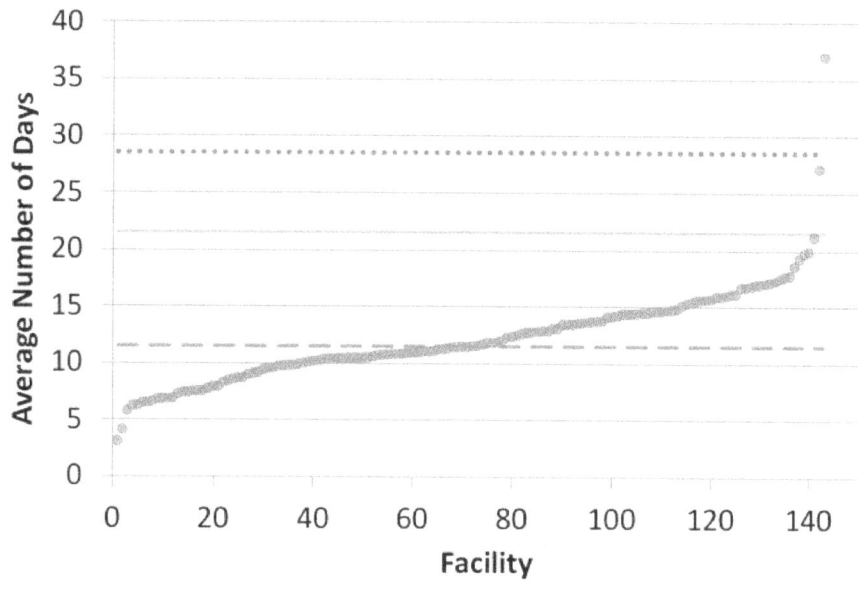

Figure 3.10-5 Average Days to Third Next Specialty Appointment – by Facility, FY 2014 to date

● Specialty 3rd Next — Median — High outlier ···· High extreme

2014 MHS Review Group
Source: TRICARE Operations Center (TOC), June 2014

Percent Appointments Web-Enabled for TRICARE OnLine (TOL) Booking

The FY 2014 mean was 70 percent and the median was 71 percent days. There are four low outliers and no extreme outliers (see Table 3.10-6 and Figure 3.10-6).

Table 3.10-6 Percent of Web-Enabled Appointment for TOL Booking – Summary FY14 to Date

Min	Max	Median	25 perc	75 perc	IQR	IQR *1.5	IQR *3	Low outlier	Low extreme	High outlier	High extreme
0.0	1.0	71%	0.57	0.82	0.25	0.37	0.74	0.20	(0.16)	1.19	1.55

2014 MHS Review Group
Source: TRICARE Operations Center (TOC), June 2014

Figure 3.10-6 Percent of Web-Enabled Appointments for TOL Booking – by Parent Facility, FY 2014 to date

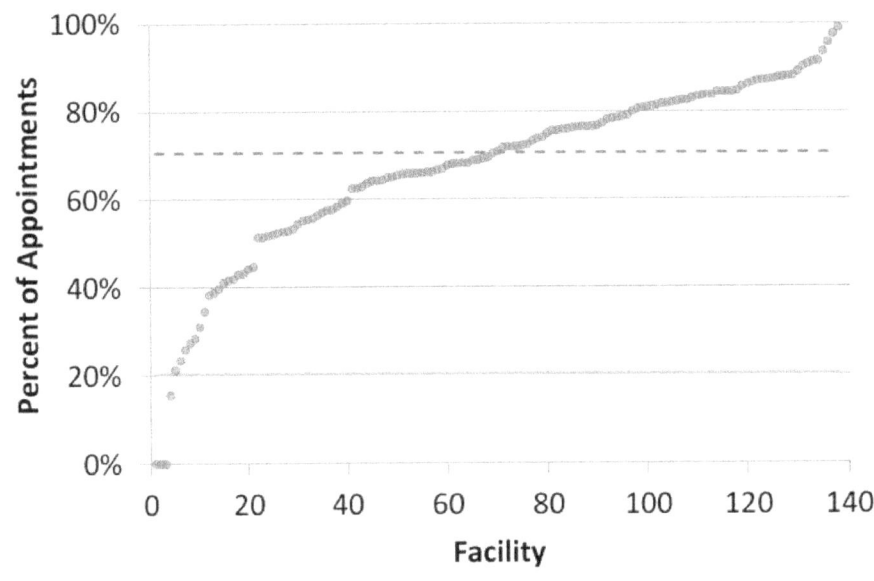

2014 MHS Review Group
Source: TRICARE Operations Center (TOC), June 2014

Patient Satisfaction With Getting Care When Needed (Service Surveys)

The FY 2014 mean was 82 percent and the median was 95 percent; 86 percent of MTFs have higher satisfaction than the mean. There are 17 low and no extreme outliers (see Table 3.10-7 and Figure 3.10-7).

Table 3.10-7 Percent Satisfied with Access to Care – By Parent Facility, November 2013 – May 2014

Min	Max	Median	25 perc	75 perc	IQR	IQR *1.5	IQR *3	Low outlier	Low extreme	High outlier	High extreme
76%	99%	95%	91%	96%	6%	8%	16%	82%	74%	104%	113%

2014 MHS Review Group
Source: Air Force Services Delivery Assessment (SDA); Army Provider Level Satisfaction Survey (APLSS); Patient Satisfaction Survey (PSS), June 2014

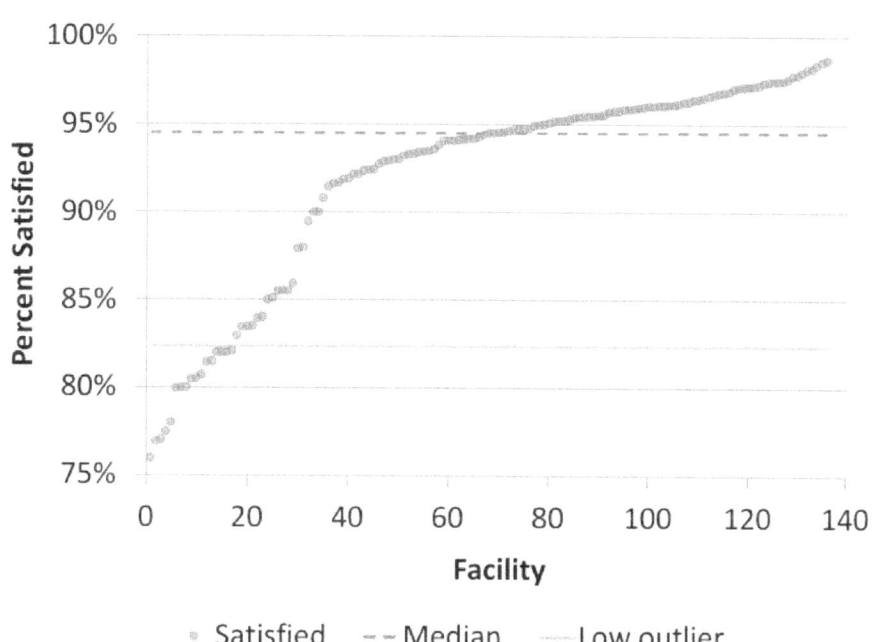

Figure 3.10-7 Percent Satisfied with Access to Care – By Parent Facility, November 2013 – May 2014

2014 MHS Review Group
Source: Air Force Services Delivery Assessment (SDA); Army Provider Level Satisfaction Survey (APLSS); Patient Satisfaction Survey (PSS), June 2014

Patient Satisfaction with Access to Care (TROSS)

The FY 2014 mean was 60 percent and the median was 61 percent; 60 percent of MTFs have higher satisfaction than the mean. There is one high outlier and two low outliers; there are no extreme outliers (see Table 3.10-8 and Figure 3.10-8).

Table 3.10-8 TROSS – Percent Satisfied with Access to Care – Summary, FY 2013

Min	Max	Median	25 perc	75 perc	IQR	IQR*1.5	IQR*3	Low outlier	Low extreme	High outlier	High extreme
36%	89%	61%	56%	68%	12%	18%	36%	38%	20%	86%	104%

2014 MHS Review Group
Source: Department of Defense TRICARE Outpatient Satisfaction Survey (TROSS), June 2014

Figure 3.10-8 TROSS – Percent Satisfied with Access to Care – by Facility, FY2013

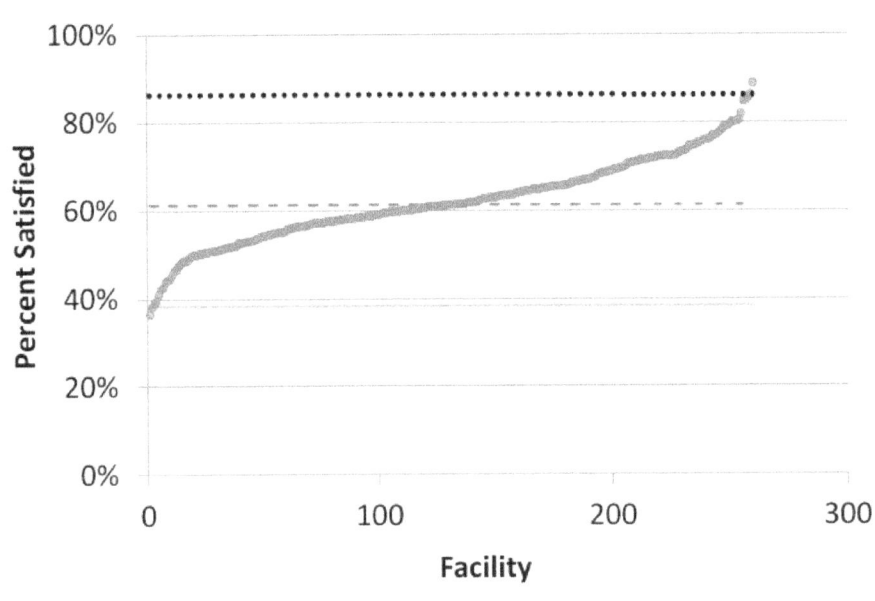

2014 MHS Review Group
Source: Department of Defense TRICARE Outpatient Satisfaction Survey (TROSS), June 2014

Appendix 3.11
Correlation Analyses

The higher the Primary Care Manager (PCM) Continuity the lower the average number of days to third next acute appointments. Correlation: -0.296138 Test Stat: -3.60240 P-value: 0.00044207 (see Figure 3.11-1).

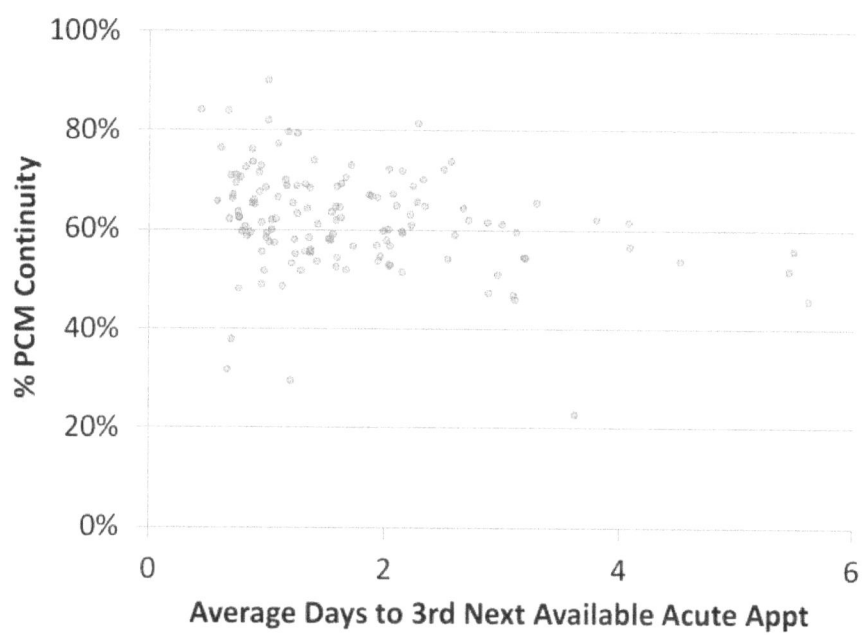

Figure 3.11-1 Correlation between PCM Continuity and Average Number of Days to Third Next Available Acute Appointment

2014 MHS Review Group
Source: TRICARE Operations Center (TOC), June 2014

The higher the PCM Continuity the lower the average number of days to third next routine appointments. Correlation: -0.307779 Test Stat: -3.75851 P-value: 0.0002535 (see Figure 3.11-2).

Figure 3.11-2 Correlation between PCM Continuity and Average Number of Days to Third Next Routine Appointment

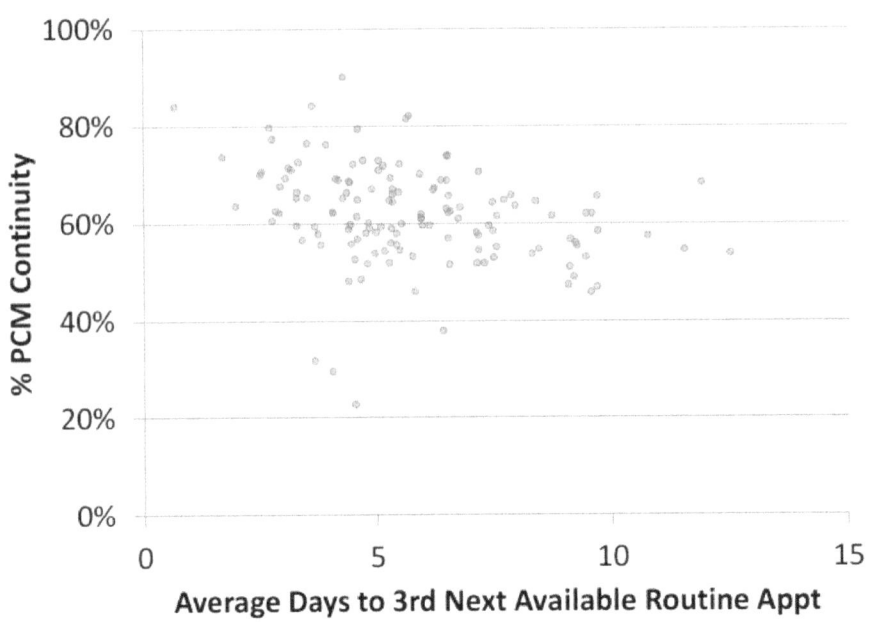

2014 MHS Review Group
Source: TRICARE Operations Center (TOC), June 2014

The lower the average number of days to an acute appointment, the higher the patient satisfaction with getting care when needed. Correlation: -0.262694 Test Stat: -3.150303 P-value: 0.0020119 (see Figure 3.11-3).

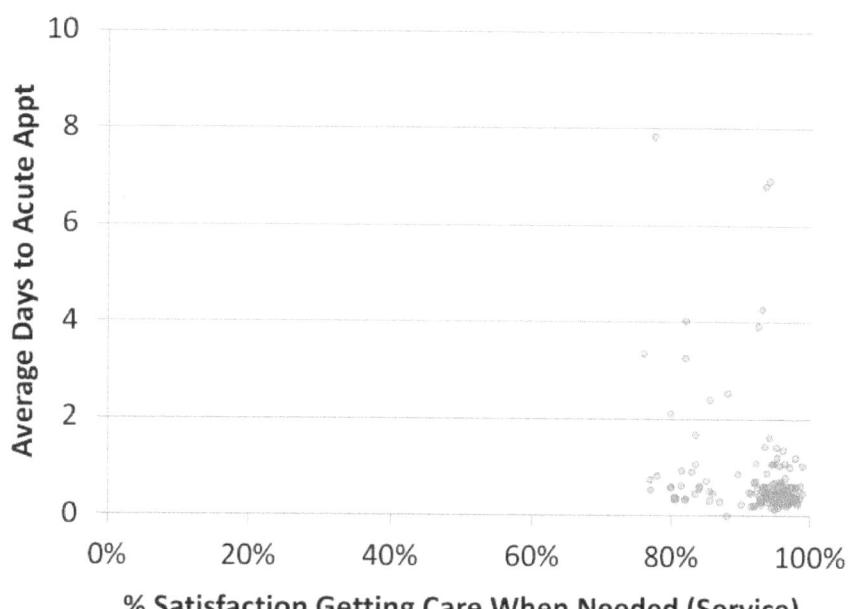

Figure 3.11-3 Correlation between Average Number of Days to Acute Appointment and Satisfaction with Getting Care When Needed (Service Surveys)

2014 MHS Review Group
Source: TRICARE Operations Center (TOC); Air Force Services Delivery Assessment (SDA); Army Provider Level Satisfaction Survey (APLSS); Patient Satisfaction Survey (PSS), June 2014

The lower the average number of days to third next acute appointments, the higher the patient satisfaction with getting care when needed. Correlation: -0.272474 Test Stat: -3.290956 P-value: 0.0012766 (see Figure 3.11-4).

Figure 3.11-4 Correlation between Average Number of Days to Third Next Available Appointment and Satisfaction with Getting Care When Needed

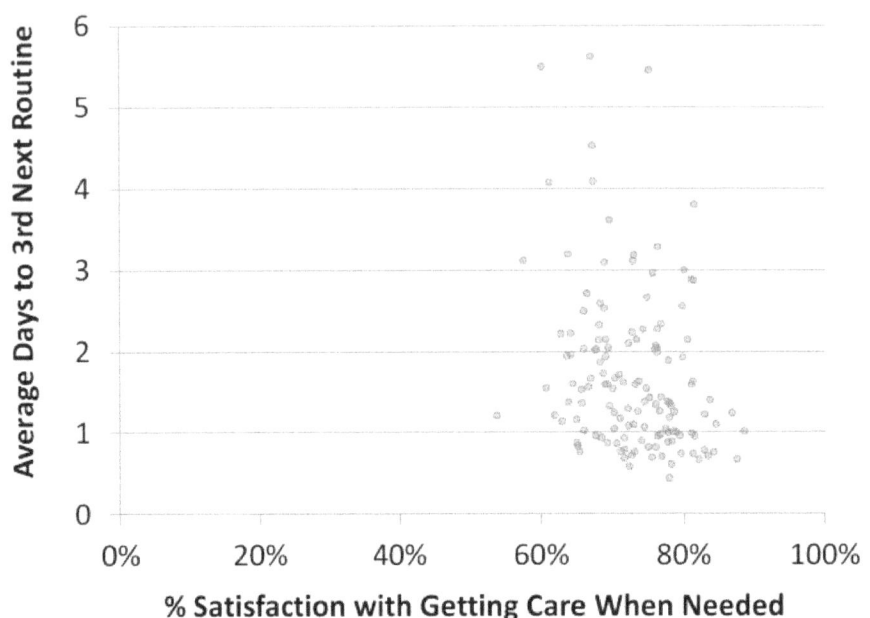

2014 MHS Review Group
Source: TRICARE Operations Center (TOC) and TRICARE Outpatient Satisfaction Survey (TROSS), June 2014

The lower the average number of days to third next routine appointments, the higher the patient satisfaction with getting care when needed. Correlation: -0.278075 Test Stat: -3.363605 P-value: 0.0010015 (see Figure 3.11-5).

Figure 3.11-5 Correlation between Average of Days to Third Next Available Routine Appointment and Satisfaction with Access to Care

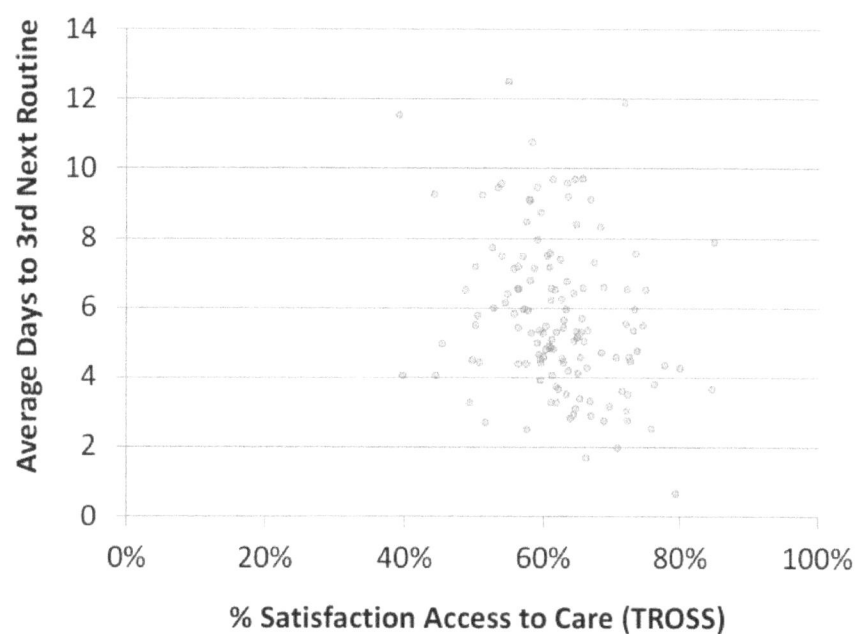

2014 MHS Review Group
Source: TRICARE Operations Center (TOC) and TRICARE Outpatient Satisfaction Survey (TROSS), June 2014

Appendix 3.12
TROSS and HCSDB Questions and Benchmarks

Table 3.12-1 TROSS and HCSDB Questions and Benchmarks – Access When Needed

TROSS Question	Question in Composite (if applicable)	Rating Scale for Satisfied
C1: Access to Care Composite	Q8: Received appt as soon as needed for urgent care	Almost Always, Always
	Q10: Received appt as soon as needed for routine care	Almost Always, Always
	Q13: Answer to medical question same day (calls during office hours)	Almost Always, Always
	Q15: Answer to medical question as soon as needed (calls after office hours)	Almost Always, Always
	Q16: Answer to time spent in the waiting room and exam room. See provider within 15 minutes	Almost Always, Always
Q3a: See Provider When Needed	Q3a: Answer to saw provider when needed	Agree, Strongly Agree

2014 MHS Review Group
Source: Department of Defense Tricare Outpatient Satisfaction Survey, July 2014

HCSDB: HCSDB is sent randomly to all MHS-eligible users and non-users, independent of whether they had a recent encounter. Respondents include those enrolled to TRICARE Prime (MTF and network enrollees) and non-enrolled beneficiaries who may receive care in MTFs or through the purchased care component. For this report, only the HCSDB results for Prime enrollees are presented (Note: Prime beneficiaries enrolled to the network are presented in the purchased care section). Beneficiary responses to two composite questions that address the beneficiary's ability to get care quickly and get needed care are evaluated, which are displayed in Table 3.12-2.

Table 3.12-2 TROSS and HCSDB Questions and Benchmarks – Getting Care Quickly and Getting Care When Needed

Composite #	Question	Rating Scale for Satisfied
Get Care Quickly Composite	Q7: In the last 12 months, when you needed care right away, how often did you get care as soon as you needed?	Usually, Always
	Q10: In the last 12 months, how often did you get an appointment for a check-up or routine care at a doctor's office or clinic as soon as you needed?	Usually, Always
Getting Needed Care - Composite	Question 37: In the last 12 months, how often did you get an appointment to see a specialist as soon as you needed?	Usually, Always
	Question 45: In the last 12 months, how often was it easy to get the care, tests, or treatment you needed?	Usually, Always

2014 MHS Review Group
Source: Health Care Survey of DoD Beneficiaries, July 2014

TROSS and HCSDB metrics are compared to benchmarks established by AHRQ through the Consumer Assessment of Healthcare Providers and Systems (CAHPS). CAHPS publicly reports the results of patient satisfaction questions by percentile. Based on these percentiles, benchmarks are identified and used to compare the MHS to the national level of patient satisfaction with ATC. The percentiles for FY 2013 are displayed in Table 3.7 in this report (Note that the percentiles change annually). The MHS compares to the CAHPS 75th percentile for its TROSS questions and the 50th percentile for its HCSDB questions. There is no benchmark for the TROSS question asking whether the patient gets care when needed.

Table 3.12-3 CAHPS Percentiles (Benchmark Highlighted), TROSS and HCSDB

Percentile grouping	TROSS FY 2013 Access to Care Composite	HCSDB FY 2013 Get Care Quickly Composite	HCSDB FY 2013 Get Care When Needed Composite
	%	%	%
90% or greater	69	89	89
75%-90%	60	88	87
50%-74%	47	86	85
25%-49%	34	84	82
<25%	<34	<83.5	<81.9

2014 MHS Review Group
Source: Consumer Assessment of Healthcare Providers and Consumers (CAHPS), June 2014

This page left intentionally blank.

APPENDIX 4. QUALITY OF CARE

Appendix 4.1
Summaries of Statute, Regulation, Instructions, and Other Guidance

DoD Policies

10 United States Code (USC), Sections 1079 and 1102: The U.S. Code is the codification by subject matter of the general and permanent laws; it is divided into 51 titles. Section 1079(o) provides the Secretary with authority to establish a Peer Review Organization (PRO) program using the Medicare PRO program as a model, and excludes from TRICARE coverage care not considered medically or psychologically necessary per the PRO. Section 1102 addresses the confidentiality, as well as authorized disclosures, of medical quality assurance (MQA) records created by or for DoD as part of a MQA program.

Code of Federal Regulations (32 CFR), Part 199: Part 199 of the Code of Federal Regulations contains the regulations published in the Federal Register relating to the CHAMPUS/TRICARE program. Section 199.15 establishes rules and procedures for the CHAMPUS Quality and Utilization Review Peer Review Organization program. In specific, it establishes rules and procedures to review the quality, completeness and adequacy of purchased care provided, as well as its necessity, appropriateness and reasonableness. In accordance with 32 CFR 199.4(a)(10), all benefits under the CHAMPUS program are subject to review under the CHAMPUS Quality and Utilization Review PRO program. All quality assurance and utilization review requirements for the basic CHAMPUS program, as set forth in 199.4 and 199.15, are applicable to Prime, Standard, and Extra under the TRICARE program in accordance with 199.17(j).

DoDM 6010.51, The TRICARE Operations Manual: The manual is written and maintained by the Defense Health Agency. The manual provides instructions and requirements for claims processing and health delivery under TRICARE. It is an integral part of the managed care support contracts. Specifically, Chapter 7, Section 4 defines the requirements for purchased care contractors to operate a CQMP, which results in demonstrable quality improvement in the health care provided beneficiaries, and in the processes and services delivered by the contractor. Chapter 17, Section 3 describes that for active duty members, a referral from an MTF or an authorization from a service point of contact shall be deemed to constitute direction to bypass provider certification.

DoDM 6025.13, Medical Quality Assurance (MQA) and Clinical Quality Management in the Military Health System (MHS) Manual: This manual reissues DoD 6025.13-R)) as a DoD manual in accordance with the authority in DoD Directive (DoDD) 5124.02 and DoD Instruction (DoDI) 6025.13 and the guidance in DoDI 5025.01. It implements policy, assigns responsibilities, and provides procedures for managing DoD MQA and clinical quality management.

DoDI 6025.13, Medical Quality Assurance (MQA) and Clinical Quality Management in the Military Health System (MHS) Instructions: The corresponding DoD Instructions primarily reissues DoD Directive (DoDD) 6025.13 as a DoD Instruction (DoDI) in accordance with the authority in DoDD 5124.02 and establishes DoD policy on issues related to MQA programs and clinical quality management activities.

DoDD 5010.42, DoD-Wide Continuous Process Improvement (CPI)/Lean Six Sigma (LSS) Program: In Accordance with the authority in Section 113 of title 10, United States Code, this Directive establishes policy and assigns responsibilities to institutionalize CPI/LSS as one of the primary approaches to assessing and improving the efficiency and effectiveness of DoD processes in support of the Department's national defense mission.

DoDI 5010.43, Implementation and Management of the DoD-Wide Continuous Process Improvement/Lean Six Sigma (CPI/LSS) Program: This corresponding instruction document establishes policy, assigns responsibilities, and provides guidance for the DoD-wide implementation of the CPI/LSS.

DoDM 6440.02, Clinical Laboratory Improvement Program (CLIP) Procedures: In accordance with the authority in DoD Directive 5136.01 and the policy in DoD Instruction (DoDI) 6440.02, this manual implements policy, assigns responsibilities, and provides for standards and procedures for managing the CLIP. This manual states the minimal conditions that all laboratories must meet to be certified to perform testing on human specimens under the CLIP.

Health Affairs Policy 98-010, 1998: HA Policy 98-010, Policy for Improving Access and Quality in the Military Health System, was a memorandum issued January 08, 1998 due to media criticisms of military medicine and renewed congressional interest in the quality of care provided to beneficiaries. The memorandum identified 13 issues and requested a summary of how the office resolved each issue or planned for resolution by January 20, 1998.

Health Affairs Policy 10-008, Policy Memorandum for Military Health System Health Care Quality Assurance Data Transparency: HA Policy 10-008, dated October 20, 2010, required the MHS to make relevant quality assurance information readily available and transparent to beneficiaries, enrollees, and providers in an understandable manner.

Health Affairs Policy 09-019, Policy Memorandum for Military Health System Data Quality Management Control Program, Revised Reporting Documents: HA Policy 09-019, dated September 21, 2009, revised the Data Quality Management Control Review List and the Data Quality Statement of DoDI 6040.40 (MHS Data Quality Management Control Procedures), dated November 26, 2002. These important documents are the basis for the Military Treatment Facility (MTF) Report Format submitted monthly from MTFs. The changes recommended in the memorandum were incorporated into the DoDI through a reissuance process and were authorized in the DoDI.

Health Affairs Policy 02-016, Military Health System Definition of Quality in Health Care: HA Policy 02-016, dated May 09, 2002, responded to the Healthcare Quality Initiatives Review Panel's recommendation to promulgate a definition of "quality" concerning health care and related services within the MHS to orient current and future measurement initiatives. The definition of quality health care was adopted by the TRICARE Clinical Quality Forum (TCQF).

Executive Order 13410, Promoting Quality and Efficient Health Care in Federal Government Administered or Sponsored Health Care Programs: To ensure that Federal health care programs promote quality and efficient delivery of health care through the use of health IT, transparency regarding health care quality and price, and better incentives for program beneficiaries, enrollees, and providers.

Health Affairs Memorandum, Policy for Comprehensive Pain Management: The memorandum, dated March 2011, resulted from a requirement within NDAA FY 2010 Section 711, that the MHS develop a comprehensive pain management policy and that all Services provide education/training to their health care providers on acute chronic pain education, use evidence-based recommendations for pain care, and make educational/training materials available to beneficiaries.

Health Affairs Memorandum, Partnership for Patients: In an effort to move towards achieving its quality goals, the MHS has also partnered with public and private organizations. For example, in 2011, Assistant Secretary of Defense for Health Affairs (ASD [HA]) pledged that the MHS would support the Partnership for Patients Initiative. The goal of this initiative, led by the Centers for Medicare & Medicaid Services (CMS), was to bring together hospital leaders, employers, caregivers, and patient advocates, along with State and Federal government leaders, to improve the safety, reliability and cost of hospital care review.

Army Policies

Army Regulation (AR) 40-68, Clinical Quality Management: This regulation establishes policies, procedures, and responsibilities for the administration of AMEDD Clinical Quality Management Program. It emphasizes the need to continually and objectively assess key aspects of individual and institutional performance to improve health care.

Army Medicine 2020 Campaign Plan: The Plan establishes the framework through which the AMEDD will achieve end sate of a responsive and reliable health service in support of all those entrusted to its care.

Medical Command (MEDCOM) Cir 40-15, Pain Assessment Documentation: This circular provides policy and implementing instructions for U.S. Army Medical Command (MEDCOM) Form 734-R (Medical Record–Pain Assessment). This form is to be completed by patients and will facilitate inpatient, health record (HREC), enhanced ambulatory record (EAR), and outpatient treatment record (OTR) documentation by cueing practitioners to document key aspects in their assessment and treatment of acute and chronic pain patients on the standard form (SF) 600 (Health Record-Chronological Record of Medical Care) (HREC, outpatient, EAR) or SF 509 (Medical Record–Progress Notes) (inpatient).

Medical Command (MEDCOM) Cir 40-13, Depression Outpatient Forms: This circular provides policy and implementing instructions for use of the depression outpatient forms prescribed by this circular: U.S. Army Medical Command (MEDCOM) Form 717-R, Depression Outpatient Documentation and MEDCOM Form 723-R, Behavioral Health Referral/Response Documentation. These forms will facilitate OTR documentation by cueing MTF practitioners to document key aspects in their assessment and treatment of depressed patients.

Medical Command (MEDCOM) Cir 40-12, Tobacco Cessation Out-Patient Forms: This circular provides policy and implementing instructions for use of the tobacco cessation outpatient form prescribed by this circular: U.S. Army Medical Command (MEDCOM) Form 709-R (Tobacco Cessation Documentation). This form will facilitate OTR documentation by cueing practitioners to document key aspects in their assessment and treatment of patients who use tobacco products.

Medical Command (MEDCOM) Cir 40-6, Low Back Pain Documentation: This circular provides policy and implementing instructions for use of the low back pain forms prescribed by this circular: U.S. Army Medical Command (MEDCOM) low back pain documentation form. This form will facilitate OTR documentation by cueing practitioners to document assessment and treatment of patients with low back pain.

The Office of the Surgeon General (OTSG)/ Medical Command (MEDCOM) Policy 14-046, Transition of Care Process for Preventing Readmissions: This policy defines the minimum standards for transitions of care related to the hospital in-patient and ED admission and discharge process for a Patient Centered Medical Home (PCMH).

Navy Policies

BUMEDINST 6010.13, Quality Assurance (QA) Program: This overarching instructional document for Navy Medicine establishes policy, publishes procedures, and assigns responsibility for Quality Assurance and Risk Management activities in Navy fixed (shore-based with permanent structures) and non-fixed (moveable shore or fleet-based) medical and dental treatment facilities in accordance with DoD Directive 6025.13.

BUMEDINST 6000.2E, Accreditation of Fixed Medical Treatment Facilities: This instructional document establishes policy, publishes procedures, and assigns responsibility for the accreditation of Navy Medicine's medical treatment facilities.

NavMed West Instructions 6010.1C, Policy and Procedures for Reporting Regional Quality Assurance and Accreditation to Navy Medicine West: This instructional document establishes policy, assigns responsibility and publishes regional guidelines for communicating selected Quality Assurance (QA) activities to Navy Medicine West (NMW), and outlines reporting guidelines for selected QA activities to NMW.

NavMed East Instructions 6010.1A, Policy and Procedures for Reporting Regional Quality Assurance and Accreditation Initiatives to Navy Medicine East: This instructional document establishes policy, assigns responsibility and publishes regional guidelines for communicating selected QA activities to the Navy Medicine East (NME) region, and outlines reporting guidelines for selected QA activities to NME.

BUMED INSTRUCTION 5220.5, Navy Medicine Continuous Process Improvement/ Lean Six Sigma (CPI/LSS): This instructional document recognizes Continuous Process Improvement CPPI/LSS as an essential approach for improving organizational performance and achieving strategic and operational priorities at all levels of the enterprise. This instruction establishes policy and provides guidance to institutionalize and fully implement CPI/LSS throughout Navy Medicine in alignment with the DoD and Department of the Navy.

Air Force Policies

Air Force Instruction (AFI) 44-171, Patient-Centered Medical Home and Family Health Operations: This instruction defines and implements standards for Air Force Family Health Clinic business practices and supports to execute the PCMH concept and meet the following goals: optimal patient-centered care for enrolled patients using evidence-based clinical practice grounded in established population health principles, patient and staff satisfaction, and continuous process improvement of PCMH execution. It is consistent and aligns with DHA policy 09-015, Policy Memorandum Implementation of the Patient-Centered Medical Home Model of Primary Care in MTFs. The AFI is the culmination of published policy memoranda on optimizing primary care and executing the principles of PCMH from 2004 to 2010. The AFI defines specific roles and responsibilities of policy execution/accountability from AF/SG, intermediary commands, through the individual PCMH team members. It states that once the MTF is trained on PCMH by the Air Force Medical Operations Agency PCMH implementation team, the AFI becomes effective. The AFI outlines directive and recommended guidance on clinical, business, and deployment operations and identifies measures. The following measures are collected and provided by headquarters to the Medical Group commander on a monthly basis: continuity of care with PCM, technician availability, 90 available appointments/week; HEDIS® measures, RVU productivity, patient satisfaction per Service Delivery Assessment questionnaires, use of Purchased Care emergency room/urgent primary care clinics, and case mix index. The AFI recommends that the measures be reviewed with the clinic staff on a monthly basis. The AFI states the AF Inspection Agency will inspect MTF compliance of policy criteria.

Air Force Policy Directive 44-1, Medical Operations: This policy establishes the policies that the Air Force Medical Service (AFMS) will use to ensure that the highest standards of practice are applied to all aspects of health care rendered to eligible beneficiaries.

Air Force Instruction 44-108, Infection Prevention and Control Program: This instruction describes procedures for preventing and controlling health care-associated infections (HAIs) in patients, visitors, volunteers and staff within any health care setting such as MTFs, LSMTFs, AESs, Air Reserve Component Medical Units, and Dental Clinics.

Air Force Instruction 44-102, Medical Care Management: This overarching instructional document implements Air Force Policy Directive AFPD 44-1, Medical Operations, and provides guidance for the organization and delivery of medical care. It implements various publications of DOD recognized professional organizations, The Joint Commission, the Accreditation Association for Ambulatory Health Care (AAAHC), and appropriate health and safety agencies. This instruction applies to all personnel assigned to or working in Air Force MTFs, Air Reserve Component (ARC) medical units and Aeromedical Evacuation units, including Reserve and Guard personnel during their active duty and Unit Training Assembly periods, civilian, volunteer personnel and trainees.

Air Force Instruction 44-119, Medical Quality Operations: This instructional policy implements AFPD 44-1, Medical Operations, DoDD 6025.13-R, Clinical Quality Management Program (CQMP) in the MHS, and outlines MTF roles and responsibilities in the area of clinical performance improvement (PI), explains patient safety and risk management (RM) programs, PI/accreditation/self-inspection requirements, credentials and privileging processes, and scope of practice in order to provide optimal health care delivery. This instruction applies to all Air Force Medical Service (AFMS) personnel and where specifically identified within this instruction for units of the Air Reserve Components (ARC) and Aeromedical Evacuation (AES).

Air Force Medical Service (AFMS) Strategic Plan, Objective E6: Reduce Variation to Create Reliability: The AFMS Strategic Plan has placed efforts to reduce variation and create reliability across the entire AFMS (and in every product line). The AFMS Strategic Objective E6: Reduce Variation to Create Reliability has facilitated the creation of work groups around various product lines in order to create standards that were implemented across the AFMS. Standards were created in the areas of Obstetrics, Intensive Care Units, Wrong Site Surgeries, Tissue Tracking, Patient Flow, and Readmissions. For each area, toolkits were developed to facilitate implementation.

Air Force Instruction 90-201, Special Management - The Air Force Inspection System: The instruction, dated August 02, 2013, provides a complete list of authorized inspections for Air Force facilities and includes a policy reference for each inspection.

Air Force Medical Service, Implementation of AFMS Support Staff Protocol (SSP): This document establishes the policies and provides guidance to SSPs (support staff protocols), as well as establishes strategies for implementation and sustainment of the SSPs. SSPs provide standardization, a key component of Patient Centered Medical Home (PCMH) success, and remain a primary objective of MTFs nursing services standards.

Air Force Medical Operations Agency, Standardized Use of Medical Readiness Decision Support System to Document TeamSTEPPS®: This memorandum standardizes documentation of TeamSTEPPS® training in the Education and Training module of MRDSS (Medical Readiness Decision Support System). TeamSTEPPS® is an evidence-based teamwork system aimed at optimizing patient outcomes by improving communication and other teamwork skills among the health care team. As per AFI 44-119, Chapter 2, the organization shall educate all personnel on patient safety concepts and implementation, which includes team training.

Surgeon General (SG) Doc 11-002, Partnership for Patients: This memorandum establishes Air Force support for and commitment to the Partnership for Patients Program.

Surgeon General (SG) Doc 10-0014, Requirement to Attend the Lean for Healthcare Course: This memorandum establishes the requirement that all Military Treatment Facility commanders must attend the Lean for Healthcare Course as a means to provide Air Force Medical Service leaders with the knowledge and tools to lead change in their organizations. Application of continuous process improvement tools in daily clinical operations requires leaders who foster and sustain a culture that constantly reduces waste and enhances quality. Lean for health care training is an excellent way to prepare leaders to translate these principles into action.

National Capital Region (NCR) Policies

6025.01 JTF Clinical Quality Manual: This Manual implements the policy guidance, procedures, and responsibilities for the administration of a Clinical Quality Management (CQM) Program (CQMP) by the Joint Task Force National Capital Region Medical (JTF CapMed) within the National Capital Region (NCR) under the guidance of DoD Instruction 6025.13, and Army Regulation 40-68. It also describes the relationships between JTF CapMed and the Military Services for quality management and administration functions for issues related to personnel assigned to inpatient Medical Treatment Facilities [(MTFs), i.e., FBCH and WRNMMC] in the NCR and the Joint Pathology Center (JPC).

Appendix 4.2
Internal and External Reports

Key Findings

The first key finding indicates the need for an enhanced MHS structure and process for disseminating and implementing study findings. Traditionally, study recommendations are presented at the Clinical Quality Forum (CQF) or the Scientific Advisory Panel (SAP), but often subsequent communication to the Services varies. In the new MHS governance structure, (see Section 2 of this report), the CQF will report its findings to the Medical Operations Group (MOG). In its role as a liaison to senior leadership, the MOG can facilitate better communication of findings and development of action plans, and ensure follow up on action plans reported to senior leadership.

A second finding was the lack of a formal mechanism to monitor internal and external study recommendations throughout the multiple layers of the organization to assess resulting change to policy or procedures. The new governance structure has greater potential for collaboration; however, a clear response system is needed to monitor positive and negative outcomes, as well as to identify ongoing research and implementation gaps.

The third finding from the internal and external study review highlights the difficulties in achieving accurate and efficient bidirectional transmission of data between outpatient and inpatient records. This concern was raised in several reports, including prenatal care, case management, and asthma studies. Collecting and analyzing appropriate metrics and information will continue to be a challenge until a new electronic health record (EHR) system linking inpatient and outpatient records is acquired.

Finally, in a number of studies reviewed, study methodology was not adequate for the study objectives and often data needed for analysis was not accessible to the authors to answer the study questions.

The 10-year retrospective review of studies and reports identified 51 studies and reports, of which 23 were potentially relevant to quality of care in the MHS. Each of the relevant studies and reports is described below.

Study Summaries

Lumetra External Review: In 2007, Congress mandated an external review of the MHS's Medical Quality Improvement Program (MQIP). The assessment was conducted from October 2007 through July 2008 to address how well DoD managed medical quality in its health care system. Lumetra made multiple recommendations, many of which were implemented following publication of the report.

Evaluation of Tobacco Use Cessation Programs (2008): The purpose of this comprehensive evaluation was to assess the overall impact and efficacy of tobacco cessation initiatives, and to evaluate the status of tobacco control and tobacco use cessation policies and programs at the Service level and at military installations. The report recommended an update to DoD policy; improvement in tracking of tobacco use prevalence, incidence, and medication costs of treating tobacco addiction; cost-benefit analysis; and a standard set of program process and outcome measures.

Evaluation of Hypertension among Beneficiaries with Diabetes Mellitus – Study Arm #1: Blood Pressure Control in the TRICARE Direct Care System (2008): The purpose of the study was three-fold: 1) examine blood pressure (BP) control observed in the TRICARE direct care component during calendar year 2007; 2) examine MHS service utilization and clinical characteristics associated with BP control; and 3) examine MHS hypertension medication regimens associated with BP control. The study recommended that a stepped-care approach of pharmacotherapy and therapeutic lifestyle change should be used to achieve BP targets, modifying the treatment plan when the targets are not achieved. It also suggested that standardized measuring regimens, BP management, and goal setting may further optimize BP control performance in the direct care system.

Evaluation of Influenza Immunization Rates among Enrolled Beneficiaries with Diagnosed Asthma, Heart Failure, and/or Acute Myocardial Infarction In the Military Health System (2008): The purpose of the study was to determine influenza immunization status and health care utilization during FY 2008 for those MTF beneficiaries with three high-risk chronic conditions (asthma, congestive heart failure [CHF], history of acute MI). The study recommended improvement in vaccination programs for high-risk patients diagnosed with asthma, CHF, or AMI to target beneficiaries with no evidence of receipt of the flu vaccine by end of November. Additionally, it recommended a future study to track availability of flu vaccine within cardiac and specialty clinics for enrolled MHS beneficiaries in high-risk categories.

Case Management Services for TRICARE Beneficiaries with Serious Mental Health Conditions - Part 1 (2010) and Part 2 (2011): The objective of the report was to describe and evaluate Case Management (CM) services among TRICARE behavioral health patients with potentially serious mental illness during FY 2010. The report made three major recommendations: 1) Develop a standard template in AHLTA to document mental health information that is essential to all providers who may provide care for beneficiaries with mental health conditions, 2) Undertake a randomized controlled trial if a definitive answer as to the effectiveness of CM in the MHS is needed; 3) Consider revising the DoD Medical Management Guide to more clearly and specifically incorporate either the AHRQ framework or the CMSA standards of practice as measurable performance objectives.

Prenatal Care Among Women with Uncomplicated Deliveries (2011): The purpose of the study was to examine compliance with the Clinical Practice Guideline (CPG) on prenatal care utilization, prenatal routine testing and pregnancy outcomes among women with uncomplicated deliveries from FY 2006 to FY 2010. The study recommended improving the coding and documentation of routine prenatal care, improving documentation of maternal Group B

Streptococcal prophylaxis in the newborn record, and developing a predictive model for prenatal appointments.

Cervical Cancer Screening Within DoD (2011): The purpose of the study was to describe DoD MHS beneficiaries and their screening for cervical cancer, including: 1) proportion of women from 18-20 years of age that are receiving PAPs and the proportion that had an abnormal test result; 2) intervals between PAPs for women between 21 and 64 years; 3) number of DoD beneficiaries that had cervical intra-epithelial neoplasia grade 2+ (CIN 2+) on a PAP and the proportion that had a 3-year negative history for CIN 2+ on a PAP; 4) among DoD beneficiaries with CIN 2+, the frequency interval of PAPs; and 5) among women with CIN 2+, the proportion of women that had appropriate follow up and the time interval for reevaluation. The report recommended emphasizing to clinicians and patients the importance of timely and appropriate follow up when PAPs are abnormal and developing a system to track results, and subsequent follow ups using the administrative database (the system could appropriately flag patient records for timely repeat PAPs or diagnostic procedures when the initial PAP results indicate necessity). Additionally, it recommended aligning PAP screening recommendations for all active duty women with the latest U.S. Preventive Services Task Force and American Congress of Obstetrics and Gynecology recommendations and to further educate providers on latest changes to cervical cancer screening recommendations within each Service.

Low Back Pain Evaluation and Treatment in the Military Health System: The purpose of the study was to collect and describe the baseline measures of key metrics and quality indicators associated with evidence-based care for the treatment and management of low back pain (LBP) in the MHS. The report recommended the implementation and use of LBP monitoring metrics and quality indicators with ongoing evaluation and monitoring at the local level of the MTF where the care is actually delivered. It also recommended the development and implementation of technological tools to facilitate adherence with guideline-concordant practice, such as an updated AHLTA template. Another recommendation was to continue the development, implementation, and use of education targeting recommended use of imaging studies in the evaluation of LBP (e.g., LBP CPG toolkit) and the design and development of proactive patient education, both inside and outside of primary care clinics.

Childhood and Adolescent Overweight / Obesity Evaluation, Recognition, and Counseling in Direct Care System Outpatient Care (2012): The purpose of the study was to investigate quality of care metrics for pediatric overweight and obese patients seeking outpatient care in MTFs and gain a more reliable understanding of BMI percentile assessments, overweight/obesity diagnosis, and counseling performed in direct care component outpatient care among patients identified as overweight or obese in Central Data Repository (CDR) data. The report made several recommendations, including: 1) Develop a MHS-wide, standardized CPG to address pediatric overweight/obesity, 2) Increase investment in nutrition specialty care across direct care outpatient clinics and/or revise TRICARE coverage policy to open access outside of the direct care component 3) Consider moving the current MHS childhood obesity quality measure on overweight/obesity diagnoses away from development to finalization, and 4) Continue developing a CDR-based methodology to adequately estimate quality of counseling as part of MHS's childhood obesity quality measures initiative.

Prenatal Care among Women with Uncomplicated Deliveries (2012): The purpose of the study was to examine prenatal care outpatient visit patterns, both routine and non-routine, among women who subsequently had an uncomplicated delivery. The report recommended improved coding and documentation of routine prenatal care, identification of reasons for the deficit of early prenatal care visits, and development of a predictive model for prenatal appointments.

Chronic Opioid Therapy Report (2012): The purpose of the report was to describe MHS chronic opioid therapy patients, and to estimate and characterize the prevalence of possible and potential opioid misuse. The report recommended validating the TROUP scoring system before applying data to MHS population, and for the MHS to operationalize a valid misuse predictive system in a real time automated risk detection program. It also recommended improving the CPGs to assist clinicians in making better decisions regarding opioid prescriptions. Additional training for clinicians to integrate a future MHS automated predictive system into an opioid pain management therapy was also a recommendation.

Evaluation of Chlamydia Trachomatis Screening for Active Duty Women (2007): The purpose of the study was to evaluate the recruit screening and annual chlamydia screening program for active duty females. Between October 2005 and April 2007, chlamydia testing and prevalence rates among active duty women, younger than age 25 and who entered the services during FY 2005, were calculated to determine compliance with the service policies regarding annual testing. The report urged services to follow current policies for annual chlamydia screening and recommended to conduct a follow-up study on screening, type of testing, and frequency of other testing simultaneously with chlamydia (e.g., PAP, Human Papilloma Virus [HPV]).

Chronic Heart Failure Care Performance Measures in the Military Health System (2007): The purpose of the study was to examine baseline MHS chronic heart failure data for 10 measures, 7 of which were being followed and reported by the IHI in its 2006 "Protecting 5 Million Lives from Harm" campaign. These measures included left ventricular systolic (LVS) function assessment, ACE inhibitor or ARB at discharge (D/C), anticoagulant at D/C for chronic heart failure patients with A-fib, smoking cessation advice and counseling, D/C instructions, and flu and pneumococcal immunizations. The other three measures included 30-day readmission rates, use of beta-blocker medications for chronic health care patients, and 90-day visit to ED or admission rate for heart failure after ED D/C for heart failure. The report recommended that DoD examine practices to improve counseling for weight monitoring, as this procedure can have a significant impact on hospital admissions and readmissions. Additionally, increasing the rate at which appropriate beta-blockers are prescribed for heart failure can also affect hospitalizations, as well as premature mortality.

Postpartum Depression in the Military Health System: The purpose of the study was to evaluate Postpartum Depression (PPD) rates among beneficiaries with liveborn deliveries. The report indicated that risk factors and differential PPD rates suggest populations may be served with improved monitoring based on certain risk characteristics. PPD may be predictable and there may be proactive means to identify for PPD.

Clinical Practice Guidelines in Military Health System (2006): The purpose of the report was to evaluate the level of CPG implementation across the MHS direct care component, and to report Primary Care Manager (PCM) attitudes regarding knowledge and use of CPGs. The report also attempted to quantify a return on investment to the MHS. The report provided the following recommendations: 1) Critically review VA/DoD CPG efforts within MHS to increase provider awareness, 2) Determine cause(s) of low provider response rate (13 percent), 3) Use survey results in context of relative provider sample size; and 4) Use study results in future CPG studies.

Military Health System Clinical Practice Guideline Implementation Evaluation- Phase 1 Quest development: The survey was developed to measure MHS health care provider attitude, awareness, knowledge, and use of CPGs, as well as identify any barriers to CPG use. The data was used to determine if there is a relationship between quality (process and outcome) of care and the availability and the provider use of CPGs.

Discharge instructions following hospitalization for heart failure (2005): The study used the data set to examine the relationship between heart failure discharge instruction documentation during a heart failure hospitalization and readmission to the hospital within 30 days. The study additionally examined 60- and 90-day re-hospitalizations for heart failure at all MTFs, pre-existing comorbidities, utilization of services following the index hospitalization and mortality of heart failure patients, and MTF services for heart failure patients. In light of the large number of beneficiaries who did not receive heart failure medications following discharge and given that medications are an effective treatment, the report recommended examining heart failure medication prescription patterns at MTFs. Additionally, it recommended studying the differences in the process of care between MTFs with heart failure clinical (HFCs) and without HFCs to understand the lack of difference in readmission outcomes between the two groups of MTFs.

DoD Medical Treatment Facilities Patient Safety Indicator (PSI) 17, Birth Trauma: The purpose of this study was to investigate the high rate of birth trauma in FY 2003 by measuring birth trauma in administrative data and in data abstracted from hospital inpatient birth records for FY 2004. The two methods of measuring birth trauma were then compared for agreement in identifying birth trauma. The study found that the percentage agreement between the administrative data identification of birth trauma and the medical record identification of trauma was 21.65 percent and 24 MTFs had percentage agreement of 25 percent or less. The study concluded that birth trauma coding at MTFs was not of sufficient quality at that time to allow the AHRQ birth trauma PSI to be calculated using SIDR data. The birth trauma rate at MTFs for FY04 using medical records data was below the AHRQ benchmark, indicating that the quality of care for infants born at MTFs is high. Recommendations were to: 1) implement ongoing obstetric coding audits across all MTFs delivering babies, and based on those audit findings, establish an appropriate ongoing system-wide training program to elevate coding proficiency to 100 percent accuracy; and 2) monitor birth trauma coding at MTFs to ensure standardization before collecting and publishing birth trauma rates.

Obstetric Utilization and Quality of Care (KePRO, Purchased Care only): The purpose of the study was to better understand the Purchased Care obstetrical practices and resulting maternal and infant outcomes related to elective induction or cesarean section between 37 and 39 completed weeks of gestation. Two of The Joint Commission's Perinatal Care (PC) Core Measures dealing with Elective Delivery (PC01) and Cesarean Section (PC02) were evaluated in this study as well as ACOG standard requiring 39 completed weeks of gestation prior to elective delivery. The report recommended that regional differences in elective delivery and C-section rates may warrant further investigation and that a study with a larger sample size would facilitate better understanding the drivers of regional differences. Because The Joint Commission's measure guidelines stipulate inclusion of factors that are not found in the administrative claims data (e.g., weeks of gestation, parity, and delivery position), only a fraction of the selected charts qualified for each clinical inclusion measure. As such, a large sample size would provide greater strength to future study conclusions.

30-Day Readmissions (KePRO, Purchased Care only) (2013): The purpose of the study was to evaluate best-practice discharge process and to identify potential drivers of unscheduled hospital readmissions among TRICARE's Prime beneficiaries who had a primary discharge diagnosis of Heart Failure (HF), Acute Myocardial (AMI) Infarction, or Pneumonia (PN). The report recommended for a prospective randomized study to assess the impact of one or more such discharge initiatives, such as patient education and arranging for post-discharge follow-up appointments, on re-hospitalization rates.

TRICARE Low Back Pain (KePRO, Purchased Care only) (2012): This focused study was conducted to better understand the diagnosis, treatment, and outcomes associated with TRICARE enrollees suffering from low back pain who received care in the Purchased Care environment. The study identified provider adherence to evidence-based practice guidelines including screening for red flag conditions, the rate of imaging procedures commonly used in the assessment of LBP for patients with positive or negative red flag condition screenings, and the magnitude and scope of physical therapy as part of low back pain treatment. The report indicated that while the final sample of 1,475 records does provide enough information to highlight general trends in the population as a whole on the use of imaging studies in LBP, comparisons between regions would benefit from a larger, more representative sample taken from each region.

A Report to Congress: Study Incidence of Breast Cancer among Members of Armed Services (2014): DoD submitted the report in accordance with the National Defense Authorization Act for Fiscal Year 2013 (HR 4310), section 737. The findings from the report reflected the MHS's commitment to implement policies and laws that are most likely to improve the quality and effectiveness of breast care to include prevention, early detection, and awareness of risks for breast cancer among all MHS eligible beneficiaries. The foundation of this commitment was the design and delivery of a comprehensive breast care benefit that continuously assesses each component of the breast care experience and that draws on evidenced-based clinical practices, cutting-edge cancer diagnostics, treatment technologies, and evidence from high-priority clinical cancer trials. DoD's internal efforts and considerations are ongoing and have not required changes to law or policy for implementation. The report also indicated that within the current policy, legislative framework, and future directions for research, the military health benefit continue to support a comprehensive consideration of promising technologies and treatments for breast cancer preventive care and treatments.

Views of Quality of Care in MTF and Civilian Systems Among TRICARE Prime Beneficiaries: The Survey of TRICARE Prime Beneficiaries was conducted to examine how their experiences with the MHS varied by where the care was received, MTF versus PCM assignment. Beneficiaries assigned to civilian PCM as opposed to MTF were more likely to rate higher the quality of care at both civilian and military facility. The results indicated that the survey should be repeated to include questions as to why beneficiaries rate as they do and determine potential MTF improvements to perceived quality of care. It also recommended determining if prior (pre-TRICARE) health insurance experience affected beneficiary perception of quality of care.

Volume of Complex Procedures and Conditions at Military Treatment Facilities: The study examined the average annual volume of complex surgical procedures and medical conditions with a high risk of mortality across MTFs guided by the assumption that greater volume among MTF surgeons and staff can promote and improve clinical skills necessary to safely treat patients with complex conditions. The report recommended measuring availability and productivity of surgeons in MTFs and determining if PCM are referring Inpatient Quality Indicators (IQI) procedures to MTF or civilian hospitals.

Appendix 4.3
Quality of Care Education and Training

Air Force Training

The Air Force has several methods of providing training related to quality care, each geared to the various levels of leadership, supervisors and staff. Formal training is offered in multiple locations with oversight provided by the Air Education Training Command (AETC), the USAF School of Aerospace Medicine (USAFSAM), or AFMOA. In the Air Force, there are currently 107 courses addressing quality of care, among the over 228 formal courses identified. There are 48 courses in particular that dedicated 787 total hours to the study of quality.

The Air Force provides resources and training on quality of care and key quality programs to Airmen and personnel. Although Air Force medics of all ranks receive extensive quality training during their professional development, there is no specific policy requiring or defining that training. Formal courses designed for senior leaders provide the education and skills required to lead organizations in providing quality health care. Instruction on quality totaled over 52 hours in these courses with 875 personnel attending within the last three years. Medical Group (MDG) Commanders attend the AF Medical Service Group Commanders' Course, the University of Tennessee Lean Healthcare Leader's Course, and the MDG Commander Aerospace Medicine Workshop. Additionally, the Chief of Medical Staff Symposium, the Nursing Practice Oversight Council, both Intermediate Executive Skills Courses and the Chief Aeromedical Services & Advanced Flight Surgeon Symposium are required for personnel identified for leadership positions within AF MTFs. MDG Commanders and Group Superintendents also attend an additional 4-16 hours of training at the AFMS annual Leadership Symposium.

Airmen in mid-level leadership roles receive 8-12 hours of combined quality and patient safety training, whereas staff serving as Chief of Quality or Chief of the Medical Staff, attend Quality Systems Program Assessment Review (QSPAR) Symposium receiving up to 40 hours of accredited quality education. Dental leaders receive 4 hours of annual quality and patient safety instruction at the annual Dental Leadership Course. Finally, a majority of Airmen participate in accreditation preparation and receive training in The Joint Commission or AAAHC performance standards.

Training on quality in formal courses is also incorporated within various entry-level and advanced training courses for supervisors and staff. There are 48 courses with a total of 787 hours specifically dedicated to Quality. There were 14,925 members trained in those courses from FY11-FY13.

Medical Airmen also completed training with alternate methods using Computer-Based Training (CBT) through USAFSAM and SWANK. There are 51 courses offered through these platforms that specifically provided Quality training. Additionally, there are nine CBT courses available and tracked within the Advanced Distributive Learning System (ADLS). This system is the AF corporate solution for tracking training online. There were 68,515 instances that members accessed these courses in the last two years.

At the MTFs, those responsible in monitoring HEDIS® or ORYX® measure of care performance, receive targeted instruction, whereas National Surgical Quality Program (NSQIP®) participants attend annual conferences to learn from established sites. Likewise, all Air Force hospitals participate in the National Perinatal Information Center (NPIC) program and train personnel on interpretation of perinatal outcome data. Furthermore, in an effort to enhance care quality at MTFs, the Air Force has invested in simulation technology for Obstetrics providers, with modules covering various obstetrics topics.

Army Training

Army training efforts concerning topics related to quality of care is provided through a multi-tiered system and defined as training that focuses on evidence based practices and objective measures of performance such as: Joint Commission ORYX® Core Measures Set, National Perinatal Information Center Data, Healthcare Effectiveness Data and Information Set (HEDIS®) Measures, Patient Surveys, Primary Care Manager (PCM) Continuity, Accreditation, and Certification.

Annually, the Army Medical Command issues training requirements. Current mandatory quality of care training includes ten hours of initial (on-boarding) training, followed by approximately eight hours of training, to be conducted every three years. Furthermore, Individual Regional Medical Commands and MTFs may require additional periodic training at the discretion of Commander; often based on performance measures and command inspection findings. In an effort to ensure compliance with Army policies, the Army Digital Training Management System is used to monitor the training status of Army commanders, supervisors and staff. In the event of lack of compliance with training requirements, facility training office notifies noncompliant staff member and their supervisors. Furthermore, to ensure visibility of compliance levels, individual and unit training status levels are briefed to the commanders monthly.

The Army Medical Department Center and School (AMEDD CS) is the entity providing centralized training to commanders, supervisors, and staff. Since 2011, AMEDD CS has provided an average of 10,300 hours of advanced level "quality of care" training annually to 1,555 supervisory and command personnel. This is in addition to the MEDCOM universal mandatory training requirements.

Training efforts to enhance quality of care are supported via a robust MEDCOM LSS PI program. During the last four years, 420 personnel have completed Green Belt training and 198 Black Belt Training. There are 35 Master Black Belt trained personnel in MEDCOM to provide guidance and advice in process improvement. Improvement projects are shared via posting to the Army "PowerSteering" web site. Process improvement projects have focused on improving the Patient Centered Medical Home experience to improving the quality of care provided to Army health system beneficiaries.

Navy Training

BUMEDINST 6010.13 says, "Individuals responsible for QA program management must by afforded educational opportunities commensurate with their responsibilities. Education may be provided within the military our through civilian sponsored services. QA education for key program managers must be sufficient in scope and frequency to enable effective program oversight." Providing safe, quality care is paramount to Navy Medicine. Navy Medicine offers the following training specific to quality to its MTF personnel:

1. Annual Joint Commission/Navy training. Audience includes staff working in patient safety, quality improvement, risk management, and the medical staff.
2. In 2012, all MTF quality staff had access to the Institute for Healthcare Improvement (IHI) open school. Numerous quality courses were offered; the ability to track course completion was not available.
3. Each year the Nurse Corps selects and sends one officer to The Joint Commission for a one-year fellowship. Follow-on tours are at the regions or Medical Centers (MEDCEN). Fellows survey each MTF in their AOR in between TJC triennial survey (and as needed) to assess compliance with standards. This initiative helps to provide an assessment of quality and sharing of best practices.
4. Navy has a robust Lean Six Sigma program. Navy Medicine's Lean Six Sigma program was launched in 2006 pursuant to higher authority directives from the Deputy Secretary of Defense, Secretary of the Navy, and Secretary of Defense. Navy Medicine's Lean Six Sigma program is structured to provide both training and mentoring throughout the Navy Medicine enterprise. The Bureau of Medicine and Surgery (BUMED) Office of Strategy Management serves as the Program Executive Office responsible for setting policy, development of standard operating procedures, training support, curriculum management, staff certification, financial validation, website development, and software management for the program. In addition, BUMED directs coordination and alignment with other process improvement entities at the BUMED, Tri-Service, and Department of the Navy levels.
    a. The Lean Six Sigma governing structure includes senior military members that serve as the Regional Black Belts, providing oversight and direction of the Lean Six Sigma activities at the respective region; and Master Black Belt's that serve as process experts and technical advisors on project management, tool selection, and statistical analysis.
    b. As of 1 July 2013, the Lean Six Sigma program has achieved a 1:11.4 program Return on Investment with more than $239 million in cost avoidance and cost savings. All enterprise projects launched in FY 14 align with one of the BUMED Strategic Planning goals of Readiness, Value and Jointness.
    c. As of July 2014, 340 Lean Six Sigma projects have been completed with a validated cost avoidance/cost savings of more than $239 million. There are currently 45 active Lean Six Sigma projects in progress that target improving patient safety, quality of care, clinical efficiency, and standardization throughout the Navy Medicine enterprise.

d. Navy Medicine has a total of eleven staff members that provide full time support to the Lean Six Sigma program; BUMED-5 total; NME-3 total; NMW-3 total. The staff serves as Regional Black Belts, Master Black Belts, Black Belts, and administrative support staff for training, software management, program communication and logistics.
e. The Lean Six Sigma training curriculum provides participants advanced knowledge on value stream mapping of the current and future state, risk prioritization, continuous process flow, Failure Mode Effects Analysis (FMEA), data analysis, statistical process control, mistake proofing, visual cuing and process standardization. A total of 2,815 Navy Medicine staff have been trained including 1,140 Champions, 185 Black Belts and 1,490 Green Belts. Additionally, 30,969 CEUs and 3677 CMEs have been awarded. The goal of the training program has been to infuse a culture of continuous improvement throughout the Navy Medicine enterprise.

5. Other available training is addressed in the safety working group but also ties into quality. It includes TapRooT®, AHRQ TeamSTEPPS®, and Systems Engineering Initiative for Patient Safety (SEIPS) training.

Ongoing Bureau of Medicine and Surgery Patient Safety/Quality Management/Risk Management Department provides training in the following:
1. Monthly infection prevention video teleconferences (VTC)
2. Bi-monthly patient safety/risk/quality management VTCs
3. Quarterly VTCs for the Executive Committee of the Medical Staff and medical staff coordinators.
4. Training/education is provided to the Senior Nurse Executives as needed/requested.

Additional training is provided by the MTF to staff; the specifics of MTF training are not available at the headquarters level. There is no standardization of quality training requirements for the Navy.

Purchased Care Education and Training

The contractors are required to maintain qualified and experienced key personnel to meet the requirements of their contract. This is accomplished through the Clinical Quality Management Program plan, which provides the staff qualifications and responsibilities required.

Appendix 4.4
Data Review: Supporting Data and Figures

Accreditation and Certifications – Supporting Tables and Figures

Table 4.4-1 Number of Accreditations and Certifications by Type and Service

Service	TJC	AAAHC	Lab & Blood Bank[3]	Radiology & Nuclear Medicine	Subspecialties	Advanced Medical and Dental Education
Air Force	13	63	110	70	23	47
Army	30	-	42	23	6	29
Navy	27	-	62	1	9	27
NCR	2	-	7	5	3	7
Total	72	63	221	99	41	110

2014 MHS Review Group

HEDIS® Measures of Performance - Supporting Tables and Figures

Table 4.4-2 HEDIS® rating based on NCQA benchmark

HEDIS® rating based on NCQA benchmark	
Star Rating	Percentile
★★★★★	At or above the 90th Percentile
★★★★	Between the 75th and 89th Percentile
★★★	Between the 50th and 74th Percentile
★★	Between the 25th and 49th Percentile
★	Below the 25th Percentile

2014 MHS Review Group
Source: MHS Population Health Portal, June 2014

---

[3] Reported number of accredited laboratories at MTFs, not the number of accredited MTFs.

Table 4.4-3 Percent of Eligible Patients Receiving Select Care Measures, External Comparison: MHS vs. HEDIS® (2010 - 2013)

HEDIS® Measures	2010	2011	2012	2013	% Change in Rate (12 to 13)	HMO Nat'l Avg. (12)	HEDIS® Benchmark Status (13)
Antidepressant Medication Management: Acute Phase	64.98	66.22	65.68	68.51	2.83	69.1	★★★
Antidepressant Medication Management: Continuation Phase	41.64	43.27	42.68	46.08	3.4	53.6	★★
Use of Appropriate Medications for People With Asthma: Overall Rate	97.29	96.42	95.78	94.71	-1.07	91.2	★★★★
Breast Cancer Screening	70.57	69.09	69.13	68.88	-0.26	70.3	★★
Cervical Cancer Screening	79.87	79.69	78.75	76.87	-1.88	75.5	★★
Chlamydia Screening	67.34	64.3	60.82	59.72	-1.11	45.1	★★★★
Cholesterol Management for Patients with Cardiovascular Conditions (LDL-C Control)	55.36	56.55	56.7	59.57	2.87	59.9	★★
Cholesterol Management for Patients with Cardiovascular Conditions (LDL-C Screening)	77.97	76.38	78.15	77.56	-0.59	88.3	★
Colorectal Cancer Screening	67.61	68.7	68.1	69.82	1.72	63.3	★★★★
Diabetes HbA1c <=9	76.82	76.82	77.24	78.2	0.96	71.5	★★★
Comprehensive Diabetes Care: HbA1c <7 percent for a Selected Population	52.21	53.27	53.39	53.53	0.14	43.2	★★★★★
Comprehensive Diabetes Care: Good Glycemic Control (HbA1c <8 percent)	69.38	69.6	69.23	70.38	1.15	61.3	★★★★
Diabetes HbA1c Screening	83.87	83.78	84.4	84.89	0.49	87.2	★
Comprehensive Diabetes Care: LDL Cholesterol Control (<100 mg/dL)	53.67	54.91	52.99	55.8	2.81	48.4	★★★★
Comprehensive Diabetes Care: LDL Cholesterol Screening	80.13	80.12	80.41	80.69	0.29	85.4	★
Follow-Up After Hospitalization for Mental Illness: Within 30 Days Post-Discharge	74.92	77.23	78.46	74.84	-3.62	76.0	★★
Follow-Up After Hospitalization for Mental Illness: Within 7 Days Post-Discharge	55.38	59.6	62.79	58.46	-4.33	57.9	★★
Well-Child Visits (Ages 0–15 Months): Six or More Well-Child Visits	62.7	68.75	73.86	79.15	5.3	78.2	★★

Green – indicates positive change with statistical significance
Red – indicates negative change with statistical significance
No color – indicates lack of statistical significance
2014 MHS Review Group
Source: MHS Population Health Portal, June 2014

Table 4.4-4 Service Level & Purchased Care HEDIS® Performance (2013)

HEDIS Measures	Air Force	Army	Navy	NCR	TRO
Antidepressant Medication Management: Acute Phase	★★★★★	★★	★★★	★★★★	★★★
Antidepressant Medication Management: Continuation Phase	★★★	★	★★	★★★	★★★
Use of Appropriate Medications for People With Asthma: Overall Rate	★★★★★	★★★★★	★★★★	★★★★★	★★★
Breast Cancer Screening	★★★	★★★★	★★★★	★★★	★
Cervical Cancer Screening	★★★	★★★★★	★★★★★	★★★★	★
Chlamydia Screening	★★★★	★★★★★	★★★★★	★★★★	
Cholesterol Management	★★	★★	★★★★	★★★	
Cholesterol Screening	★	★	★★	★	★
Colorectal Cancer Screening	★★★★	★★★★★	★★★★★	★★★★★	★★★
Comprehensive Diabetes Care: Poor Glycemic Control (HbA1c >9 percent)— Lower rates signify better performance	★★	★★★	★★★★	★★★★	
Comprehensive Diabetes Care: HbA1c <7 percent for a Selected Population	★★★★★	★★★★★	★★★★★	★★★★★	
Comprehensive Diabetes Care: Good Glycemic Control (HbA1c <8 percent)	★★★★	★★★★	★★★★★	★★★★★	
Comprehensive Diabetes Care: HbA1c Screening	★★	★★	★★★	★★	★
Comprehensive Diabetes Care: LDL Cholesterol Control (<100 mg/dL)	★★★★	★★★★	★★★★★	★★★★	
Comprehensive Diabetes Care: LDL Cholesterol Screening	★★	★★★	★★★★	★★	★
Follow-Up After Hospitalization for Mental Illness: Within 30 Days Post-Discharge	★★	★★★★	★★★	★★	★
Follow-Up After Hospitalization for Mental Illness: Within 7 Days Post-Discharge	★★	★★★★	★★★★	★★	★
Well-Child Visits (Ages 0–15 Months): Six or More Well-Child Visits	★★	★★	★★	★★	★★

2014 MHS Review Group
Source: MHS Population Health Portal, June 2014

Table 4.4-5 HEDIS® Measures: CONUS – OCONUS

HEDIS® Measures (CONUS/OCONUS)	2013 OCONUS (percent of Patients)	Change in Rate (2012 to 2013) OCONUS	2013 Star Rating OCONUS	2013 CONUS (percent of Patients)	Percent Change in Rate (2012 to 2013) CONUS	2013 Star Rating CONUS
Antidepressant Medication Management: Acute Phase	64.01	3.79	★★	68.75	2.79	★★★
Antidepressant Medication Management: Continuation Phase	40.77	4.58	★	46.37	3.35	★★
Use of Appropriate Medications for People With Asthma: Asthma Medication Rate	95.33	-1.43	★★★★★	94.68	-1.06	★★★★
Breast Cancer Screening	65.8	-3.58	★	68.95	-0.18	★★
Cervical Cancer Screening	84.6	-4.51	★★★★★	76.44	-1.76	★★
Chlamydia Screening in Women: Total Rate	66.11	1.28	★★★★★	59.12	-1.33	★★★★
Cholesterol Management for Patients with Cardiovascular Conditions: LDL Control (<100 mg/dL)	60.04	11.49	★★	59.56	2.78	★★
Cholesterol Management for Patients with Cardiovascular Conditions: LDL Cholesterol Screening	84.99	3.83	★	77.47	-0.67	★
Colorectal Cancer Screening	67.82	-4.7	★	69.86	1.77	★★★★
Comprehensive Diabetes Care: Poor Glycemic Control (HbA1c >9 percent)—Lower rates signify better performance	79.17	4.56	★★★★	78.16	0.89	★★★
Comprehensive Diabetes Care: HbA1c <7 percent for a Selected Population	50.14	-2.12	★★★★★	53.64	0.23	★★★★
Comprehensive Diabetes Care: Good Glycemic Control (HbA1c <8 percent)	69.31	2.7	★★★★	70.41	1.14	★★★★
Comprehensive Diabetes Care: HbA1c Screening	89.63	5.16	★★	84.79	0.4	★
Comprehensive Diabetes Care: LDL Cholesterol Control (<100 mg/dL)	54.12	12.28	★★★★	55.86	2.69	★★★★
Comprehensive Diabetes Care: LDL Cholesterol Screening	86.82	4.91	★★★	80.58	0.18	★
Follow-Up After Hospitalization for Mental Illness: Within 30 Days Post-Discharge	94.63	0.41	★★★★★	74.08	-3.78	★★
Follow-Up After Hospitalization for Mental Illness: Within 7 Days Post-Discharge	89.27	0.12	★★★★★	57.29	-4.52	★★
Well-Child Visits (Ages 0–15 Months): Six or More Well-Child Visits	80.9	8.42	★★	79.02	5.07	★★

2014 MHS Review Group
Source: MHS Population Health Portal, June 2014

Table 4.4-6 Percent of Eligible Purchased Care Patients Receiving Select Care Measures, External Comparison: MHS vs. HEDIS® (2010 – 2013)

HEDIS® Measures Purchased Care (TRO)	2010	2011	2012	2013	% Change in Rate (12 to 13)	HMO Nat'l Avg. (12)	HEDIS® Benchmark Status (13)
Antidepressant Medication Management: Acute Phase	63.61	64.77	64.75	68.78	4.03	69.1	
Antidepressant Medication Management: Continuation Phase	42.79	45.68	45.12	49.64	4.52	53.6	
Use of Appropriate Medications for People With Asthma: Overall Rate	97.2	94.75	94.4	92.68	-1.71	91.2	
Breast Cancer Screening	66.45	64.49	63.93	63.46	-0.47	70.3	★
Cervical Cancer Screening	71.9	71.38	70.13	68.9	-1.23	75.5	★
Cholesterol Screening	73.67	73.67	74.26	71.52	-2.74	88.3	★
Colorectal Cancer Screening	61.57	62.9	63.48	64.18	0.7	63.3	
Comprehensive Diabetes Care: HbA1c Screening	78.27	77.71	78.6	78.03	-0.57	87.2	★
Comprehensive Diabetes Care: LDL Cholesterol Screening	74.33	73.65	74.22	72.48	-1.73	85.4	★
Follow-Up After Hospitalization for Mental Illness: Within 30 Days Post-Discharge	63.21	61.82	61.92	57.4	-4.52	76.0	★
Follow-Up After Hospitalization for Mental Illness: Within 7 Days Post-Discharge	38.24	36.73	40.18	34.43	-5.74	57.9	★
Well-Child Visits (Ages 0–15 Months): Six or More Well-Child Visits	69.55	74.79	75.73	77.97	2.24	78.2	★★

Green – indicates positive change with statistical significance
Red – indicates negative change with statistical significance
No color – indicates lack of statistical significance
2014 MHS Review Group
Source: MHS Population Health Portal, June 2014

Table 4.4-7 Star Ratings for OCONUS from 2010 to 2013

HEDIS® Measures (OCONUS)	2010	2011	2012	2013	Change in Rate (12 to 13)	Current Rating
Antidepressant - Acute	60.98	61.54	60.23	64.01	3.79	★★
Antidepressant – Continuous	35.01	36.67	36.2	40.77	4.58	★
Asthma Appropriate Meds	96.67	97.67	96.76	95.33	-1.43	★★★★★
Breast Cancer Screening	69.02	67.22	69.38	65.8	-3.58	★
Cervical Cancer Screening	87.62	88.63	89.11	84.6	-4.51	★★★★★
Chlamydia Screening	70.3	67.62	64.84	66.11	1.28	★★★★★
Cholesterol Management	51.65	55.53	48.55	60.04	11.49	★★
Cholesterol Screening	80.92	80.58	81.16	84.99	3.83	★
Colorectal Cancer Screening	65.76	67.91	72.52	67.82	-4.7	

HEDIS® Measures (OCONUS)	2010	2011	2012	2013	Change in Rate (12 to 13)	Current Rating
Diabetes A1C <=9	74.44	74.31	74.61	79.17	4.56	★★★★
Diabetes A1C <7	46.29	48.41	52.27	50.14	-2.12	★★★★★
Diabetes A1C <8	65.21	65.62	66.61	69.31	2.7	★★★★
Diabetes A1C Screening	85.27	86.22	84.47	89.63	5.16	★★
Diabetes LDL Control	48.06	48.85	41.85	54.12	12.28	★★★★
Diabetes LDL Screening	81.94	83.82	81.91	86.82	4.91	★★★
Mental FU 30 Days	89.67	91.85	94.22	94.63	0.41	★★★★★
Mental FU 7 Days	83.37	85.05	89.15	89.27	0.12	★★★★★
Well Child >=6 Visits	59.55	63.12	72.48	80.9	8.42	★★★

Green – indicates positive change with statistical significance; Red – indicates negative change with statistical significance; No color – indicates lack of statistical significance
2014 MHS Review Group
Source: MHS Population Health Portal, June 2014

Table 4.4-8 Star Ratings for CONUS from 2010 to 2013

HEDIS® Measures (CONUS)	2010	2011	2012	2013	Change in Rate (2012 to 2013)	Current Rating
Antidepressant - Acute	65.24	66.48	65.96	68.75	2.79	★★★
Antidepressant – Continuous	42.07	43.64	43.02	46.37	3.35	★★
Asthma Appropriate Meds	97.32	96.36	95.74	94.68	-1.06	★★★★
Breast Cancer Screening	70.6	69.13	69.13	68.95	-0.18	★★
Cervical Cancer Screening	79.42	79.17	78.2	76.44	-1.76	★★
Chlamydia Screening	67.05	63.97	60.46	59.12	-1.33	★★★★
Cholesterol Management	55.41	56.57	56.77	59.56	2.78	★★
Cholesterol Screening	77.92	76.34	78.14	77.47	-0.67	★
Colorectal Cancer Screening	67.64	68.71	68.09	69.86	1.77	★★★★
Diabetes A1C <=9	76.9	76.91	77.28	78.16	0.89	★★★
Diabetes A1C <7	52.44	53.46	53.41	53.64	0.23	★★★★★
Diabetes A1C <8	69.52	69.74	69.27	70.41	1.14	★★★★
Diabetes A1C Screening	83.84	83.73	84.4	84.79	0.4	★
Diabetes LDL Control	53.86	55.11	53.17	55.86	2.69	★★★★
Diabetes LDL Screening	80.09	80.05	80.39	80.58	0.18	★
Mental FU 30 Days	74.5	76.65	77.87	74.08	-3.78	★★
Mental FU 7 Days	54.57	58.61	61.81	57.29	-4.52	★★
Well Child >=6 Visits	62.96	69.16	73.95	79.02	5.07	★★

Green – indicates positive change with statistical significance; Red – indicates negative change with statistical significance; No color – indicates lack of statistical significance
2014 MHS Review Group
Source: MHS Population Health Portal, June 2014

HEDIS® Methodological Considerations

There are mitigating factors that can account for some of the considerable lag between HEDIS® measure performance in the Purchased Care component compared to Direct Care. The Defense Enrollment

Eligibility Reporting System (DEERS) database captures information on beneficiary enrollment in TRICARE Prime and also on beneficiaries with Other Health Insurance (OHI). HEDIS® calculations are performed only on Prime enrollees and normally exclude patients with OHI. Previous MHS studies have shown that OHI documentation in DEERS, which is dependent on beneficiary self-reporting, is significantly understated resulting in an inflated denominator for various HEDIS® measures. Commercial health plans exclude beneficiaries with Primary OHI and use supplemental databases to capture clinical information about their enrolled population that would otherwise not be available. The MHS only uses financial claims data. Within the DHA, efforts are currently underway to improve the fidelity of OHI documentation and allow the regional contractors to use supplemental databases.

Quality of Care in the Purchased Care Component – Supporting Tables and Figures

Figure 4.4-1 displays the performance of TRICARE network hospitals compared to national benchmarks on Hospital Compare composite measure of performance.

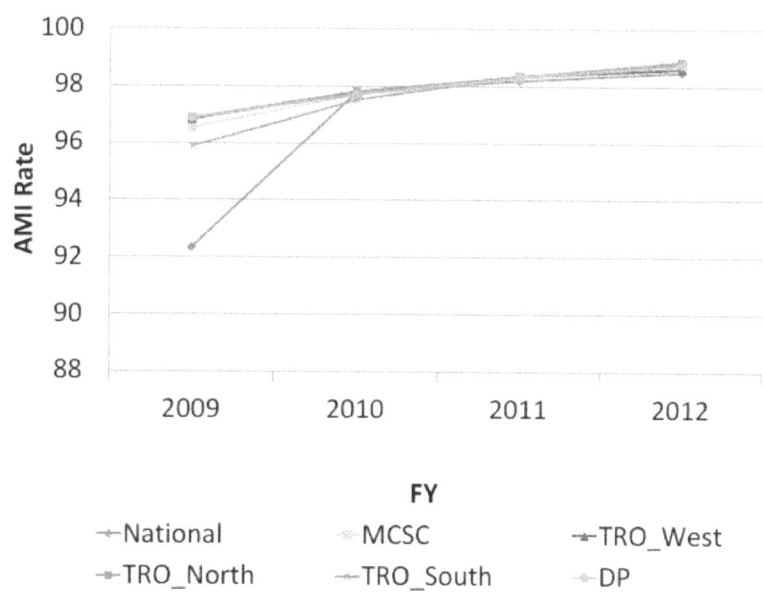

Figure 4.4-1 Hospital Compare Measures in Purchased Care Component

Figure 4.4-1a Purchased Care Acute Myocardial Infarction (AMI) Rate, FY09 – FY12

2014 MHS Review Group
Source: Centers for Medicare & and Medicaid Services, Hospital Compare Data File, June 2014; MHS Mart (M2) Comprehensive Ambulatory/Professional Encounters Record (CAPER), June 2014

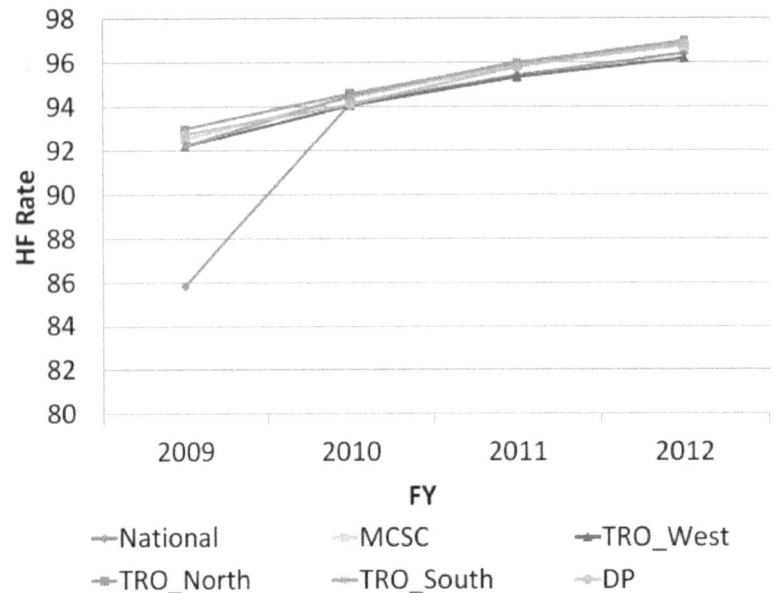

Figure 4.4-1b Purchased Care Heart Failure (HF) Rate, FY09 – FY12

2014 MHS Review Group
Source: Centers for Medicare & Medicaid Services, Hospital Compare Data File, June 2014; MHS Mart (M2) Comprehensive Ambulatory/Professional Encounters Record (CAPER), June 2014

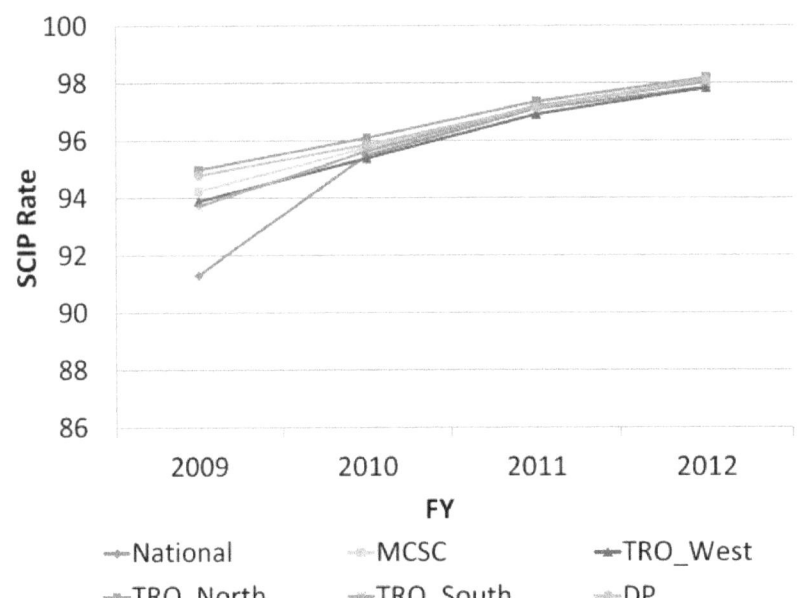

Figure 4.4-1c Purchased Care Surgical Care (SCIP) Rate, FY09 – FY12

2014 MHS Review Group
Source: Centers for Medicare & Medicaid Services, Hospital Compare Data File, June 2014; MHS Mart (M2) Comprehensive Ambulatory/Professional Encounters Record (CAPER), June 2014

Figure 4.4-1d Purchased Care Children's Asthma Care (CAC) Rate, FY09 – FY12

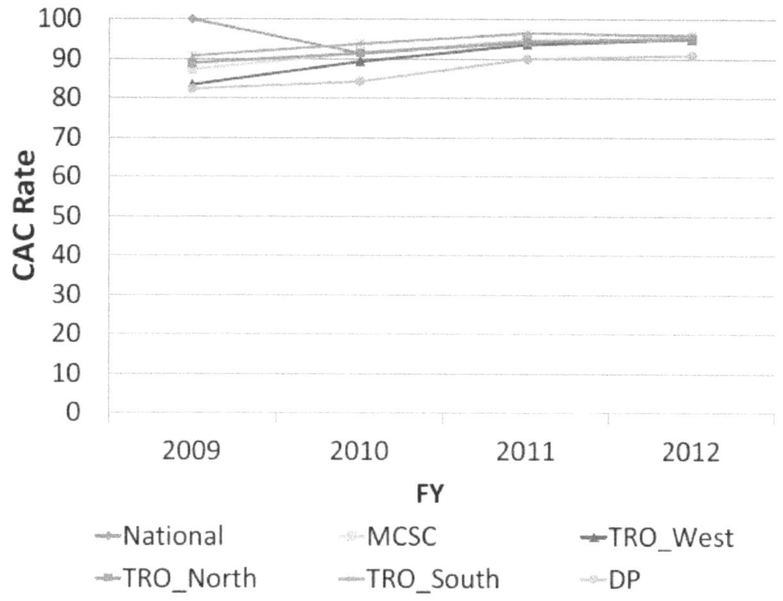

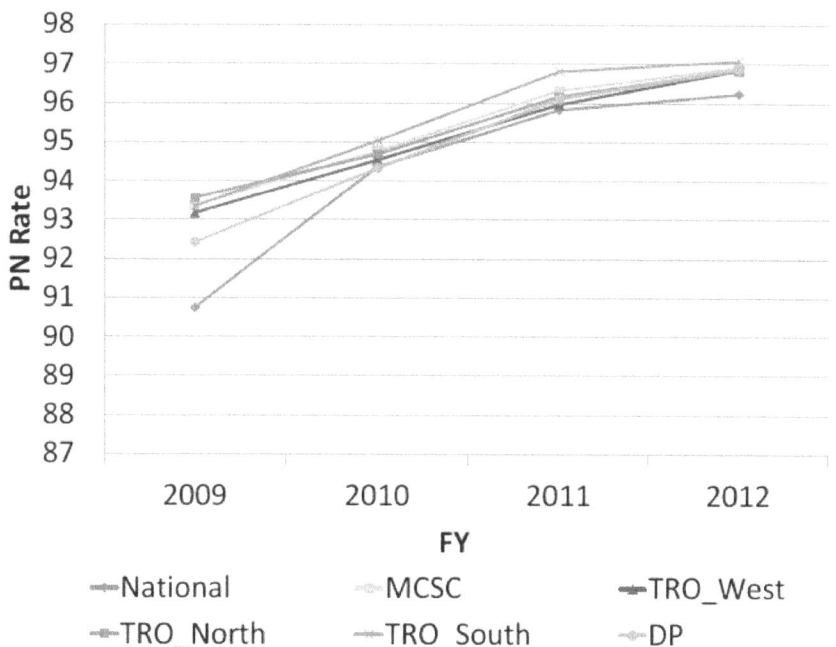

2014 MHS Review Group
Source: Centers for Medicare & Medicaid Services, Hospital Compare Data File, June 2014; MHS Mart (M2) Comprehensive Ambulatory/Professional Encounters Record (CAPER), June 2014

Figure 4.4-1e Purchased Care Pneumonia Rate, FY09 – FY12

2014 MHS Review Group
Source: Centers for Medicare & Medicaid Services, Hospital Compare Data File, June 2014; MHS Mart (M2) Comprehensive Ambulatory/Professional Encounters Record (CAPER), June 2014

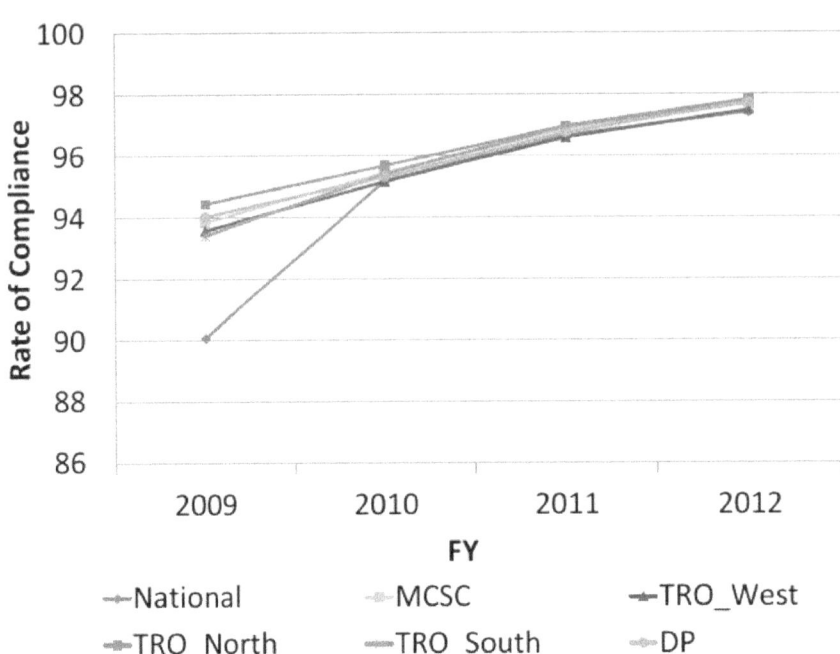

Figure 4.4-1f Purchased Overall Rate, FY09 – FY12

2014 MHS Review Group
Source: Centers for Medicare & Medicaid Services, Hospital Compare Data File, June 2014; MHS Mart (M2) Comprehensive Ambulatory/Professional Encounters Record (CAPER), June 2014

ORYX® – National Hospital Quality Measures – Supporting Tables and Figures

The figures below show 2010-2013 measures contributing to low composite measures for direct care when compared to national benchmarks.

Figure 4.4-2 TJC Oryx Core Measures

Figure 4.4-2a Primary Percutaneous Coronary Intervention (AMI-8a), FY10 – FY13

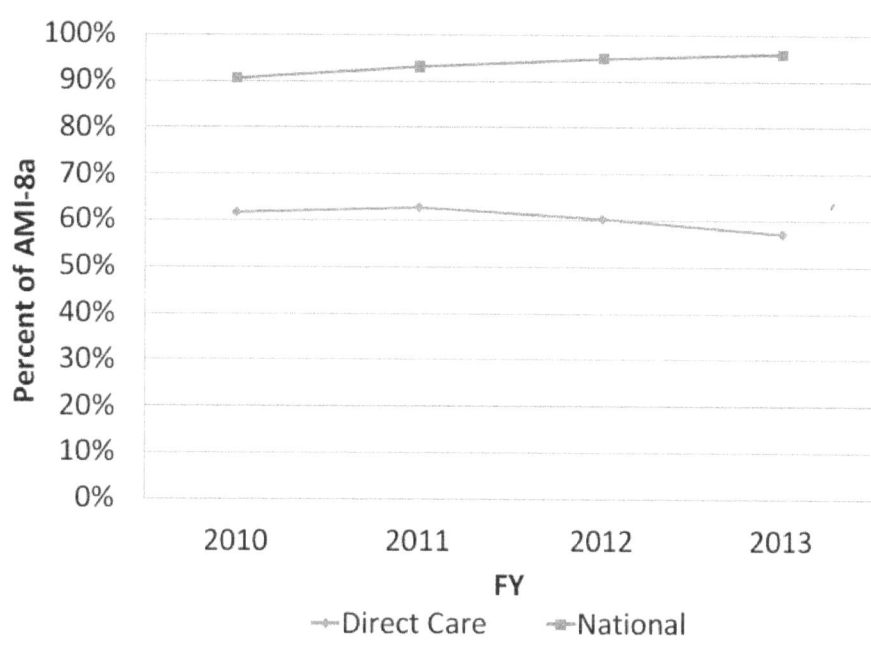

2014 MHS Review Group
Source: The Joint Commission National Hospital Accrediting Agency, July 2014. Data are displayed by fiscal year because the original data were provided in that form.

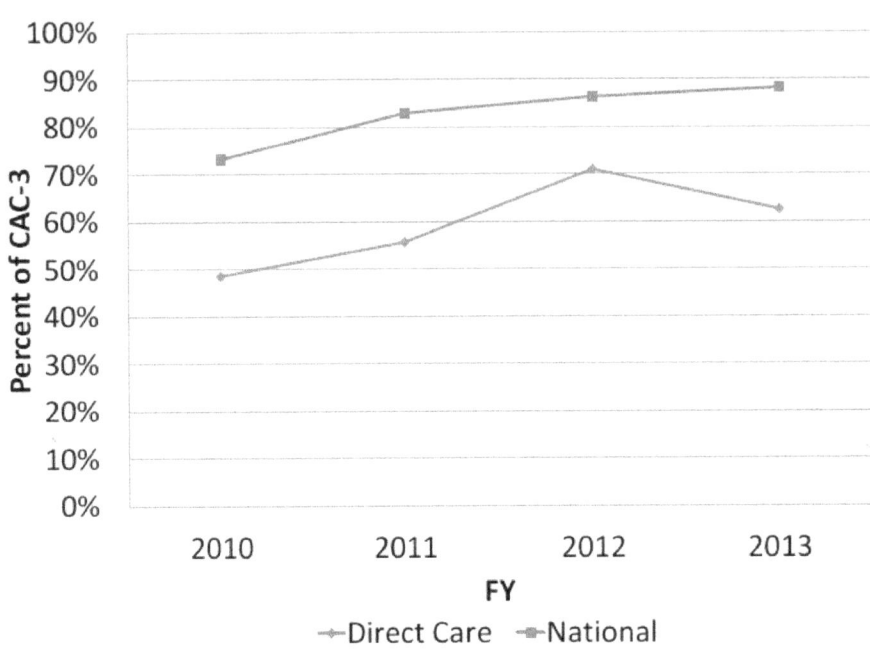

Figure 4.4-2b Home Management Plan of Care Given to Patient/Caregiver (CAC-3), FY10 – FY13

2014 MHS Review Group
Source: The Joint Commission National Hospital Accrediting Agency, July 2014. Data are displayed by fiscal year because the original data were provided in that form.

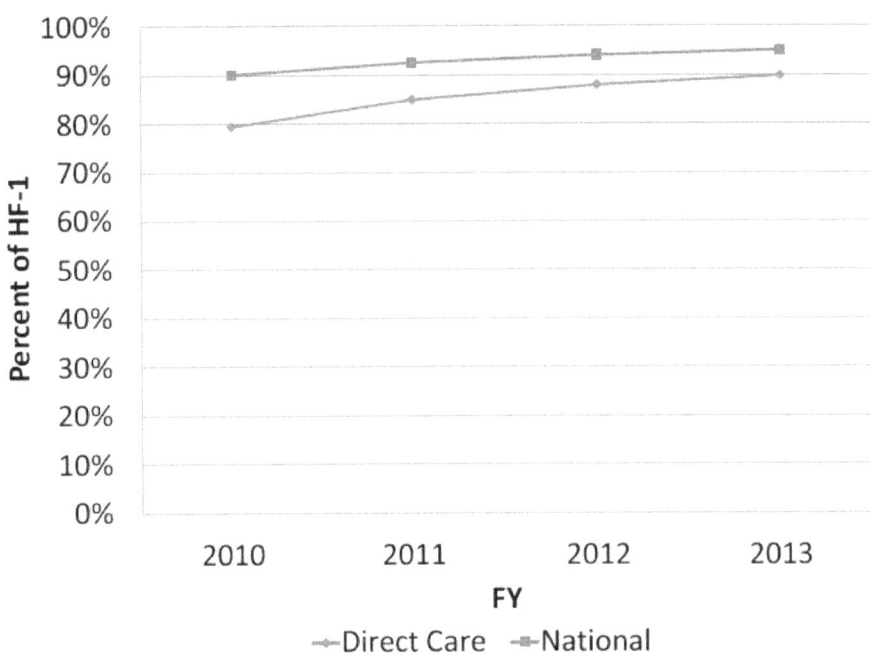

Figure 4.4-2c Discharge Instructions (HF-1), FY10 – FY13

2014 MHS Review Group
Source: The Joint Commission National Hospital Accrediting Agency, July 2014. Data are displayed by fiscal year because the original data were provided in that form.

Figure 4.4-2d Blood Cultures Performed in the ED prior to Initial Antibiotic in Hospital (PN-3b), FY10 – FY13

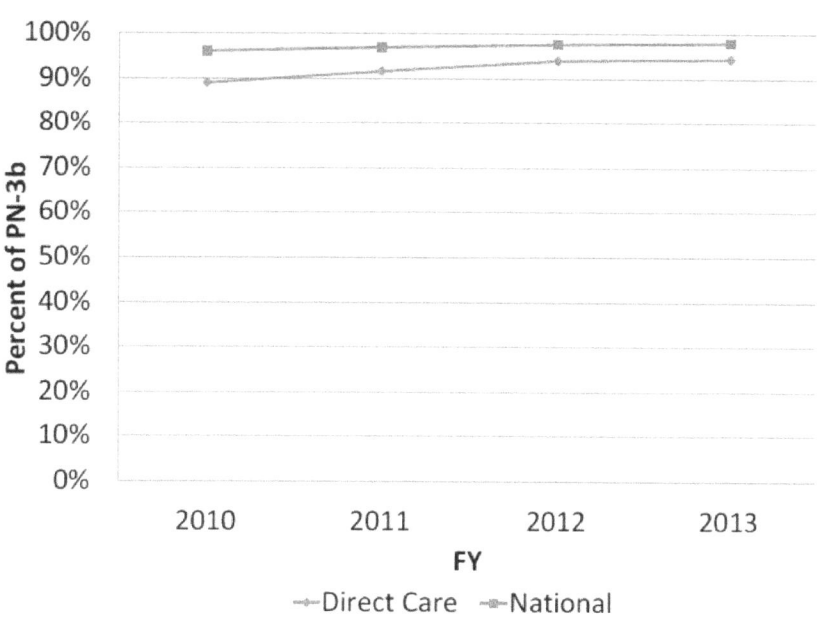

2014 MHS Review Group
Source: The Joint Commission National Hospital Accrediting Agency, July 2014. Data are displayed by fiscal year because the original data were provided in that form.

Figure 4.4-2e Surgery Patients on Beta-Blocker Therapy prior to Arrival Who Received a Beta-Blocker During the Perioperative Period (SCIP-Card2), FY10 – FY13

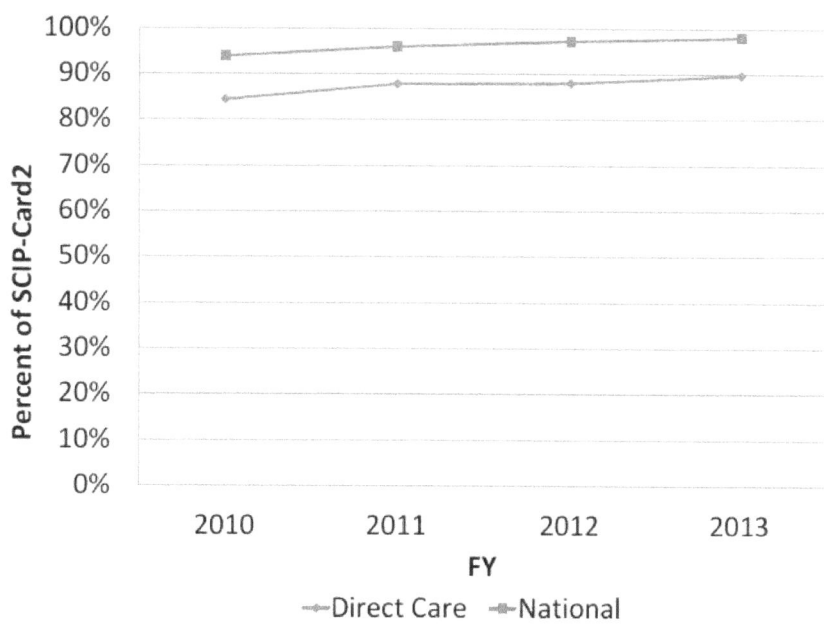

2014 MHS Review Group
Source: The Joint Commission National Hospital Accrediting Agency, July 2014. Data are displayed by fiscal year because the original data were provided in that form.

Figure 4.4-2f Prophylactic Antibiotic Selection for Surgical Patients (SCIP-2a), FY10 – FY13

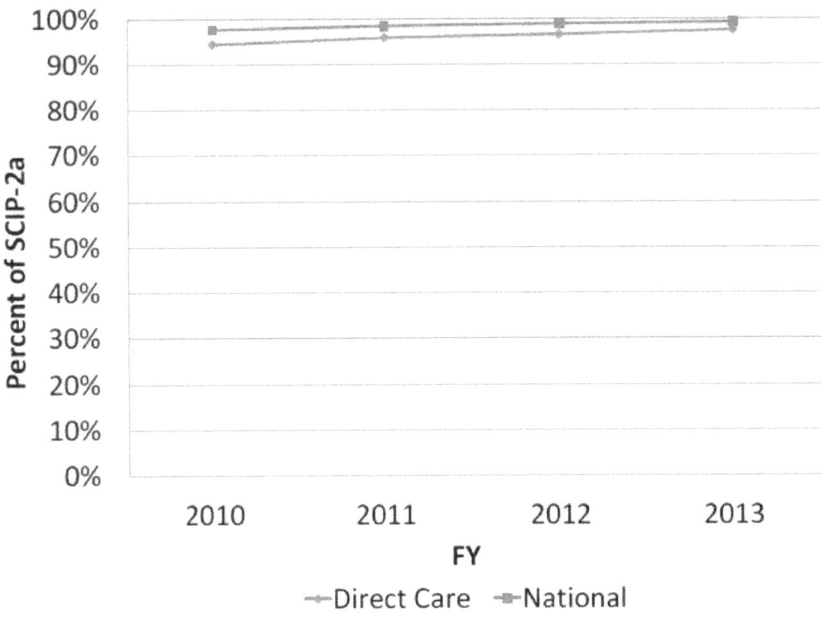

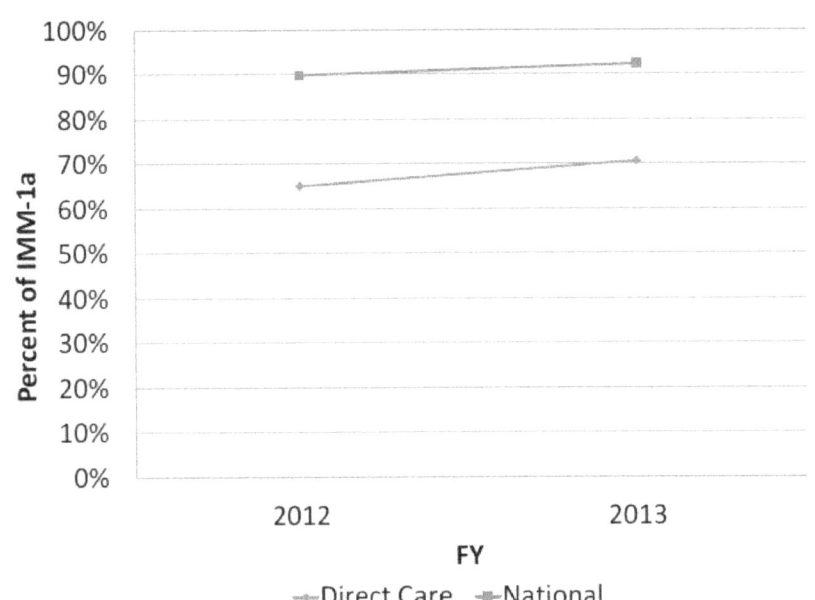

2014 MHS Review Group
Source: The Joint Commission National Hospital Accrediting Agency, July 2014. Data are displayed by fiscal year because the original data were provided in that form.

Figure 4.4-2g Pneumococcal Immunization (IMM-1a), FY12 – FY13

2014 MHS Review Group
Source: The Joint Commission National Hospital Accrediting Agency, July 2014. Data are displayed by fiscal year because the original data were provided in that form.

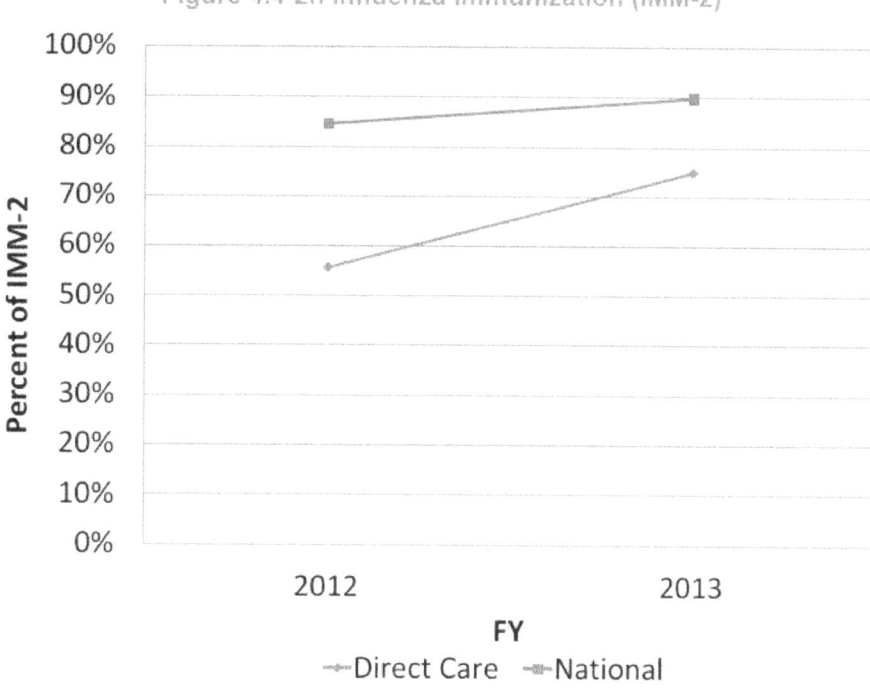

Figure 4.4-2h Influenza Immunization (IMM-2)

2014 MHS Review Group
Source: The Joint Commission National Hospital Accrediting Agency, July 2014. Data are displayed by fiscal year because the original data were provided in that form.

The table below provides more information on TJC definitions for common cause and special cause variation.

Table 4.4-9a ORYX® TJC Definitions

Common cause variation is the noise within the process and is characterized by:

    Phenomena constantly active with the process,

    Predictable variation within given limits,

    Expected variation within a historical experience base,

    Lack of significance in individual high or low values.

Unexpected special cause variation is characterized by:

    New, unanticipated, emergent, or previously neglected phenomena within the system,

    Variation inherently unpredictable,

    Unexpected variation outside the historical experience base, and

    Evidence of some inherent change in the system or our knowledge of it.

2014 MHS Review Group
Source: The Joint Commission National Hospital Accrediting Agency, February 2011

Table 4.4-9b ORYX® Index Score Criteria

Index Score	Meaning
3	Perfect score: meets measure 100% of time
2	> 3 standard deviations above the national average
1	Within +/- 3 standard deviations from the national average
0	> 3 standard deviations below the national average

2014 MHS Review Group
Source: DoD Joint Commission Core Measure Database, June 2014

The control limits describe the natural variability of a process over time. A process that is in statistical control can be further analyzed to determine whether performance is at an acceptable level. The control limits are set to three standard deviations above and below the center line. The upper control limit (UCL) is calculated by adding three times the standard deviation for the quarter to the national average. The lower control limit (LCL) is calculated by subtracting three times the standard deviation for the quarter from the national average. The target performance level for MTFs is an index score of one or greater.

Table 4.4-9c Direct Care Average Index Score

Measure	FY10	FY11	FY12	FY13	Status
AMI 1	1	1	1	2	E
AMI 2	1	0	1	0	N
AMI 3	2	2	1	2	E
AMI 5	1	0	1	0	N
AMI 7a	0	1	1	1	S
AMI 8a	0	0	0	0	N
AMI 10		1	1	1	S
CAC 1a	2	2	1	3	E
CAC 2a	1	1	0	1	S
CAC 3	0	0	0	0	N
HF 1	0	0	0	0	N
HF 2	1	0	0	1	S
HF 3	1	1	1	1	S
HBIPS 1a	ND	ND	3	2	E
HBIPS 4a	ND	ND	1	2	E
HBIPS 5a	ND	ND	1	1	S
HBIPS 6a	ND	ND	0	0	N
HBIPS 7a	ND	ND	1	0	N
OP 6	1	1	0	0	N
OP 7	1	1	1	1	S
PC 1	ND	ND	2	1	S

Measure	FY10	FY11	FY12	FY13	Status
PC 2	ND	ND	2	2	E
PC 3	ND	ND	1	0	N
PC 5	ND	ND	2	2	E
PN 3a	1	1	1	1	S
PN 3b	0	0	0	0	N
PN 6a	1	1	0	0	N
PN 6b	1	1	1	1	S
SCIP 1a	0	0	0	1	S
SCIP 2a	2	0	0	0	N
SCIP 3a	0	0	1	0	N
SCIP 4	1	0	1	1	S
SCIP 6	0	0	1	1	S
SCIP 9	2	0	1	1	S
SCIP Card 2	0	0	0	0	N
SCIP VTE 2	1	0	0	0	N
STK 1	ND	ND	3	2	E
STK 2	ND	ND	3	3	E
STK 3	ND	ND	2	3	E
STK 4	ND	ND	2	3	E
STK 5	ND	ND	3	3	E
STK 6	ND	ND	2	3	E
STK 8	ND	ND	2	1	S
STK 10	ND	ND	1	2	E
VTE 1	ND	1	2	2	E
VTE 2	ND	1	1	1	S
VTE 3	ND	2	1	1	S
VTE 4	ND	2	2	3	E
VTE 5	ND	0	0	1	S
VTE 6	ND	2	2	1	S
IMM 1a	ND	ND	0	0	N
IMM 2	ND	ND	0	0	N
SUB 1	ND	ND	1	0	N
SUB 2	ND	ND	2	1	S
SUB 3	ND	ND	1	1	S
SUB 4	ND	ND	1	1	S
TOB 1	ND	ND	1	1	S
TOB 2	ND	ND	1	1	S

Measure	FY10	FY11	FY12	FY13	Status
TOB 3	ND	ND	1	1	S
TOB 4	ND	ND	2	1	S

Statistical comparison is done on rate measures only, ED measures are continuous

E = Exceeding
S = Showing improvement or meeting target
N = Needs Improvement

Index Score	Meaning
3	Perfect score: meets measure 100% of time
2	> 3 standard deviations above the national average
1	Within +/- 3 standard deviations from the national average
0	> 3 standard deviations below the national average

2014 MHS Review Group; ND indicates No Data.
Source: DoD Joint Commission Core Measure Database, June 2014

Table 4.4-10 provides a description of each measure set to include AMI, CAC, HBIPS, HF, OP, PC, PN, SCIP, STK, VTE, IMM, and SUB.

Table 4.4-10 TJC Oryx® Measures

Measure Set	Measure	Description
Acute Myocardial Infarction	AMI1	Aspirin at Arrival
Acute Myocardial Infarction	AMI2	Aspirin Prescribed at Discharge
Acute Myocardial Infarction	AMI3	ACEI or ARB for LVSD
Acute Myocardial Infarction	AMI5	Beta-Blocker Prescribed at Discharge
Acute Myocardial Infarction	AMI7a	Fibrinolytic Therapy Received Within 30 Minutes of Hospital Arrival
Acute Myocardial Infarction	AMI8a	Primary PCI Received Within 90 Minutes of Hospital Arrival
Acute Myocardial Infarction	AMI10	Statins Prescribed at Discharge
Children's Asthma Care	CAC1a	Relievers for Inpatient Asthma (age 2 years through 17 years) – Overall Rate
Children's Asthma Care	CAC2a	Systemic Corticosteroids for Inpatient Asthma (age 2 years through 17years) – Overall Rate
Children's Asthma Care	CAC3	Home Management Plan of Care (HMPC) Document Given to Patient/Caregiver

Measure Set	Measure	Description
Hospital-Based Inpatient Psychiatric Services	HBIPS1a	Admission Screening for Violence Risk, Substance Use, Psychological Trauma History and Patient Strengths Completed - Overall Rate
Hospital-Based Inpatient Psychiatric Services	HBIPS4a	Patients Discharged on Multiple Antipsychotic Medications - Overall Rate
Hospital-Based Inpatient Psychiatric Services	HBIPS5a	Patients Discharged on Multiple Antipsychotic Medications with Appropriate Justification - Overall Rate
Hospital-Based Inpatient Psychiatric Services	HBIPS6a	Post Discharge Continuing Care Plan Created - Overall Rate
Hospital-Based Inpatient Psychiatric Services	HBIPS7a	Post Discharge Continuing Care Plan Transmitted to Next Level of Care Provider Upon Discharge - Overall Rate
Heart Failure	HF1	Discharge Instructions
Heart Failure	HF2	Evaluation of LVS Function
Heart Failure	HF3	ACEI or ARB for LVSD
Hospital Outpatient Department	OP6	Prophylactic Antibiotic Initiated Within One Hour Prior to Surgical Incision
Hospital Outpatient Department	OP7	Prophylactic Antibiotic Selection for Surgical Patients
Perinatal Care	PC1	Elective Delivery
Perinatal Care	PC2	Cesarean Section - Overall Rate
Perinatal Care	PC3	Antenatal Steroids
Perinatal Care	PC5	Exclusive Breast Milk Feeding
Pneumonia	PN3a	Blood Cultures Performed Within 24 Hours Prior to or 24 Hours After Hospital Arrival for Patients Who Were Transferred or Admitted to the ICU Within 24 Hours of Hospital Arrival
Pneumonia	PN3b	Blood Cultures Performed in the Emergency Department Prior to Initial Antibiotic Received in Hospital
Pneumonia	PN6a	Initial Antibiotic Selection for Community-Acquired Pneumonia (CAP) in Immunocompetent Patients – ICU Patients
Pneumonia	PN6b	Initial Antibiotic Selection for Community-Acquired Pneumonia (CAP) in Immunocompetent Patients – Non-ICU Patients
Surgical Care Improvement Project	SCIP1a	Prophylactic Antibiotic Received Within One Hour Prior to Surgical Incision - Overall Rate
Surgical Care Improvement Project	SCIP2a	Prophylactic Antibiotic Selection for Surgical Patients - Overall Rate
Surgical Care Improvement Project	SCIP3a	Prophylactic Antibiotics Discontinued Within 24 Hours After Surgery End Time - Overall Rate

Appendix 4. Quality of Care

Measure Set	Measure	Description
Surgical Care Improvement Project	SCIP4	Cardiac Surgery Patients with Controlled 6 A.M. Postoperative Blood Glucose
Surgical Care Improvement Project	SCIP6	Surgery Patients with Appropriate Hair Removal
Surgical Care Improvement Project	SCIP9	Urinary Catheter Removed on Postoperative Day 1 (POD 1) or Postoperative Day 2 (POD 2) with Day of Surgery Being Day Zero
Surgical Care Improvement Project	SCIPCard2	Surgery Patients on Beta-Blocker Therapy Prior to Admission Who Received a Beta-Blocker During the Perioperative Period
Surgical Care Improvement Project	SCIPVTE2	Surgery Patients Who Received Appropriate Venous Thromboembolism Prophylaxis Within 24 Hours Prior to Surgery to 24 Hours After Surgery
Stroke	STK1	Stroke Patients with DVT Prophylaxis
Stroke	STK2	Discharged on Antithrombotic Therapy
Stroke	STK3	Anticoagulation Therapy for Atrial Fibrillation/Flutter
Stroke	STK4	Thrombolytic Therapy
Stroke	STK5	Antithrombiotic Therapy by End of Hospital Day Two
Stroke	STK6	Discharged on Statin Medication
Stroke	STK8	Stroke Education
Stroke	STK10	Assessed for Rehabilitation
Venous Thromboembolism	VTE1	VTE Prophylaxis
Venous Thromboembolism	VTE2	ICU VTE Prophylaxis
Venous Thromboembolism	VTE3	VTE Patients With Anticoagulation Overlap Therapy
Venous Thromboembolism	VTE4	VTE Patients Receiving UFH with Dosages/Platelet Count Monitoring by Protocol or Nomogram
Venous Thromboembolism	VTE5	VTE Discharge Instructions
Venous Thromboembolism	VTE6	Incidence of Potentially Preventable VTE
Immunization	IMM1a	Pneumococcal Immunization (PPV23) - Overall Rate
Immunization	IMM2	Influenza Immunization
Substance Use	SUB1	Alcohol Use Screening
Substance Use	SUB2	Alcohol Use Brief Intervention Provided or Offered
Substance Use	SUB3	Alcohol and Other Drug Use Disorder Treatment Provided or Offered at Discharge

Measure Set	Measure	Description
Substance Use	SUB4	Alcohol and Drug Use: Assessing Status after Discharge
Tobacco Treatment	TOB1	Tobacco Use Screening
Tobacco Treatment	TOB2	Tobacco Use Treatment Provided or Offered
Tobacco Treatment	TOB3	Tobacco Use Treatment Provided or Offered at Discharge
Tobacco Treatment	TOB4	Tobacco Use: Assessing Status after Discharge

2014 MHS Review Group
Source: DoD Joint Commission Core Measure Database, June 2014

Table 4.4-11 shows direct care performance (N=55) on 16 core measures for 4Q2012-3Q2013.

Appendix 4. Quality of Care

Table 4.4-11 MTF ORYX® Core Measure Status for 4Q 2012 – 3Q2013

MTF	AMI	CAC	HF	HBIPS	OP	PC	PN	SCIP	STK	VTE	IMM	SUB	TOB
31 MDG - Aviano AB	---	---	---	---	---	S	---	S	---	N	N	---	---
96 MDG - Eglin AFB	S	E	E	---	---	S	E	E	---	E	---	---	---
3 MDG - Elmendorf AFB	S	---	E	---	---	S	E	E	---	S	---	---	---
81 MDG - Keesler AFB	S	E	E	---	E	S	E	E	---	---	---	---	---
48 MDG - Lakenheath AB	---	E	---	---	S	S	S	E	---	N	---	---	---
1 MDG - Langley AFB	S	E	S	---	N	S	E	E	---	S	---	---	---
35 MDG - Misawa AB	---	E	---	---	---	S	N	E	---	N	S	---	S
366 MDG - Mountain Home AFB	---	---	E	---	---	S	N	E	---	N	N	---	---
99 MDG - Nellis AFB	S	E	S	N	---	S	E	E	---	E	---	---	---
51 MDG - Osan AB	---	---	---	---	---	---	S	N	---	S	N	N	S
60 MDG - Travis AFB	S	E	S	S	---	S	E	S	---	E	---	---	---
88 MDG - Wright-Patterson AFB	S	---	E	---	---	S	S	S	---	E	---	---	---
374 MDG - Yokota AB	---	E	---	---	---	S	N	S	---	N	---	---	S
Bassett ACH	---	E	S	---	---	S	S	E	---	S	---	---	---
Bayne-Jones ACH	---	E	E	---	---	S	S	E	---	S	---	---	---
Wm Beaumont AMC	S	E	E	E	---	N	S	S	---	E	---	---	---
Blanchfield ACH	S	E	E	---	---	S	E	E	---	---	---	---	---
Brooke AMC	S	E	E	S	N	S	S	S	E	N	---	N	N
Darnall ACH	N	E	E	S	---	S	S	S	---	---	---	---	---
D. Eisenhower AMC	S	E	E	S	---	---	S	S	---	E	---	---	---
Evans ACH	---	E	S	---	---	S	S	N	---	E	---	---	---
Ireland ACH	---	E	S	---	---	S	S	S	---	S	---	---	---
Irwin ACH	---	E	---	---	E	S	S	S	---	---	---	---	---
Keller ACH	---	E	---	---	---	S	S	S	---	N	N	---	---
Madigan AMC	S	E	S	S	---	S	S	S	---	E	---	---	---
Martin ACH	S	E	E	S	---	S	S	E	---	E	---	---	---
Moncrief ACH	---	---	---	S	E	---	N	E	---	S	---	---	---
Reynolds ACH	S	E	E	---	---	N	S	S	---	---	---	---	---
Tripler AMC	S	E	E	S	---	S	S	S	---	E	---	---	---
Winn ACH	N	E	E	E	E	S	S	S	---	---	---	---	---
Brian Allgood Medical Center	---	E	---	S	---	S	S	S	---	S	---	---	---
Landstuhl AMC	S	E	E	E	---	S	E	E	---	---	---	---	---
Weed ACH	---	E	---	---	---	N	N	E	---	N	N	---	---
Womack AMC	S	E	S	S	---	S	E	S	---	E	---	---	---
Gen L. Wood ACH	N	E	E	E	---	N	E	E	---	S	---	---	---
NH Beaufort	---	---	---	---	E	---	S	S	---	N	N	---	---
NH Bremerton	S	E	E	---	---	S	E	E	---	S	N	---	---
NH Camp LeJeune	S	E	S	S	---	S	E	S	---	S	---	---	---
NH Camp Pendleton	---	E	E	---	S	S	E	E	---	---	---	---	---
USNH Guam	---	---	E	---	---	S	E	E	---	E	---	---	---
USNH Guantanamo Bay	---	---	---	---	---	S	N	S	---	N	N	---	S
NH Jacksonville	S	E	E	---	---	N	E	S	---	---	---	---	---
NH Lemoore	---	E	---	---	---	N	N	E	---	N	---	N	S
USNH Naples	---	---	---	---	---	N	---	E	---	N	---	---	---
NH Oak Harbor	---	---	---	---	---	N	---	E	---	N	---	---	---
USNH Okinawa	N	E	E	S	---	S	E	E	---	S	---	S	---
NH Pensacola	S	---	S	---	---	S	E	E	---	E	---	---	---
NMC Portsmouth	S	E	E	S	---	N	S	S	---	---	---	---	S
USNH Rota	---	E	E	---	---	N	---	S	---	N	S	---	---
NMC San Diego	S	E	E	S	---	S	E	E	---	E	---	---	---
USNH Sigonella	---	---	---	---	---	S	---	S	---	N	N	---	S
NH Twentynine Palms	---	S	---	---	---	S	S	E	---	N	---	---	S
USNH Yokosuka	N	E	E	---	---	S	S	E	---	E	---	---	S
Ft Belvoir Community Hospital	S	S	E	S	---	S	E	S	---	E	---	---	---
Walter Reed NMMC - Bethesda	S	E	E	S	---	S	E	E	---	E	---	---	---

Bold MTFs have no composite measures needing improvement when statistically compared to national benchmarks

E = Excelling   S = Showing improvement or meeting target   N = Need improvement

2014 MHS Review Group; Source: DoD Joint Commission Core Measure Database: June 2014

Table 4.4-12 shows TJC Direct Care Top Performers for 2010-2012. These facilities maintained a composite rate of 95 percent.[4]

Table 4.4-12 Military Treatment Facility Joint Commission Top Performers (2010 – 2012)[5]

MTF	SCIP	PN	VTE	HF
2010				
Bayne-Jones Army Community Hospital	x			
Moncrief Army Community Hospital		x		
2011				
Weed Army Community Hospital			x	
Irwin Army Community Hospital	x			
Bayne-Jones Army Community Hospital	x		x	
Keller Army Community Hospital (VTE)			x	
2012				
Naval Hospital Pensacola	x		x	
96th Medical Group	x	x	x	
81st Medical Group	x			x
48th Medical Group RAF Lakenheath			x	

2014 MHS Review Group
Source: DoD Joint Commission Core Measure Database, June 2014

---

[4] Note: Only 49/55 DoD facilities are eligible for recognition. The 2013 list will be published November 8, 2014. Surgical Care and VTE measures are the top two measures receiving recognition.
[5] Ibid.

Appendix 4. Quality of Care

Table 4.4-13 below shows TJC ORYX® comparison of Direct Care to 3 external health systems.

Table 4.4-13 TJC Oryx® MTF to External Health System Comparison

Measure	National	DoD	HS3	HS2-1	HS2-4	HS2-2	HS1-1	HS1-2	HS1-3	HS1-4	HS1-5	HS1-6	HS1-7	HS1-8	HS1-9	HS1-10	HS1-11	HS1-12	HS1-13	HS1-14
AMI1	99.4%	99.8%	ND	99.7%	99.2%	100.0%	100.0%	100.0%	100.0%	100.0%	100.0%	99.4%	100.0%	100.0%	100.0%	99.3%	100.0%	100.0%	100.0%	100.0%
AMI2	99.3%	97.0%	ND	100.0%	99.6%	100.0%	100.0%	100.0%	100.0%	100.0%	100.0%	99.7%	100.0%	100.0%	100.0%	100.0%	100.0%	100.0%	100.0%	100.0%
AMI3	98.0%	98.0%	ND	100.0%	100.0%	100.0%	100.0%	100.0%	100.0%	100.0%	100.0%	99.1%	100.0%	100.0%	100.0%	100.0%	100.0%	100.0%	100.0%	100.0%
AMI5	99.2%	96.3%	ND	100.0%	100.0%	100.0%	100.0%	100.0%	100.0%	100.0%	100.0%	99.5%	100.0%	100.0%	100.0%	100.0%	100.0%	100.0%	100.0%	100.0%
AMI7a	57.0%	50.0%	ND	ND	ND	ND	100.0%	100.0%	ND	100.0%	100.0%	ND	ND	ND	100.0%	100.0%	ND	ND	50.0%	ND
AMI8a	95.9%	57.1%	ND	100.0%	94.2%	100.0%	100.0%	100.0%	ND	100.0%	100.0%	100.0%	ND	ND	ND	ND	ND	ND	ND	ND
AMI10	98.5%	98.1%	ND	100.0%	100.0%	100.0%	100.0%	100.0%	100.0%	100.0%	100.0%	99.7%	100.0%	100.0%	100.0%	100.0%	100.0%	100.0%	100.0%	100.0%
HF1	95.0%	89.8%	ND	ND	ND	ND	100.0%	98.5%	98.6%	99.4%	100.0%	98.3%	100.0%	100.0%	100.0%	100.0%	99.8%	100.0%	100.0%	98.5%
HF2	99.5%	98.9%	ND	100.0%	99.7%	100.0%	ND	ND	ND	ND	ND	ND	ND	ND	ND	ND	ND	ND	ND	ND
HF3	97.3%	96.2%	ND	96.9%	96.9%	100.0%	100.0%	100.0%	100.0%	100.0%	100.0%	98.9%	100.0%	100.0%	100.0%	100.0%	99.4%	100.0%	100.0%	100.0%
PN3a	98.4%	95.2%	ND	100.0%	95.8%	100.0%	100.0%	100.0%	100.0%	100.0%	99.4%	100.0%	100.0%	100.0%	100.0%	100.0%	100.0%	100.0%	100.0%	100.0%
PN3b	98.0%	94.4%	ND	ND	ND	ND	100.0%	98.4%	99.4%	100.0%	100.0%	96.8%	100.0%	98.4%	99.4%	100.0%	100.0%	98.7%	95.0%	98.5%
PN6a	92.5%	78.2%	ND	92.3%	90.0%	100.0%	100.0%	100.0%	100.0%	100.0%	ND	90.0%	100.0%	100.0%	100.0%	100.0%	100.0%	100.0%	100.0%	100.0%
PN6b	96.9%	96.3%	ND	100.0%	99.2%	99.4%	100.0%	100.0%	95.5%	100.0%	100.0%	100.0%	100.0%	100.0%	100.0%	100.0%	100.0%	100.0%	100.0%	98.9%
SCIP1a	98.8%	98.1%	ND	99.3%	98.8%	97.4%	99.2%	98.8%	98.2%	99.6%	99.7%	99.5%	100.0%	100.0%	99.7%	99.7%	99.3%	99.3%	99.6%	99.0%
SCIP2a	99.1%	97.4%	ND	99.5%	99.8%	99.0%	99.2%	99.7%	98.8%	99.6%	100.0%	98.5%	100.0%	100.0%	100.0%	99.3%	100.0%	99.7%	99.6%	99.7%
SCIP3a	98.0%	96.5%	ND	98.1%	98.3%	98.5%	100.0%	97.6%	98.4%	99.2%	100.0%	99.3%	100.0%	100.0%	99.4%	99.3%	99.6%	100.0%	99.6%	99.7%
SCIP4	96.7%	95.3%	ND	94.4%	98.7%	96.0%	ND	ND	ND	99.7%	100.0%	97.9%	ND	ND	ND	ND	ND	ND	ND	ND
SCIP6	99.9%	99.7%	ND	100.0%	99.7%	99.7%	100.0%	99.8%	100.0%	99.6%	99.4%	99.9%	99.0%	100.0%	100.0%	99.8%	99.8%	100.0%	100.0%	100.0%
SCIP9	97.6%	98.4%	ND	99.4%	93.3%	98.4%	98.8%	98.0%	98.9%	99.6%	99.4%	99.1%	100.0%	100.0%	99.4%	99.7%	100.0%	100.0%	100.0%	99.3%
SCIPCard2	97.9%	89.7%	ND	99.7%	98.1%	99.7%	100.0%	99.3%	97.7%	99.1%	99.1%	98.3%	100.0%	100.0%	100.0%	97.3%	99.3%	100.0%	97.8%	99.2%
SCIPVTE2	98.2%	96.2%	ND	96.3%	97.5%	97.8%	100.0%	99.7%	99.5%	100.0%	100.0%	99.8%	100.0%	100.0%	99.7%	99.3%	100.0%	99.8%	100.0%	99.7%
PC1	5.0%	4.6%	7.4%	ND	ND	ND	ND	ND	ND	ND	ND	ND	ND	ND	ND	ND	ND	ND	ND	ND
VTE1	91.6%	95.7%	82.6%	91.6%	90.3%	86.8%	ND	ND	ND	ND	ND	ND	ND	ND	ND	ND	ND	ND	ND	ND
VTE2	95.0%	97.2%	92.1%	100.0%	97.3%	94.5%	ND	ND	ND	ND	ND	ND	ND	ND	ND	ND	ND	ND	ND	ND

National, DoD and Wisconsin Collaborative rates are aggregated by FY 2013. Institutions rates are aggregated by CY 2013.
Blue indicates lowest rate in the measure comparison.
Gold represents highest score
Red letters indicate limited reporting by other institutions.
HS-A, HS-B used since original values did not match de-identification key values
2014 MHS Review Group
Source: DoD Joint Commission Core Measure Database, June 2014

Thirty Day Readmissions - Supporting Figures and Tables

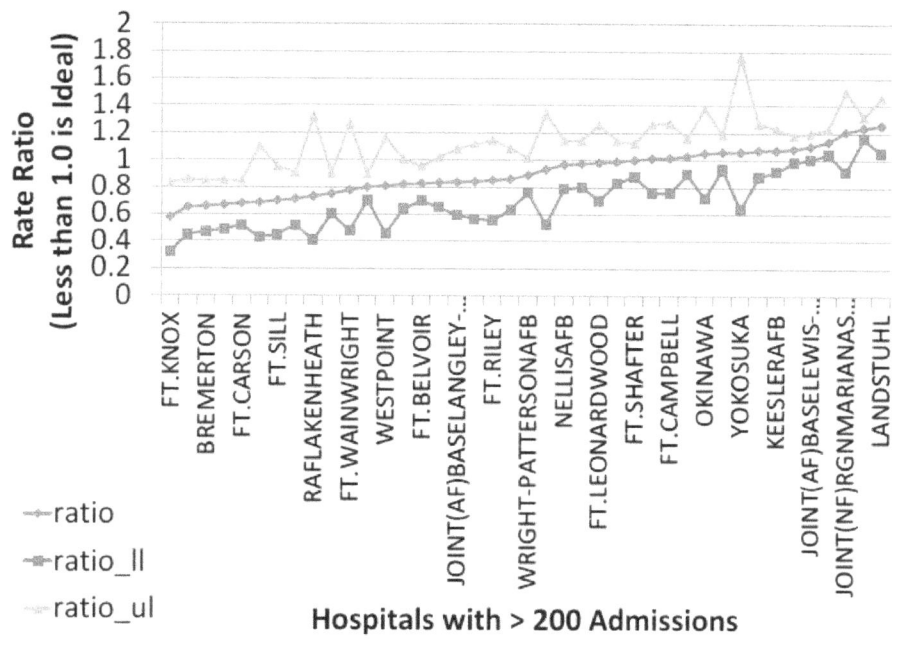

Figure 4.4-3 Thirty-Day Risk-Adjusted Readmission Rate Ratio (Observed/Expected)

2014 MHS Review Group
Source: DoD Joint Commission Core Measure Database, June 2014

Military Health System Perinatal Care - Supporting Figures and Tables

The MHS has 52 MTFs that provide inpatient obstetrical care. The nine perinatal and neonatal centers are Naval Medical Center San Diego, Naval Medical Center Portsmouth, U.S. Naval Hospital Okinawa, Walter Reed National Military Medical Center, Tripler Army Medical Center, Madigan Army Medical Center, Darnall Army Community Hospital, and San Antonio Military Medical Center. Landstuhl Army Regional Medical Center and Okinawa are the two OCONUS facilities.

The Defense Health Agency (DHA) oversees the National Capital Region-Medical Directorate (NCR-MD) that includes two MTFs, Walter Reed National Military Medical Center and Ft. Belvoir Community Hospital. These two facilities make up the rates and averages in the NCR. NCR has been impacted with an issue of inadequate number of coders resulting in a large number of un-coded charts. This has resulted in significant inaccuracy in data from administrative claims data pulls from the Standard Inpatient Data Record (SIDR). When this issue was discovered in 2012, the decision was made to remove the NCR-MD from the MHS averages until the coding issue was rectified. In the data presented in this report, NCR-MD data is represented in the MHS data in the following charts/graphs: Operative Vaginal Deliveries - Vacuum Extraction; Operative Vaginal Deliveries – Forceps; Postpartum Readmissions to Delivery Site; Inborn Readmissions to Birth MTF; Patient Safety Indicator (PSI) 17; PSI 18; PSI

19; Postpartum Hemorrhage; Vaginal Delivery Coded for Shoulder Dystocia; Inborn Mortality greater than or equal to 500 grams.

National Perinatal Information Center (NPIC) – Additional Information

NPIC averages are based on 86 facilities with 700,000 combined annual maternal and infant discharge data creating one of the largest repositories for hospital based perinatal clinical and financial discharge data in the country. Many of the hospitals in the NPIC database are large perinatal hospitals that provide the majority of their care in normal mother infant care settings, but care for the high risk dyads similar to the nine MHS OB specialty facilities. When the complexity of the mother or the infant exceeds the capabilities of the facility the mother infant dyad is transferred to an appropriate level of care. This ability to transfer out of the MHS decreases the percentage of complicated patients treated in the MHS as a whole when compared to NPIC larger perinatal member facilities.

Tables 4.4-14a-c Descriptive Measures

Table 4.4-14a Total Deliveries

	2010	2011	2012	2013
ARMY (21 MTFs)	24,056	24,410	26,366	25,246
NAVY (17 MTFs)	16,440	15,516	15,974	14,975
AIR FORCE (12 MTFs)	6,402	6,353	5,935	5,654
NCRMD (2 MTFs)	2,825	2,846	2,443	2,388
MHS (52 MTFs)	49,723	49,125	50,718	48,263
CONUS (37 MTFs)	44,072	43,279	45,032	42,745
OCONUS (15 MTFs)	5,651	5,846	5,686	5,518
MEDCEN (14 MTFs)	22,961	23,907	24,216	23,759
HOSPITAL (38 MTFs)	26,762	25,218	26,502	24,504
SPECIALTY (10 MTFs)	23,021	21,705	21,839	21,685

2014 MHS Review Group
Source: National Perinatal Information Center Database, July 2014

Table 4.4-14b Percent Deliveries (MHS)

	2010	2011	2012	2013
ARMY (21 MTFs)	48%	50%	52%	52%
NAVY (17 MTFs)	33%	32%	31%	31%
AIR FORCE (12 MTFs)	13%	13%	12%	12%
NCRMD (2 MTFs)	6%	6%	5%	5%
MHS				
CONUS (37 MTFs)	89%	88%	89%	89%
OCONUS (15 MTFs)	11%	12%	11%	11%
MEDCEN (14 MTFs)	46.2%	48.7%	47.7%	49.2%
HOSPITAL (38 MTFs)	53.8%	51.3%	52.3%	50.8%
Total MHS Deliveries	49,723	49,125	50,718	48,263

2014 MHS Review Group
Source: National Perinatal Information Center Database, July 2014

Table 4.4-14c Percent C-Section

	2010	2011	2012	2013
ARMY (21 MTFs)	25.56%	25.29%	25.06%	24.84%
NAVY (17 MTFs)	26.46%	26.97%	25.33%	26.24%
AIR FORCE (12 MTFs)	25.62%	26.49%	27.60%	27.61%
NCRMD (2 MTFs)	30.65%	28.46%	29.23%	31.45%
CONUS (37 MTFs)	26.35%	26.27%	25.67%	25.86%
OCONUS (15 MTFs)	24.67%	25.38%	25.47%	26.44%
MEDCEN (14 MTFs)	26.74%	27.15%	26.58%	27.04%
HOSPITAL (38 MTFs)	25.65%	25.23%	24.79%	24.85%
SPECIALTY (10 MTFs)	26.88%	27.34%	26.57%	27.18%
MHS (52 MTFs)	26.15%	26.16%	25.64%	25.93%
NPIC	35.20%	35.10%	34.70%	34.80%

2014 MHS Review Group
Source: National Perinatal Information Center Database, July 2014

Figures for Comparative Measures

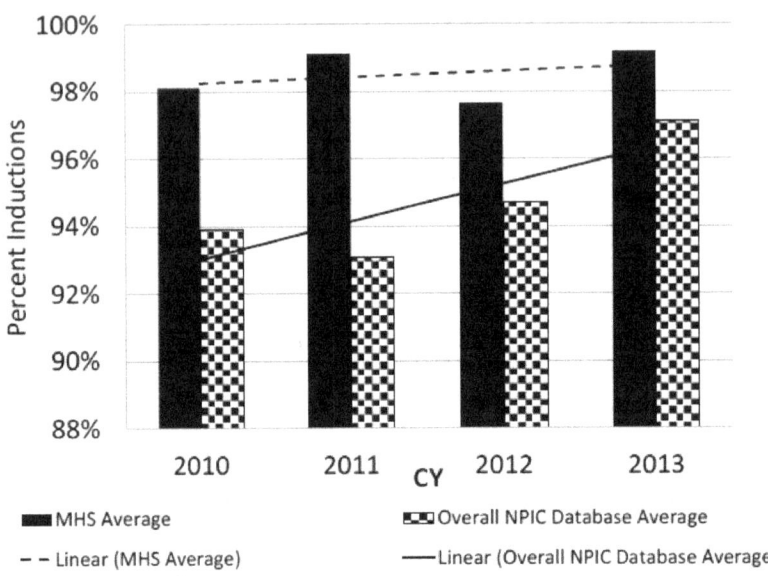

Figure 4.4-4a MHS Level-Induction of Labor at Less Than 37 Weeks Gestation with Medical Indication, CY10 – CY13

2014 MHS Review Group
Source: National Perinatal Information Center/Quality Analytic Services (NPIC/QAS), July 2014

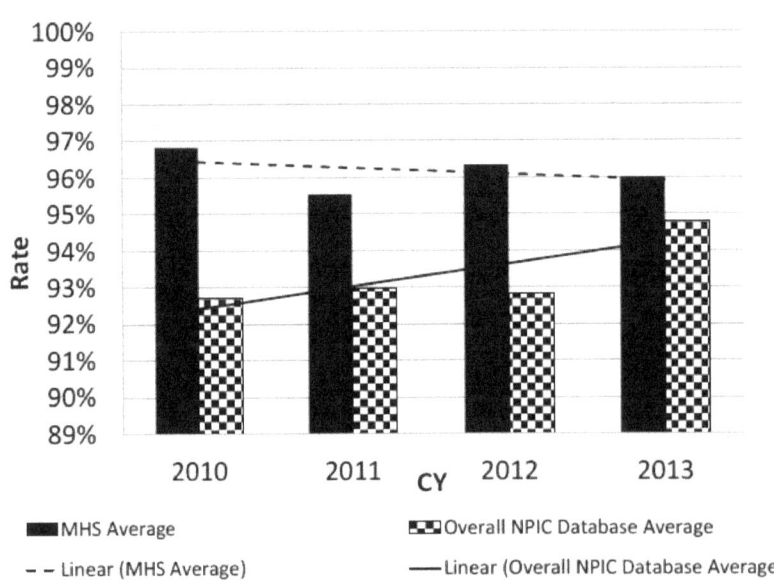

Figure 4.4-4b MHS Level C-Section at Less Than 37 Weeks Gestation with Medical Indication, CY10 – CY13

2014 MHS Review Group
Source: National Perinatal Information Center/Quality Analytic Services (NPIC/QAS), July 2014

Figure 4.4-5 MHS Level Patient Safety Indicator (PSI) 18, CY10 – CY13

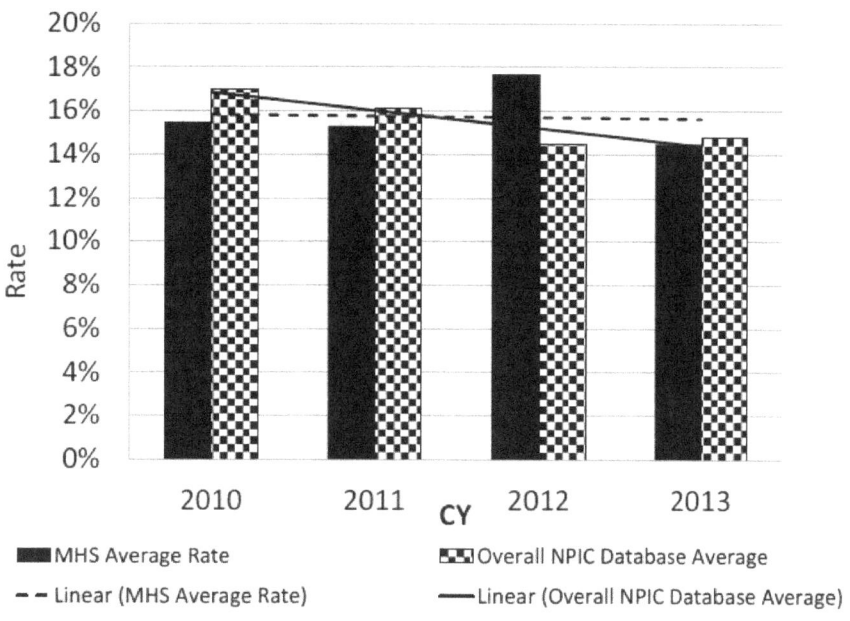

2014 MHS Review Group
Source: National Perinatal Information
Center/Quality Analytic Services (NPIC/QAS), July 2014

Figure 4.4-6 Annual Rate of PSI 19 Obstetric Trauma-Vaginal Delivery without Instruments, CY10 – CY13

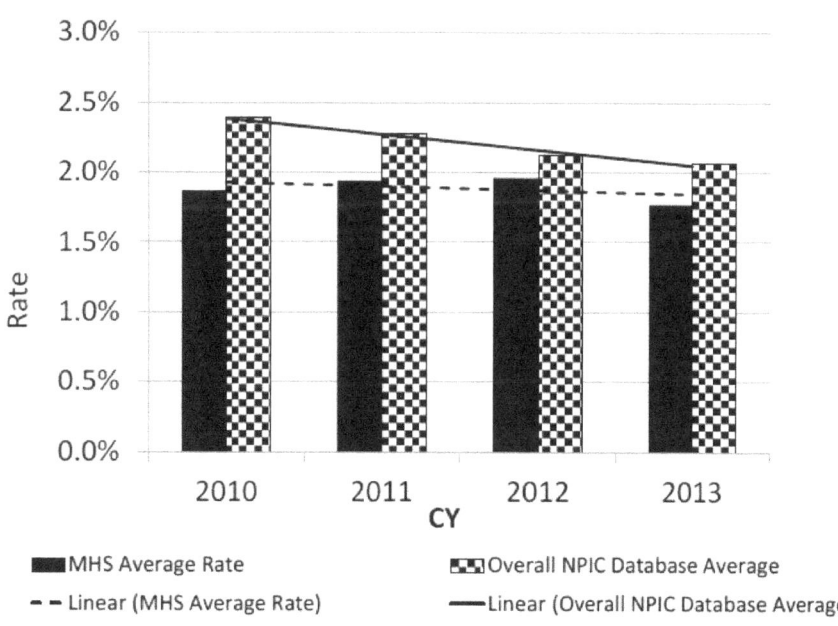

2014 MHS Review Group
Source: National Perinatal Information
Center/Quality Analytic Services (NPIC/QAS), July 2014

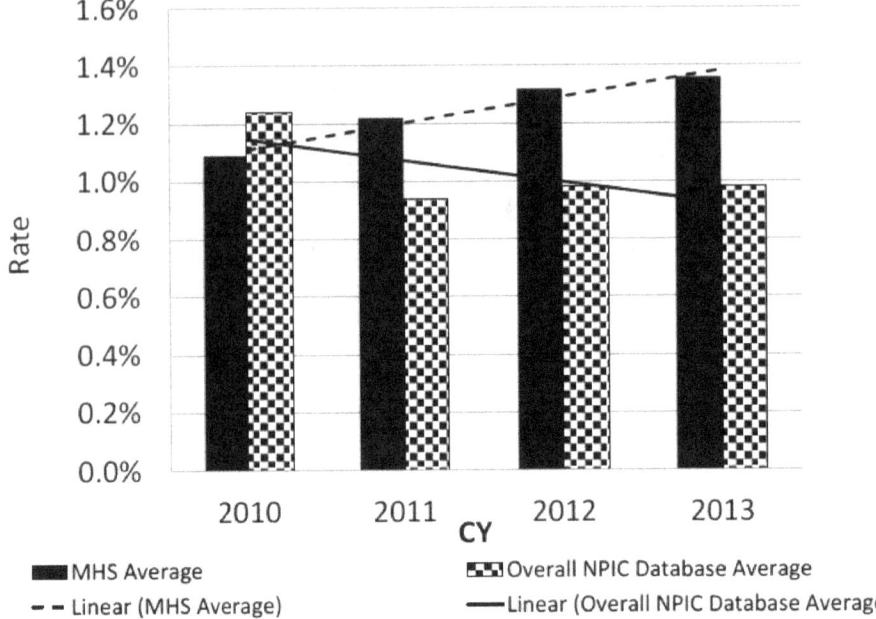

Figure 4.4-7 Annual Rate of Postpartum Readmissions to Delivery Site, CY10 – CY13

2014 MHS Review Group
Source: National Perinatal Information Center/Quality Analytic Services (NPIC/QAS), July 2014

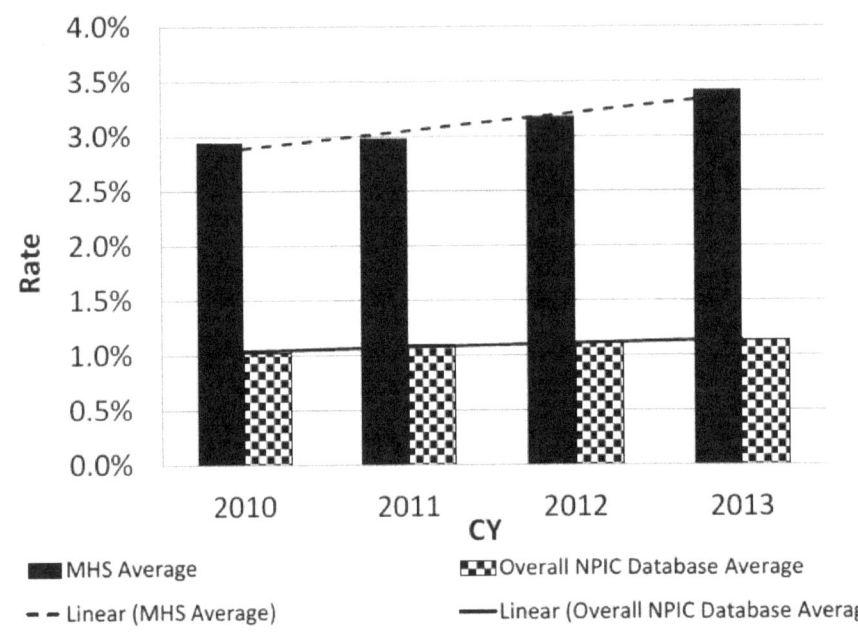

Figure 4.4-8 Annual Percent of Inborn Readmissions to Birth Site, CY10 – CY13

2014 MHS Review Group
Source: National Perinatal Information Center/Quality Analytic Services (NPIC/QAS), July 2014

Figure 4.4-9 Annual Rate of Vaginal Deliveries Coded with Shoulder Dystocia by Branch of Service, CY10 – CY13

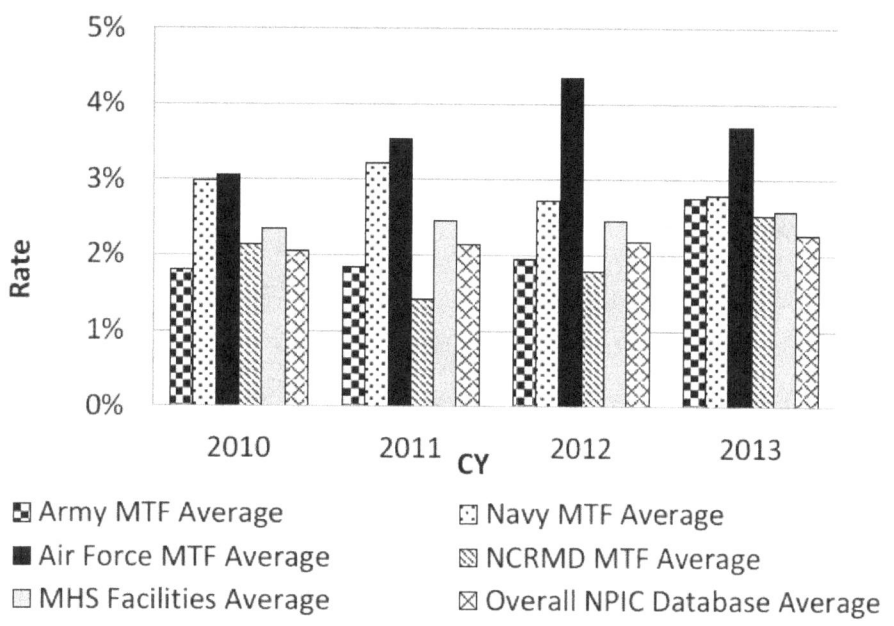

2014 MHS Review Group
Source: National Perinatal Information Center/Quality Analytic Services (NPIC/QAS), July 2014

Figure 4.4-10 Annual Rate of Postpartum Hemorrhage by Branch of Service, CY10 – CY13

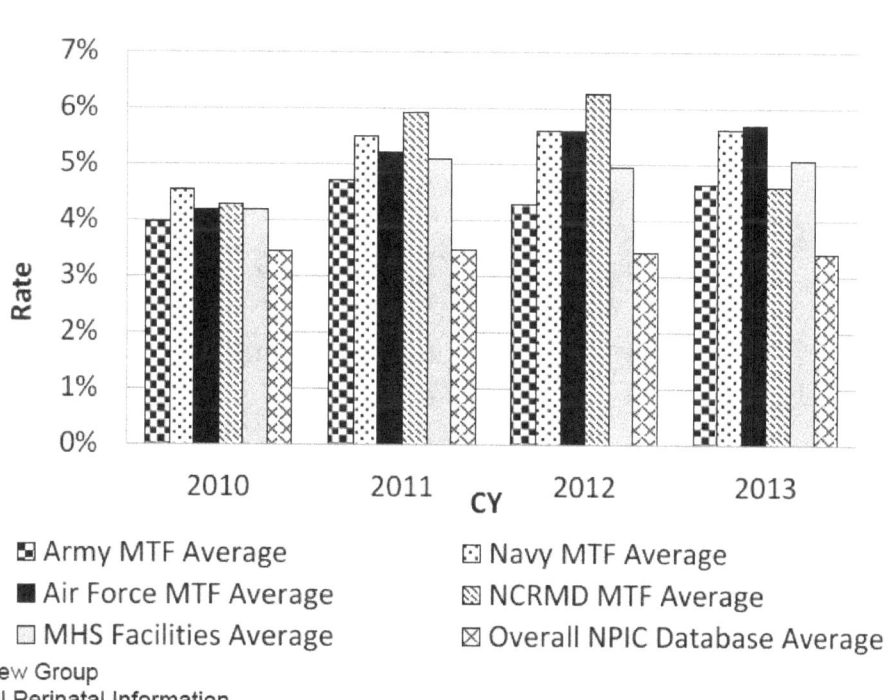

2014 MHS Review Group
Source: National Perinatal Information Center/Quality Analytic Services (NPIC/QAS), July 2014

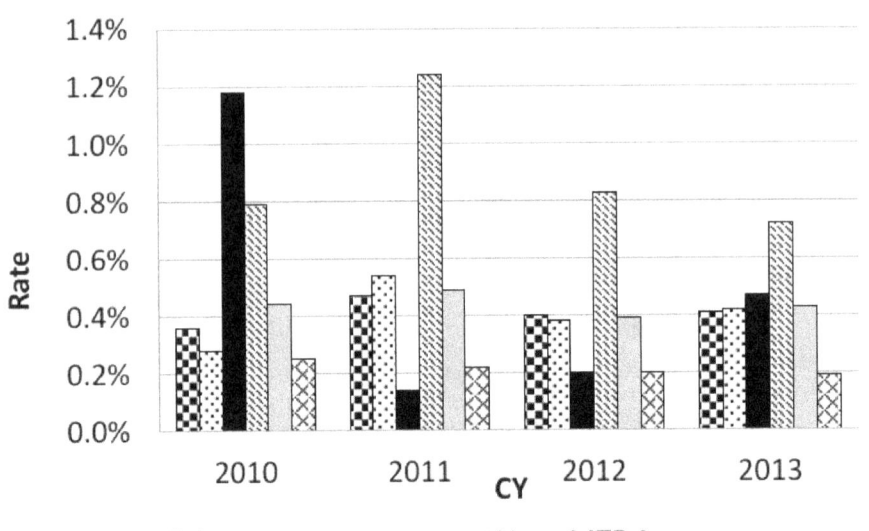

Figure 4.4-11 Annual Rate of PS1 17 Injury to Neonate by Branch of Service, CY10 – CY13

2014 MHS Review Group
Source: National Perinatal Information Center/Quality Analytic Services (NPIC/QAS), July 2014

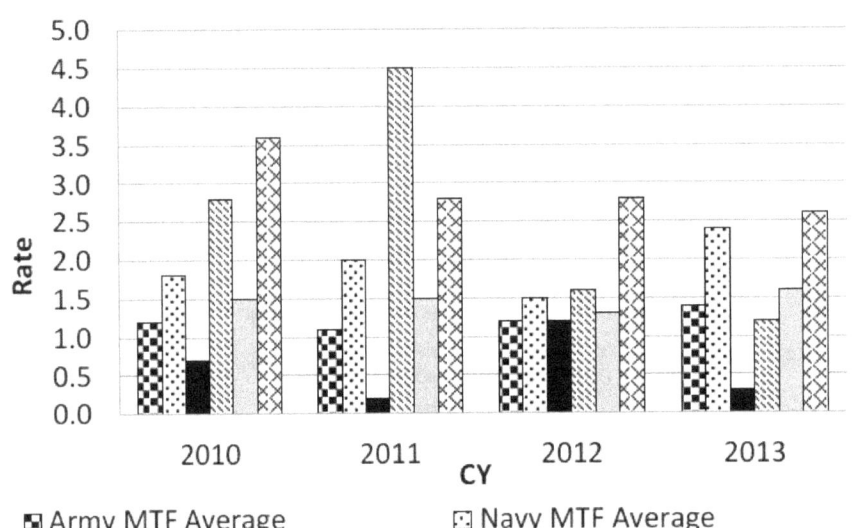

Figure 4.4-12 Inborn Mortality Rate (per 1,000 live births) ≥ 500 Grams by Branch of Service, CY10 – CY13

2014 MHS Review Group
Source: National Perinatal Information Center/Quality Analytic Services (NPIC/QAS), July 2014

Table 4.4-15 Facility Level Data

Military Treatment Facilities by Select Maternal and Neonatal Birth Outcome Measures, CY2010-CY2013

MTF	Volume	Measures** with ≥2 Elevated Yrs	Postpartum Hemorrhage Above/At/Below NPIC Avg				Score***	PSI17 Birth Trauma Above/At/Below NPIC Avg				Score***	Vaginal Delivery with Coded Shoulder Dystocia Above/At/Below NPIC Avg				Score***
			CY10	CY11	CY12	CY13	CY10-13	CY10	CY11	CY12	CY13	CY10-13	CY10	CY11	CY12	CY13	CY10-13
Army																	
Tripler	VH	PPH	-	△	△	△	3	-	-	-	-	0	♦	♦	♦	♦	-4
Darnall	VH	PPH,BT	△	-	△	△	3	△	△	△	△	4	-	-	♦	-	-1
Womack	VH	PPH	-	△	△	△	3	♦	-	-	♦	-2	♦	♦	♦	♦	-4
Madigan	VH	PPH,BT	△	△	△	△	4	-	-	-	-	3	-	-	♦	-	-2
Evans	VH		-	-	-	△	1	-	-	-	-	0	♦	-	-	-	-1
Blanchfield	H	SD	△	-	-	-	1	♦	-	-	-	-1	△	△	△	△	4
Brook	H		♦	♦	-	-	-2	N/A	-	-	△	1	N/A	♦	♦	-	-2
Beaumont	H		♦	-	♦	-	-2	-	-	-	△	1	♦	♦	♦	♦	-4
Winn	M	SD	-	-	-	-	0	♦	-	♦	-	-3	-	-	△	△	2
Irwin	M	PPH	△	△	△	-	3	-	-	-	-	1	-	-	-	-	0
Landstuhl	M		-	△	-	-	1	-	-	-	-	0	-	-	-	♦	-1
Martin	M	PPH,BT	△	-	△	△	3	△	-	-	△	2	-	△	-	-	1
Bassett	M	PPH	△	△	△	-	3	-	-	-	-	0	-	-	-	-	0
Bayne-Jones	M	PPH,SD	△	-	△	△	4	-	-	-	-	0	-	△	-	△	2
Reynolds	M	SD	♦	♦	-	-	-2	-	-	-	-	0	△	△	-	-	2
Leonard Wood	M		-	-	♦	♦	-2	-	-	-	-	0	-	-	-	-	0
Ireland	M		-	-	△	△	1	♦	-	-	♦	-3	△	-	-	-	1
Seoul	M		-	-	-	-	0	-	-	-	-	0	♦	-	-	-	-1
Weed	L		♦	-	-	-	-1	-	-	♦	-	-1	-	-	-	-	0
Keller	L		-	-	-	-	0	♦	-	-	♦	-2	-	♦	♦	-	-2
Vincenza	L		-	-	-	-	0	♦	♦	♦	-	-3	♦	♦	-	-	-2
Air Force																	
Langley	H	PPH,BT,SD	-	△	△	△	3	△	-	-	△	2	△	△	△	△	4
Eglin	M	PPH,SD	△	△	-	△	3	N/A	♦	-	♦	-2	N/A	△	△	-	2
Elmendorf	M	PPH,SD	-	△	-	△	2	△	-	-	-	1	-	-	△	△	2
Mike O'callagan	M	PPH	♦	-	-	△	1	-	-	♦	♦	-2	-	-	-	-	0
Lakenheath	M		-	-	-	-	0	♦	-	-	♦	-3	-	-	-	△	1
Keesler	M		♦	-	-	-	-1	N/A	-	-	♦	-1	N/A	-	-	-	0
Wright Patterson	M	PPH	-	△	△	-	2	-	-	-	-	0	-	-	-	-	0
Mountain Home	L		-	-	-	△	1	♦	-	-	♦	-3	♦	-	♦	△	-1
Yokota AB	L		-	-	-	-	0	N/A	♦	-	-	-1	N/A	-	-	-	0
Misawa	L	PPH	△	△	-	-	2	♦	♦	♦	♦	-4	-	-	-	-	0
Aviano	L	PPH	-	△	-	-	2	-	-	-	-	0	-	-	-	-	0
David Grant	L	PPH,SD	-	△	△	-	3	-	♦	-	♦	-2	△	-	△	-	2
Navy																	
Portsmouth	VH	BT	♦	-	-	-	0	-	△	△	-	2	-	-	-	♦	-1
San Diego	VH	PPH,SD	△	△	△	△	4	-	△	-	-	1	△	△	-	-	2
Camp Lejune	H	PPH,SD	△	△	△	△	4	-	-	-	△	1	△	△	△	△	4
Camp Pendleton	M	PPH,BT	△	△	△	△	4	-	-	△	-	2	-	-	-	-	0
Okinawa	M	PPH	♦	-	△	-	1	-	-	-	-	0	-	-	-	-	0
Jacksonville	M		-	♦	-	△	0	-	-	-	♦	-1	-	△	-	-	1
Bremerton	M	PPH	△	△	△	-	3	-	-	-	-	0	-	-	△	-	1
Twenty Nine Palms	M		♦	-	♦	-	-2	-	-	-	-	0	-	-	-	-	0
Yokosuka	M	PPH	-	△	△	△	3	-	-	△	-	1	-	△	-	-	1
Pensacola	M	PPH,SD	-	△	△	△	3	-	-	-	-	0	△	△	△	-	3
Guam	M	PPH	-	△	△	-	3	♦	-	-	-	-1	△	-	-	-	1
Lemoore	M		-	-	-	-	0	-	-	♦	♦	-2	♦	-	-	-	-2
Oak Harbor	L		♦	♦	-	-	-2	-	-	-	-	0	-	-	-	-	0
Naples	L		-	-	-	-	0	-	♦	♦	♦	-3	-	-	-	-	0
Sigonella	L		-	△	-	-	1	♦	-	♦	-	-2	-	-	-	-	0
Rota	L		♦	-	-	♦	-2	♦	♦	♦	♦	-4	♦	♦	♦	-	-3
Guantanamo Bay	L		-	-	-	♦	-3	N/A	♦	♦	♦	-3	N/A	♦	♦	♦	-3
NCR-MD																	
Dewitt	M	BT	-	-	-	-	0	△	△	△	△	4	-	♦	-	-	-1
WR NMMC	M	PPH	△	△	△	△	4	-	-	-	-	1	-	-	-	♦	-1

Legend for Volume in Annual Deliveries: VH (very high) >= 2,000; H (high): 1,500 - 1,999; M (medium): 300 - 1,499; L (low): 1-299

♦ indicates MTF average was at least two standard deviations below the NPIC average (counts as -1 towards score),
- indicates the MTF average was within two standard deviations of the NPIC average (counts as 0 towards score),
△ indicates the MTF average was at least two standard deviations above the NPIC average (counts as 1 towards score)
N/A indicates that data were not available from these MTFs in CY 2010

** PPH=Postpartum Hemorrhage, BT=Birth Trauma, SD=Shoulder Dystocia
*** Lower score is better

2014 MHS Review Group
Source: National Perinatal Information Center Database. Prepared by: Defense Health Agency, July 2014

National Surgical Quality Improvement Program (NSQIP®) - Supporting Figures and Tables

Background

The National Surgical Quality Improvement Program (NSQIP®), administered by the American College of Surgeon (ACS), is a voluntarily reported, data-driven, outcome-based program to measure the quality of surgical care. The data are adjusted for the type of surgery and how complicated the patients are to allow comparisons between facilities.

The focus of ACS NSQIP® is to assist hospitals with assessing and improving the quality of surgical care while decreasing costs. NSQIP® use abstracted actual clinical data rather than administrative data. Clinical data are more detailed, informative and capture more complications than does administrative data. NSQIP® uses a rigorous, validated sampling and measurement process, as well as validated case-mix and risk adjustment procedures that have been detailed and published elsewhere).[6]

The primary outcome measures for NSQIP® are mortality and morbidity 30 days following surgery, risk adjusted for a patient's pre-operative co-morbidities. Primary outcomes assessed are death and morbidity derived from cardiac events, pneumonia, unplanned intubation, Deep Vein Thrombosis (DVT)/Pulmonary Embolism (PE), Renal Failure, Surgical Site infection (SSI), Urinary Tract Infection (UTI), and Return to Operating Room (ROR). NSQIP® reports these measures for each sub-specialty program supported by each facility.

The process is as follows:
1. Hospitals abstract actual clinical data
2. ACS NSQIP® analyzes data
3. ACS NSQIP® reports data back to hospitals twice yearly
4. Hospitals act on their data
5. Hospitals monitor interventions with data.

NSQIP® is a national standard for surgical quality improvement with well-defined measures, data collection processes, and robust analytics that has been in use by the MHS since 2009. Currently, 507 hospitals participate in the program out of more than 5,000 community hospitals in the United States. Participation involves a significant investment of time, people, money, and a cultural commitment to performance improvement.

Inpatient Mortality Measures - Supporting Figures and Tables

Due to the availability of other process-focused quality measures, data on inpatient mortality has played a limited role in the overall MHS quality program. Inpatient mortality has traditionally not been viewed as an accurate reflection of care quality. Considerable research over the last decade has focused on the how best to use mortality measures in the assessment of inpatient care quality. What has emerged is a consensus among leading civilian organizations that the

---

[6] Available at: http://site.acsnsqip.org/program-specifics/data-collection-analysis-and-reporting/.

judicious use of risk adjusted mortality measures can serve a valuable role in identifying trends warranting further investigation.

Experience of Care Summary[7] - Supporting Figures and Tables

Rating of Health Care:

- MHS beneficiary overall ratings of their health care (the percentage rating 8, 9, or 10 on a 0–10 scale) increased from 66 percent in FY 2010 to 70 percent in FY 2013.
- The increased ratings between FY 2011 and FY 2012 were statistically significant when compared to the previous fiscal year.
- Among MHS beneficiaries, ratings by those using civilian outpatient care remained at 80 percent from FY 2010 to FY 2013, while ratings by those using MTF-based care increased from 56 percent in FY 2010 to 61 percent in FY 2013.
- Between FY 2010 and FY 2012, the increases were statistically significant when compared to the previous fiscal year.

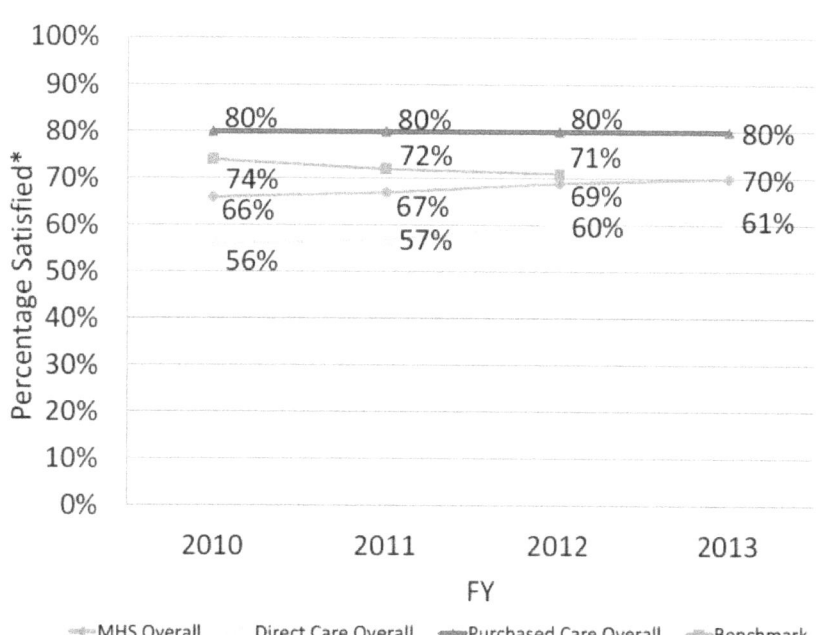

Figure 4.4-13 Overall Rating of Health Care, FY10 – FY13

*"Percentage Satisfied" for Overall Rating of Health Care is a score of 8, 9, or 10 on a 0-10 scale where 10 is best.
2014 MHS Review Group
Source: DHA Business Support Directorate Defense Health Cost Assessment and Program Evaluation (DHCAPE) TROSS survey results of 11/15/2013, July 2014

Rating of Health Plan:

- Beneficiary overall rating of the health plan among MHS beneficiaries (the percentage rating 8, 9, or 10 on a 0–10 scale) has *slightly increased* from 69 percent in FY 2010 to

---

[7] Bannick, R.R, Marshall, K. MHS Quality of Care/Experience of Care and Access to Care from DHCAPE.

71 percent in FY 2013. The FY 2011 rating (71 percent) was statistically significantly *higher* compared with FY 2010.
- Health plan ratings by those receiving outpatient care at civilian facilities has also *remained stable* around 78 percent, while plan ratings for MTF-based facilities *increased* from 65 percent in FY 2010 to 67 percent in FY 2013.
- During FY 2012, there was a *statistically significant decrease* from FY 2011 for beneficiaries receiving care in civilian facilities.
- Notes: There is no civilian benchmark for Rating of Health Plan.

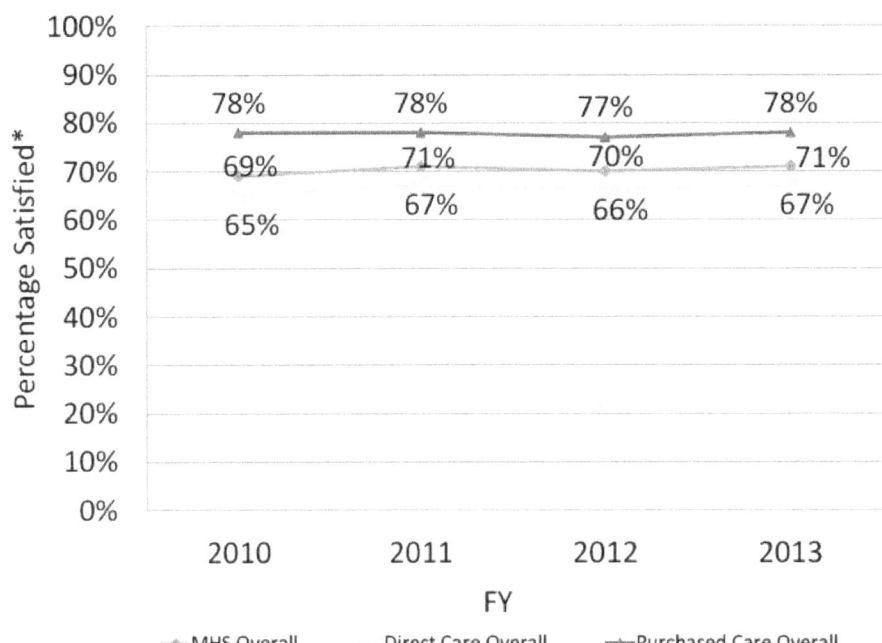

Figure 4.4-14 Overall Rating of Health Plan, FY10 – FY13

*"Percentage Satisfied" for Overall Rating of Health Care is a score of 8, 9, or 10 on a 0-10 scale where 10 is best.
2014 MHS Review Group
Source: DHA Business Support Directorate Defense Health Cost Assessment and Program Evaluation (DHCAPE) TROSS survey results of 11/15/2013, July 2014

Overall Rating of Hospital

- Overall, beneficiaries who received care within the Purchased care component for surgical and OB care rated their hospital higher than did those in the Direct care component.
- MHS beneficiaries needing surgical care, whether discharged from MTF or civilian hospitals, rated their hospital stay higher than users that make up the civilian benchmark.
- Beneficiaries who received medical services in military facilities rated their hospital higher (71 percent for 2013) than the civilian benchmark (70 percent for 2013; CMS).

Figure 4.4-15 Overall Rating of Hospital

Figure 4.4-15a Rating of Hospital in Medical Care, FY11 – FY13

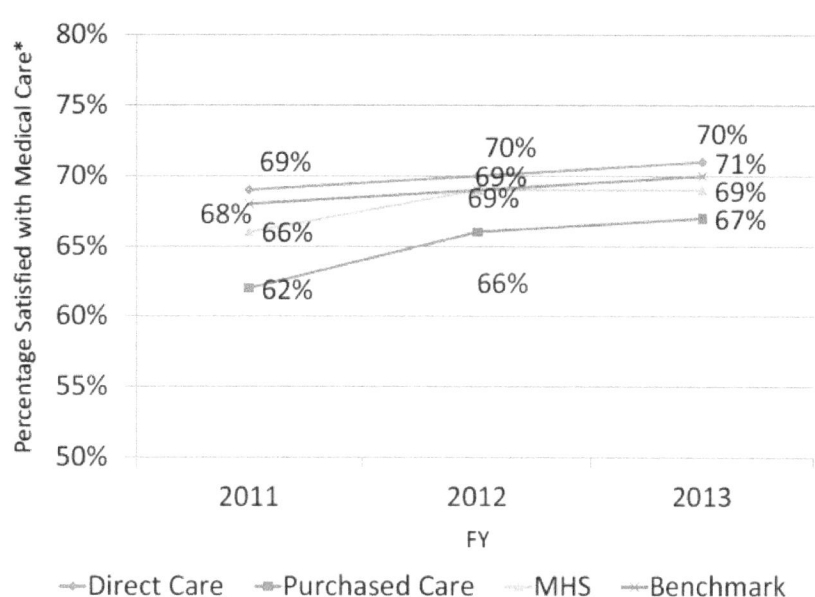

*"Percentage Satisfied" for Overall Rating of Health Care is a score of 8, 9, or 10 on a 0-10 scale where 10 is best.
2014 MHS Review Group
Source: DHA Business Support Directorate Defense Health Cost Assessment and Program Evaluation (DHCAPE) TROSS survey results of 11/15/2013, July 2014

Figure 4.4-15b Rating of Hospital in Surgical Care, FY11 – FY13

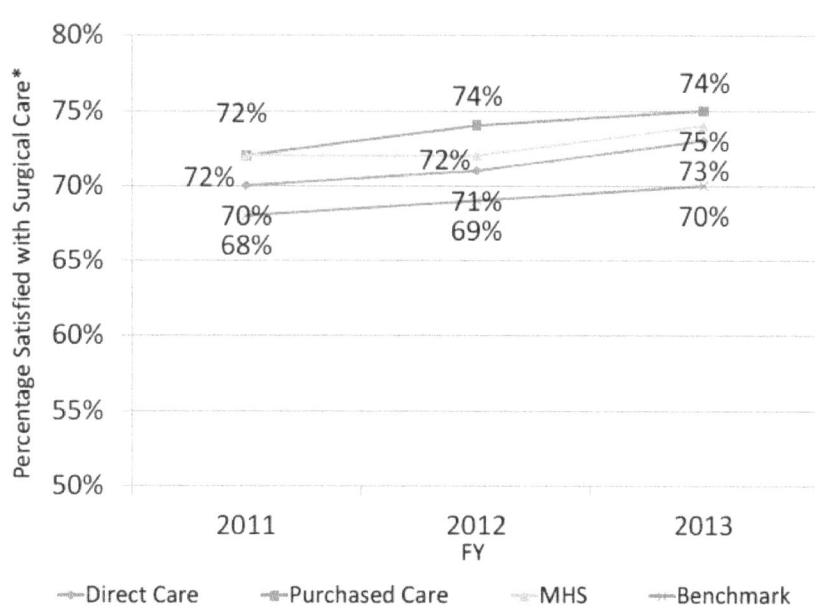

*"Percentage Satisfied" for Overall Rating of Health Care is a score of 8, 9, or 10 on a 0-10 scale where 10 is best.
2014 MHS Review Group
Source: DHA Business Support Directorate Defense Health Cost Assessment and Program Evaluation (DHCAPE) TROSS survey results of 11/15/2013, July 2014

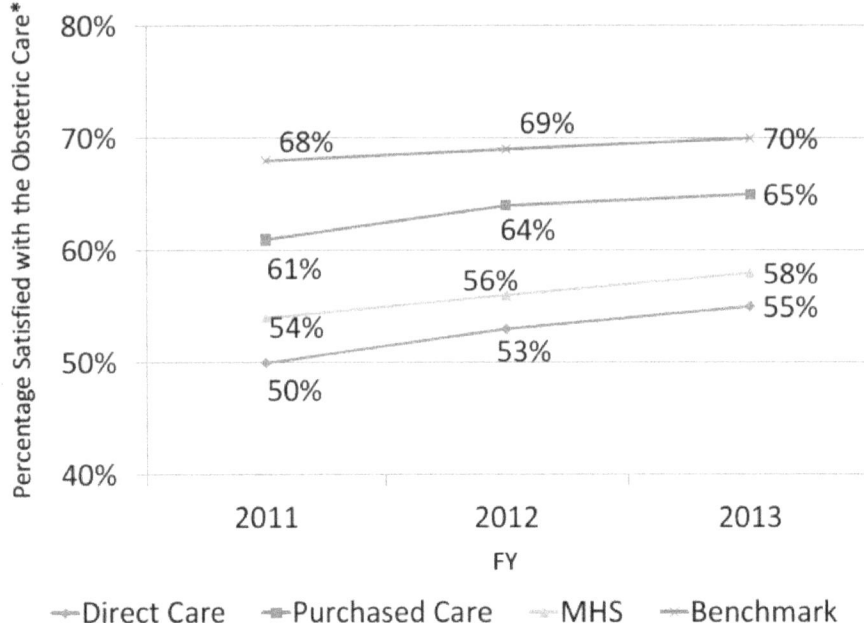

Figure 4.4-15c Rating of Hospital in Obstetric Care, FY11 – FY13

*"Percentage Satisfied" for Overall Rating of Health Care is a score of 8, 9, or 10 on a 0-10 scale where 10 is best.
2014 MHS Review Group
Source: DHA Business Support Directorate Defense Health Cost Assessment and Program Evaluation (DHCAPE) TROSS survey results of 11/15/2013, July 2014

Willingness to Recommend Hospital

- Direct care medical and surgical product lines beneficiaries' recommendation of their hospital exceeds the civilian benchmarks, while direct care obstetrics beneficiaries' falls below the civilian benchmarks. (Figure 4.4-16).
- Purchased care beneficiaries' recommendation of their hospital consistently exceeds the civilian benchmarks for surgical and OB product lines.
- Note: Percentage reporting satisfied of willingness to recommend is a score of 'always' when asked if one would recommend a hospital to family or friends.

Figure 4.4-16 Willingness to Recommend Hospital

Figure 4.4-16a Willingness to Recommend Hospital for Medical Care, FY11 – FY13

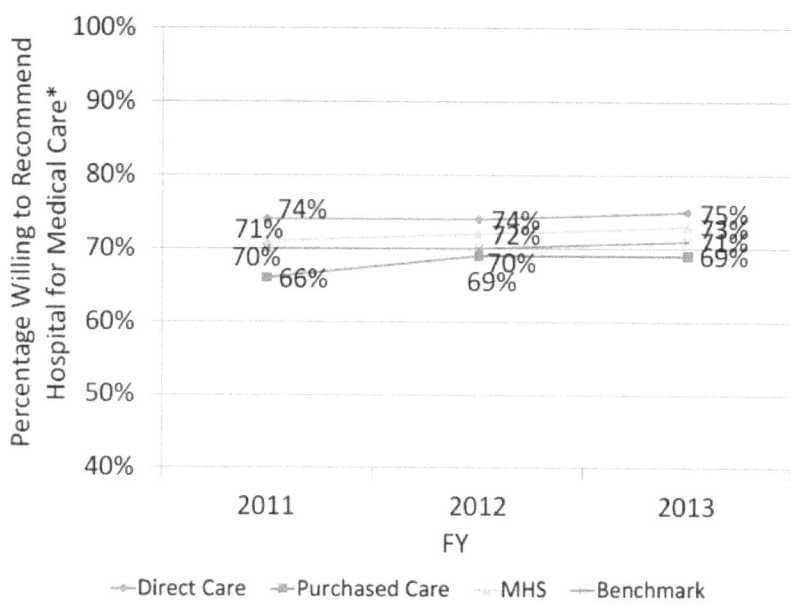

*"Percentage Reporting Satisfied" for recommendation of hospital is a score of always when asked if one would recommend a hospital to family of friends.
2014 MHS Review Group
Source: DHA Business Support Directorate Defense Health Cost Assessment and Program Evaluation (DHCAPE) TROSS survey results of 11/15/2013, July 2014

Figure 4.4-16b Willingness to Recommend Hospital for Surgical Care, FY11 – FY13

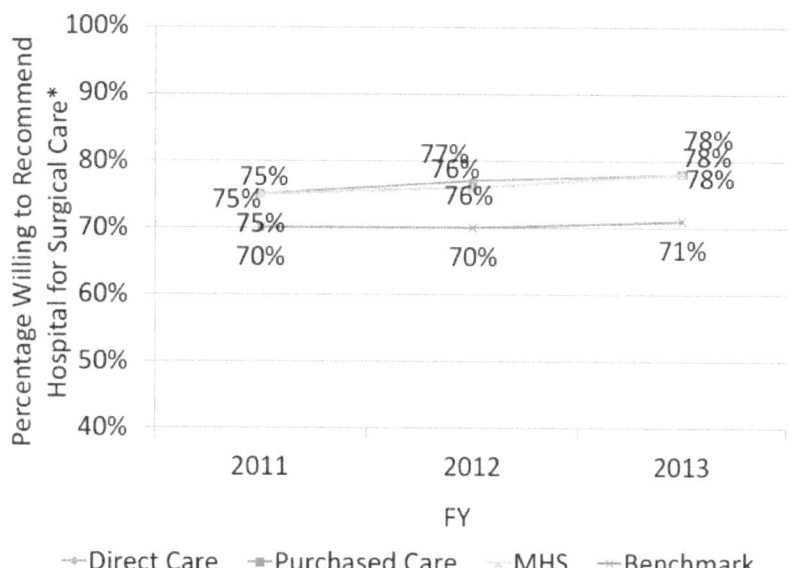

*"Percentage Reporting Satisfied" for recommendation of hospital is a score of always when asked if one would recommend a hospital to family of friends.
2014 MHS Review Group
Source: DHA Business Support Directorate Defense Health Cost Assessment and Program Evaluation (DHCAPE) TROSS survey results of 11/15/2013, July 2014

Figure 4.4-16c Willingness to Recommend Hospital for Obstetric Care, FY11 – FY13

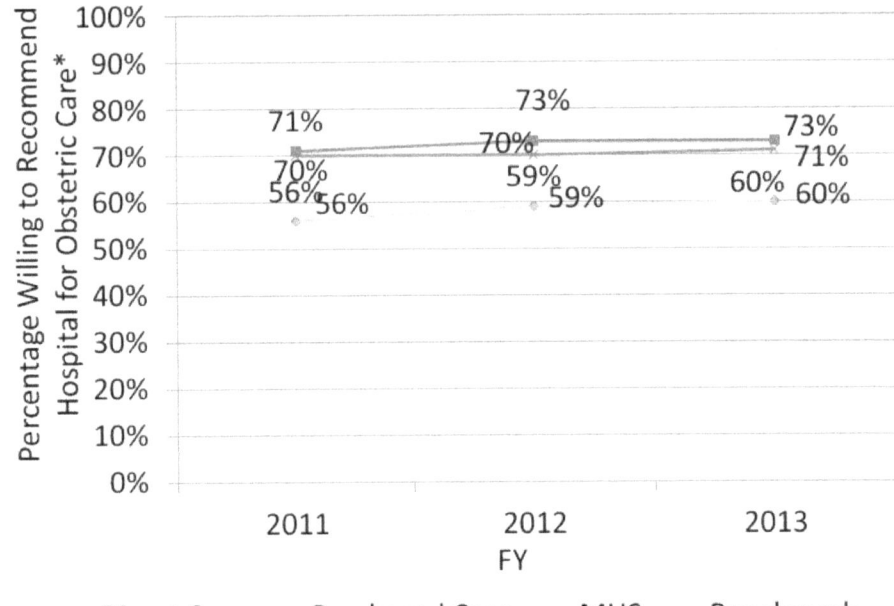

*"Percentage Reporting Satisfied" for recommendation of hospital is a score of always when asked if one would recommend a hospital to family of friends.
2014 MHS Review Group
Source: DHA Business Support Directorate Defense Health Cost Assessment and Program Evaluation (DHCAPE) TROSS survey results of 11/15/2013, July 2014

Quality of Care: Beneficiary Reported Experience and Satisfaction with Key Aspects of TRICARE and trends in satisfaction ratings

- MHS beneficiaries in the U.S. who have used TRICARE are compared with the civilian benchmark with respect to ratings of: 1) the health plan, in general; 2) health care; 3) personal physician; and 4) specialty care. Health plan ratings depend on access to care and how the plan handles various service aspects such as claims, referrals, and customer complaints.
- Satisfaction levels with health care quality and health plan increased slightly from FY 2011 to FY 2013.
- MHS satisfaction rates with health care remained below the civilian benchmarks, with the exception of health plan, which exceeded the benchmark over this period.
- Satisfaction with primary care and specialty care remained stable between FY 2011 and FY 2013.

Figure 4.4-17 Reported Experience and Satisfaction with Key Aspects of TRICARE

Figure 4.4-17a Health Plan, FY11 – FY13

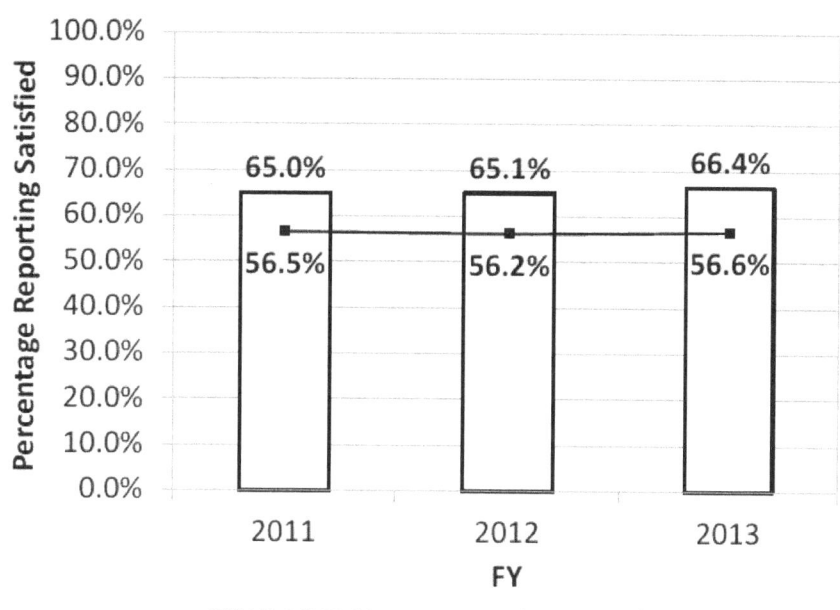

2014 MHS Review Group
Source: TRICARE Program: Access, Cost and Quality Fiscal Year 2014 Report to Congress, July 2014

Figure 4.4-17b Primary Care Physician, FY11 – FY13

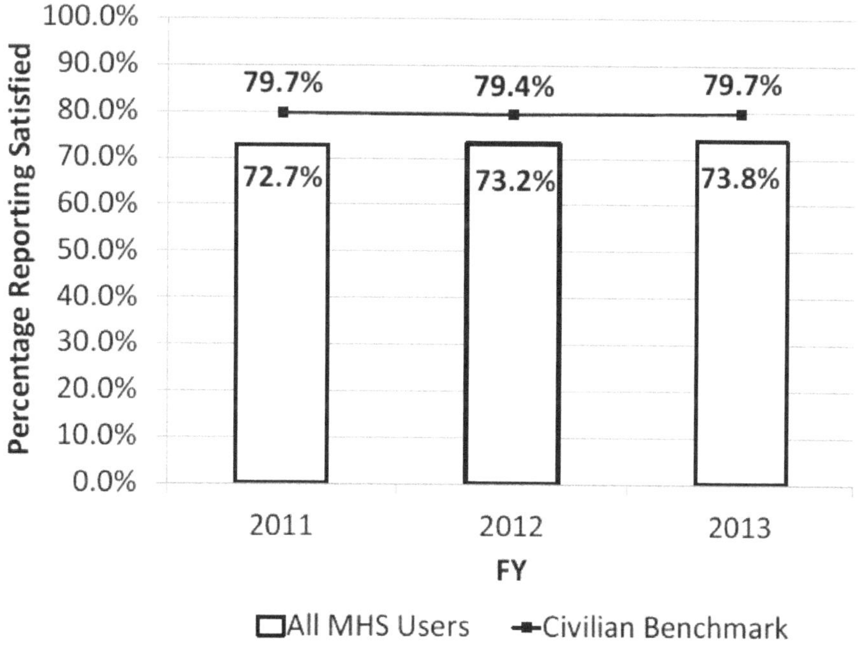

2014 MHS Review Group
Source: TRICARE Program: Access, Cost and Quality Fiscal Year 2014 Report to Congress, July 2014

August 29, 2014 — Appendix 4. Quality of Care

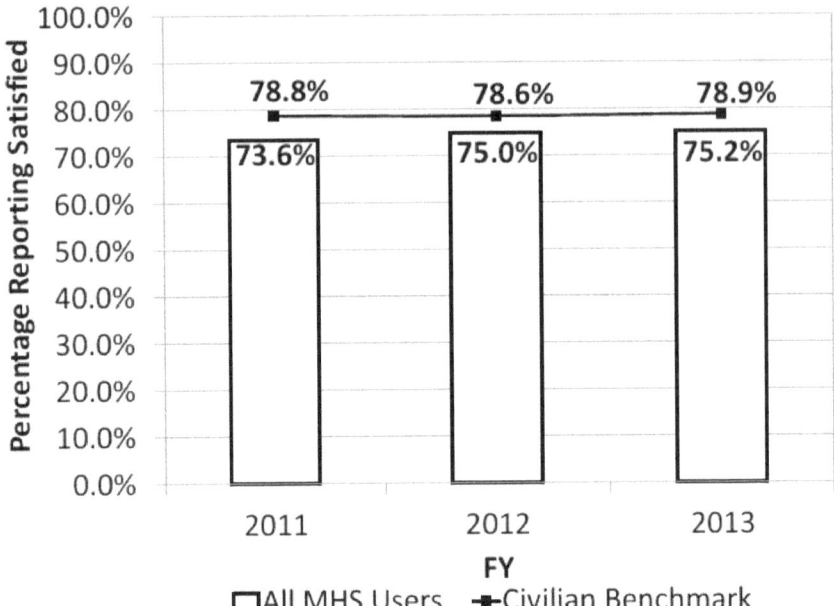

Figure 4.4-17c Specialty Physician, FY11 – FY13

2014 MHS Review Group
Source: TRICARE Program: Access, Cost and Quality Fiscal Year 2014 Report to Congress, July 2014

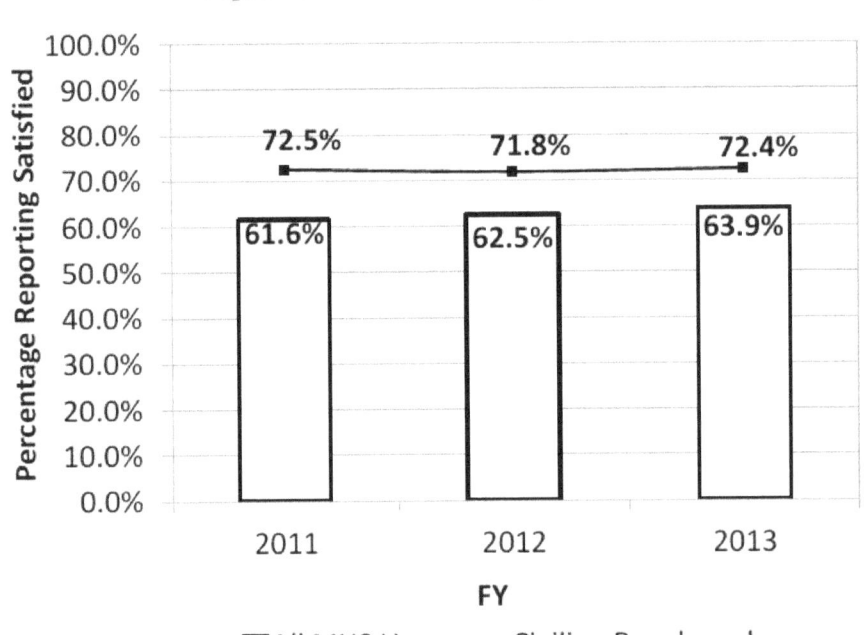

Figure 4.4-17d Health Care, FY11 – FY13

2014 MHS Review Group
Source: TRICARE Program: Access, Cost and Quality Fiscal Year 2014 Report to Congress, July 2014

Military Health System Review – Final Report
August 29, 2014

Quality of Care: Satisfaction with the Health Plan Based on Enrollment Status and trends in satisfaction with Health Plan based on enrollment status: (Figure 4.4-18 and Figure 4.4-19)

- DoD health care beneficiaries can participate in TRICARE in several ways: by enrolling in the Prime option or by not enrolling and using the traditional indemnity option for seeing participating providers (Standard) or network providers (Extra). Satisfaction levels with one's health plan across the TRICARE options are compared with commercial plan counterparts.
- Satisfaction with the TRICARE health plan remained stable for Prime enrollees and non-enrollees from FY 2011 to FY 2013. The civilian benchmark also remained stable.
- During each of the past three years (FY 2011 to FY 2013), enrolled and non-enrolled MHS beneficiaries reported higher levels of satisfaction than their civilian counterparts.

Figure 4.4-18 Trends in Satisfaction with Health Plan Based on Enrollment Status, FY11 – FY13

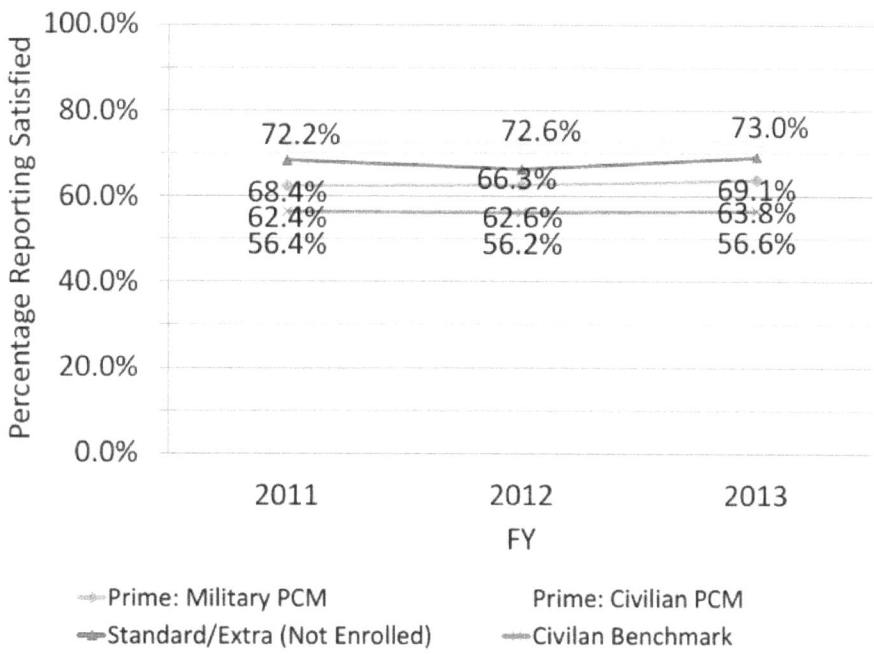

2014 MHS Review Group
Source: TRICARE Program: Access, Cost and Quality Fiscal Year 2014 Report to Congress, July 2014

Quality of Care: Satisfaction with the Health Plan by Beneficiary Category and trends in satisfaction with Health Plan by beneficiary category

- Satisfaction levels of different beneficiary categories are examined to identify any diverging trends among groups.
- Satisfaction of Active Duty beneficiaries equaled the civilian benchmark in all three years (FYs 2011–2013).
- ADFM and RETFM satisfaction ratings exceeded the civilian benchmark in all three years (FYs 2011–2013).

Figure 4.4-19 Trends in Satisfaction with Health Plan Based on Beneficiary Status, FY11 – FY13

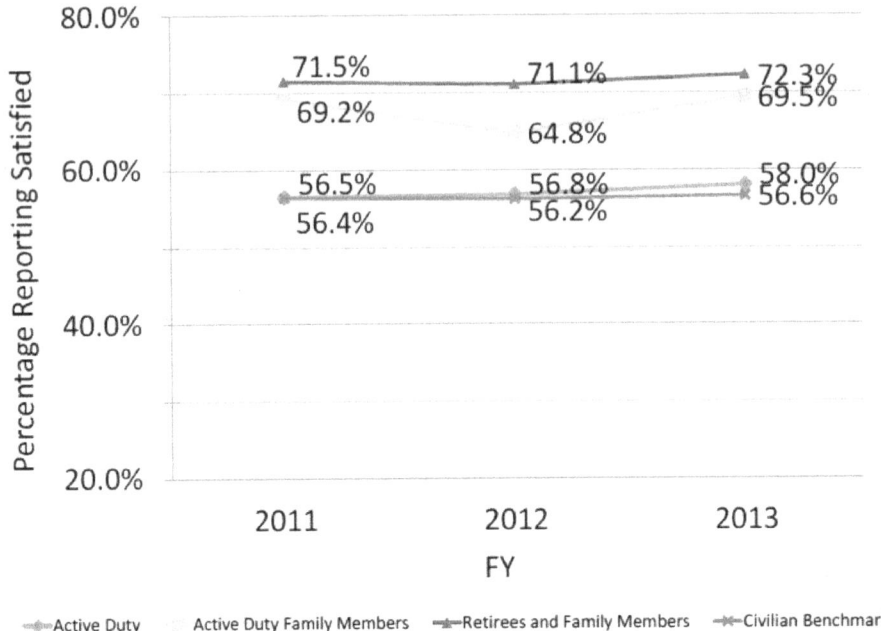

2014 MHS Review Group
Source: TRICARE Program: Access, Cost and Quality Fiscal Year 2014 Report to Congress, July 2014

Quality of Care: Satisfaction with the Health Care Based by Beneficiary Category/Enrollment Status and trends in satisfaction with TRICARE Health Care by Beneficiary Category and Enrollment Status, Figures 4.4-20a and 4.4-20b, respectively.

- Satisfaction remained stable during FY 2011- FY 2013 for active duty, ADFMs, and retirees and families.
- The satisfaction levels of active duty and their families continued to lag the civilian benchmark for all three years, but retirees and families equaled (no statistically significant difference) the benchmark over that time.
- The satisfaction of enrollees with military PCMs lagged the civilian benchmark in FY 2011 to FY 2013.
- Satisfaction levels of enrollees with civilian PCMs and satisfaction levels of non-enrollees equaled or exceeded the civilian benchmark.

Figure 4.4-20a Trends in Satisfaction with TRICARE Health Care Based on Beneficiary Category, FY11 – FY13

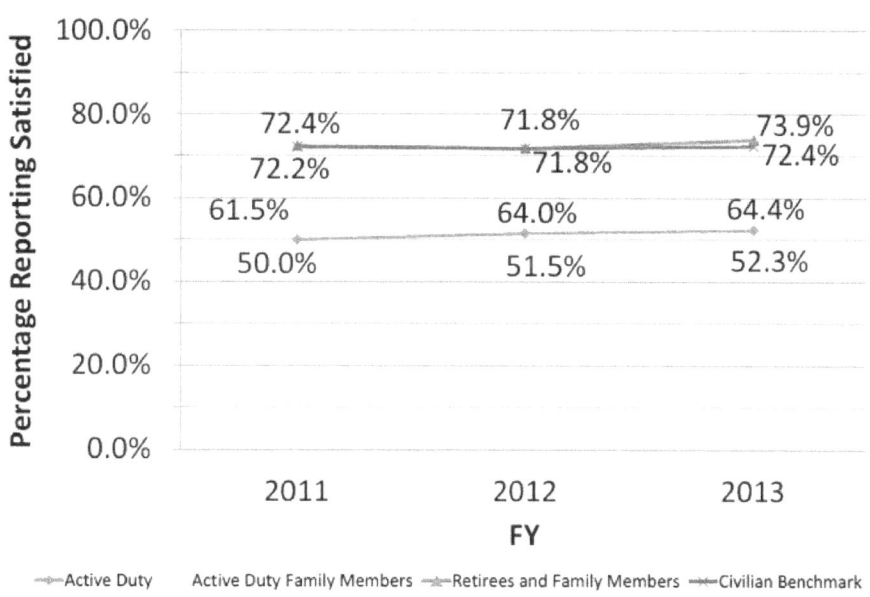

2014 MHS Review Group
Source: TRICARE Program: Access, Cost and Quality Fiscal Year 2014 Report to Congress, July 2014

Figure 4.4-20b Trends in Satisfaction with TRICARE Health Care Based on Enrollment Status, FY11 – FY13

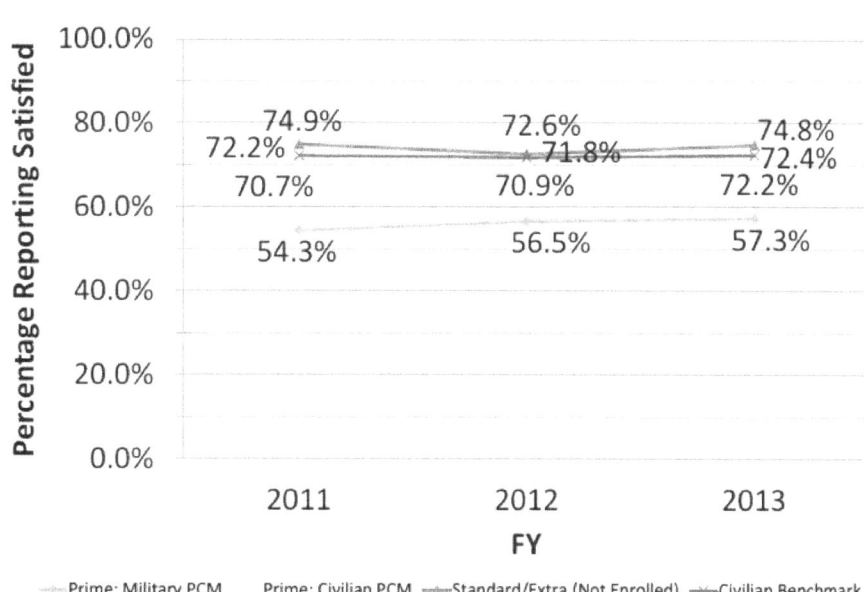

2014 MHS Review Group
Source: TRICARE Program: Access, Cost and Quality Fiscal Year 2014 Report to Congress, July 2014

Appendix 4. Quality of Care

Quality of Care: Satisfaction with one's Personal Provider Based on Enrollment of Beneficiary Category and trends in Satisfaction with one's Personal Provider by Enrollment Status Beneficiary Category (Figure 4.4-21 and Figure 4.4-22)

- Satisfaction levels of Prime enrollees (both military and civilian PCMs) remained below the civilian benchmarks. Satisfaction levels of non-enrollees are comparable to the civilian benchmark.
- Satisfaction levels by beneficiary category for active duty and their family members remained below the civilian benchmark, and remained steady over the three-year period for all beneficiary categories.

Figure 4.4-21 Trends in Satisfaction with One's Personal Provider Based on Enrollment Status, FY 11 – FY13

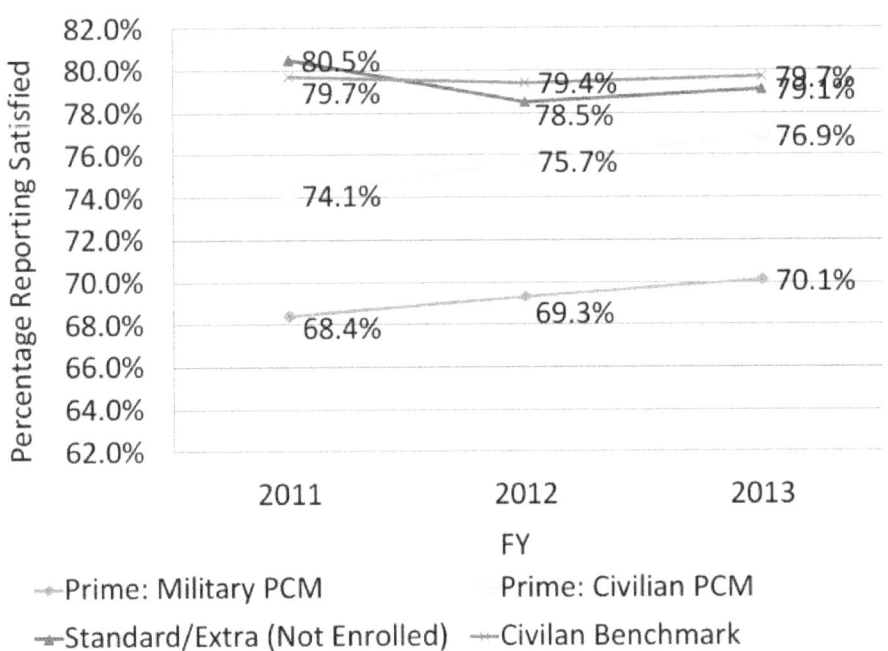

2014 MHS Review Group
Source: TRICARE Program: Access, Cost and Quality Fiscal Year 2014 Report to Congress, July 2014

Figure 4.4-22 Trends in Satisfaction with One's Personal Provider Based on Beneficiary Status, FY11 – FY13

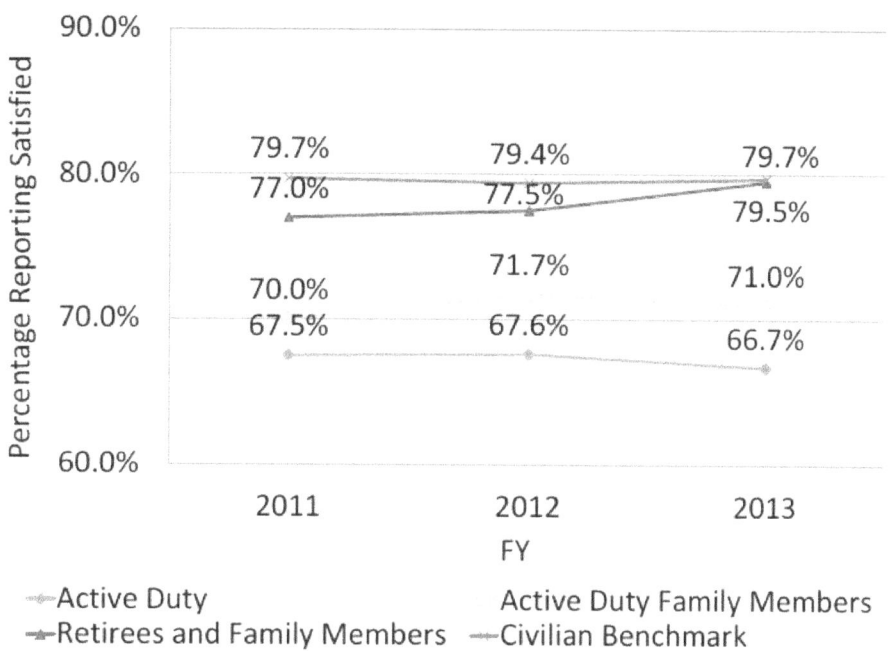

2014 MHS Review Group
Source: TRICARE Program: Access, Cost and Quality Fiscal Year 2014 Report to Congress, July 2014

This page left intentionally blank.

APPENDIX 5. PATIENT SAFETY

Appendix 5.1
Patient Safety Goals

Navy

The U.S. Navy Bureau of Medicine and Surgery (BUMED) Instruction 6010.23 does not define Patient Safety. However, it states "The goal of the PSP is to prevent injuries to patients, visitors, and personnel and to minimize the negative consequences of injuries that do occur. This is accomplished through the identification, reporting, and intensive analysis of sentinel events, adverse events, and close calls. The information reported through the PSP shall be used exclusively for improving health care system and processes that impact on medical errors and patient safety...." (p. 2)

Air Force

AFI44-19 states: "Patient safety proactively and retroactively identifies potential and actual risks to safety, identifies underlying causes and makes the necessary improvements to reduce risks. It establishes processes in response to sentinel events and adverse incidents by identifying risks through a Root Cause Analysis (RCA) and implementing process improvements. Patient safety, in collaboration with other activities including performance improvement and risk management, promotes a culture of safety in which errors are identified and reported freely without retribution. The goal is to reduce variability and vulnerability for error in processes. Safety is rooted in the daily operations of the health care organization where proactive risk identification, assessment and control are the foundation for safe and effective healthcare." (p. 28)

Army

Army MEDCOM Reg 40-68 states: "Patient safety activities are proactive and focus on reducing or avoiding misadventures during the delivery of medical/healthcare. Deliberate attention is required to improve medical systems and processes in order to prevent harm related to medical/healthcare interventions and to modify, reduce, or eliminate beneficiary exposure wherever possible. ...PS addresses incidents involving both potential harm (close call) to patients as well as those in which actual injury occurred (adverse event)." (p. 102).

Appendix 5.2
MHS Governance Related to Patient Safety

Figure 5.2-1 Central Defense Health Agency Structure

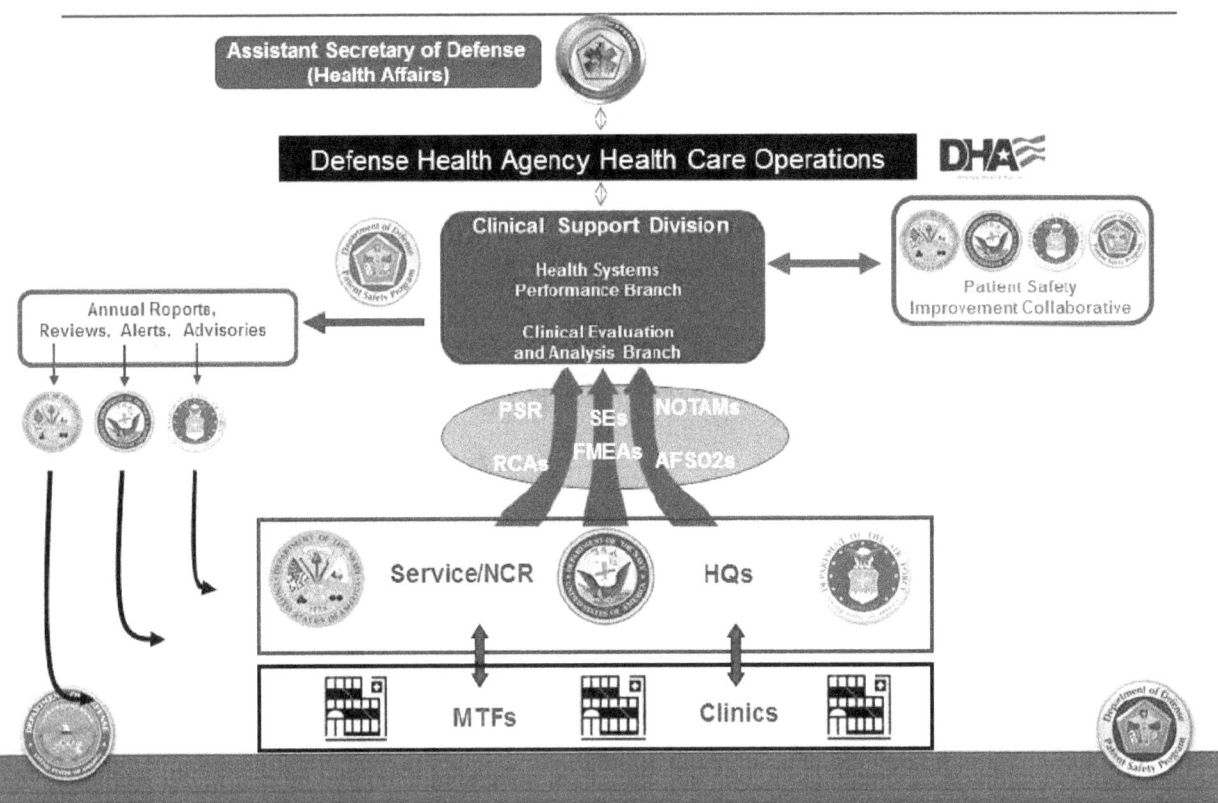

2014 MHS Review Group
Source: Basic Patient Safety Manager Course, Introduction Module, Updated February 2014

Patient Safety Program

The DoD Patient Safety Program (PSP) was mandated as part of the Floyd Spence National Defense Authorization Act of 2001 in an effort to ensure the safe delivery of care for to 9.6 million TRICARE beneficiaries across the MHS. PSP's mission was to promote a culture of safety to eliminate preventable patient harm by engaging, educating and equipping patient care teams to institutionalize evidence-based safe practices. The vision was to support the military mission by building organizational (Army, Navy, Air Force, and TRICARE Management Activity) commitment and capacity to implement and sustain a culture of safety to protect the health of the patients entrusted to our care. The PSP was aligned under the Office of the Chief Medical Officer, TRICARE Management Activity.

With the establishment of the DHA, the PSP was integrated with Clinical Quality and Risk Management. It was aligned, under the Health Systems Performance Branch and, in turn, the Clinical Support Division. It continues as a comprehensive program with the overarching goal of advancing a culture of patient safety and quality within the MHS. The PSP uses adverse event report-based information and lessons learned to produce products and services designed to reduce medical errors and assist with education and training in patient safety. The specific PSP goals are to:

- Engage members of the MHS, MTFs, military patients and their families in understanding patient safety and its role in maintaining military readiness.
- Create a learning environment and build competency within health care teams (inclusive of the patient and families) to understand, create, engage in, and promote a culture of safety.
- Use data to continuously improve patient safety in the MHS.
- Advance patient safety in collaboration with other national health care leaders.
- Ensure an efficient infrastructure to sustain patient safety activities and mandates through targeted goals and actions.

Before the establishment of the DHA, the PSP operated under the direction of the Patient Safety Planning and Coordinating Committee (PSPCC), a collaborative multi-Service body composed of patient safety, quality, and risk management experts. The objectives of the PSPCC were to:

- Improve the coordination of patient safety activities across the three Services, Armed Forces Institute of Pathology, Uniformed Services University, and the TRICARE Management Activity.
- Develop analysis plan for patient safety data and align it with national standards.
- Evaluate effectiveness of DoD patient safety training.
- Increase near miss reporting.
- Evaluate interventions to increase transparency after patient safety event.
- Increase transfer / implementation of patient safety in operational units.
- Increase patient awareness/involvement in patient safety initiatives.

Following the formation of the DHA, the DoD Patient Safety Improvement Collaborative (PSIC), formerly known as the Patient Safety Planning and Coordination Committee, was created to promote continuous improvement in the safety and quality of care delivered to MHS beneficiaries. This collaborative improves and fosters a culture of patient safety by developing, promoting, and supporting a comprehensive PSP aligned with MHS missions. The voting members of the PSIC consist of patient safety representatives from Army, Navy, Air Force, the National Capital Region, and the DHA. It also has advisory members (for example, Director, PSQAC, patient safety representative from the Senior Enlisted community, Section Chiefs from Clinical Quality, RM, Clinical Evaluation and Analysis Branch) and as well as ad hoc members. The specific goals of the PSIC are:

- Identify high-priority themed areas for enterprise-wide focused safety improvement intervention and tracking. Priority areas will be aligned with MHS strategic goals, will lead to a safer clinical environment, and likely to result in cost savings.
- Lead these focused improvement projects incorporating the translation of evidence into practice and health professions learning. These projects will involve tri-Service coordination to avoid duplication; they will be data-driven to demonstrate actual improvement.
- Promote knowledge transfer, transparency, and implementation of patient safety practices throughout the MHS.
- Coordinate the development, validation, and dissemination of patient safety activities across the MHS.
  - Support MHS/Service efforts to integrate patient safety into all health professions curriculum. Goal is to create clinical learning environments aimed at achieving safe high-quality patient care.
  - Disseminate patient safety information across the enterprise using multiple communication modalities.
  - Increase patient awareness and engagement in patient safety related initiatives.
  - Encourage leadership development in patient safety across the MHS.
  - Draft and review patient safety policy, instructions and/or directives.
  - Monitor the effectiveness of the DoD PSP, including training, education, data analysis, and research.
  - Foster interagency collaboration in the implementation of the PSP.

The PSIC reports directly to the MHS Clinical Quality Forum (CQF). There are differences in the Service approach to governance relative to how they are structured:

- Army and Navy MTFs fall under their Surgeon General (SG).
- Air Force MTFs fall under the line commands.
- The NCR MTFs fall under the DHA.

The DoD PSP consists of Service Patient Safety Representatives and their headquarters staff, MTF patient safety managers/staff, and the centralized Patient Safety Analysis Center (PSAC) and Patient Safety Operations. The PSP maintains a close working relationship with the Patient Safety and Quality Academic Collaborative (PSQAC) at the Uniformed Services University (USU).

Service Information

The centrally funded PSP is comprised of:
- DHA: Central Office – Three civilians and 29 contracted staff;
- NCR: Approximately four staff (two are MTF Patient Safety Managers [PSMs] – all civilian).
- Army: Approximately 44 staff (37 are MTF PSMs – AD and civilian).
- Navy: Approximately 40 staff (37 are MTF PSMs – AD, civilian, and contracted staff).

- Air Force: Approximately 91 staff (84 are MTF PSMs – all contracted staff).

Navy Governance

The Navy SG has direct authority and responsibility for the Quality oversight programs including Patient Safety and Quality. The Quality Oversight Programs (Patient Safety, Quality, Risk Management, Credentials, and Infection Prevention) are located within the BUMED Medical Operations Code (M3). BUMED's quality oversight programs have SMEs in each area to include a TJC trained fellow for Quality. Medical Operations Code reports directly to the SG. In addition, BUMED's Senior Strategy Board provides Execution and Oversight of BUMED Quality Projects and Regional Performance Reviews. Regional Commanders are responsible for oversight of the quality programs for their facilities. Regional Commands have a TJC trained fellow as a SME for Patient Safety and Quality Management. MTFs have Patient Safety and Quality Managers who, in conjunction with their physician advisors, implement these programs and provide recommendations to leadership. Various multidisciplinary committees support this effort at the MTF level.

Air Force Medical Service Governance

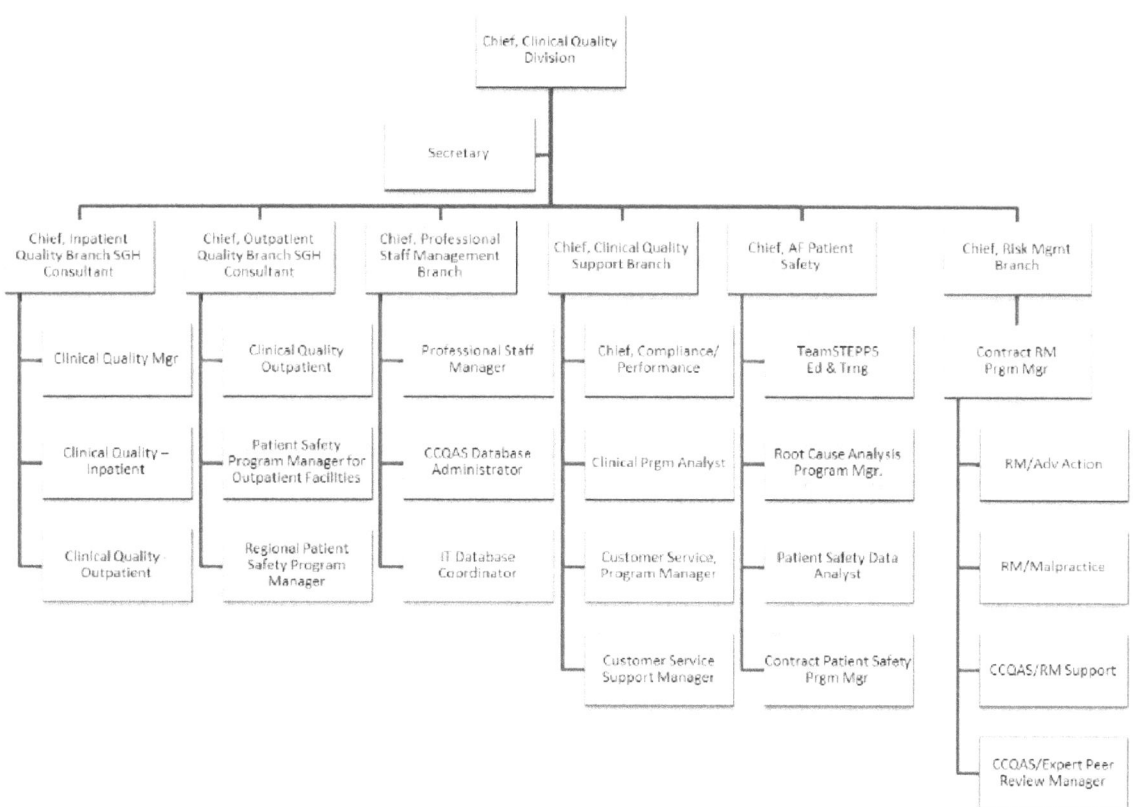

Figure 5.2-2 AFMOA/SGHQ Organizational Chart

2014 MHS Review Group
Source: Air Force Medical Operations Agency

The Air Force Medical Service (AFMS) strategic map demonstrates clear objectives to reduce the variability in system processes to drive reliable safe health care. A culture of patient safety is inherently about working relationships and effectively communicating in collaborative teams. This culture is patient focused and has an attitude of awareness and personal responsibility to apply safe practices with every patient encounter.

The Air Force SG establishes policy and delegates broad oversight responsibility for the AFMS Patient Safety Program to the Commander, Air Force Medical Operations Agency (AFMOA), Office of the Surgeon General, San Antonio, Texas. The AFMOA Commander ensures patient safety policies and processes are implemented in each MTF, including Aeromedical Evacuation sites and deployed locations. The Chief, Clinical Quality Management Division, AFMOA is responsible for delegating management of the program to the Chief Air Force PSP who executes the PSP program requirements via a centralized contract, which provides the manpower and expertise to operationalize the program within AFMOA and at each MTF. In turn, each MTF Commander is responsible to ensure the PSP is implemented and in compliance with DOD and AF policy.

The Clinical Quality Management Division patient safety team provides corporate-level expertise and guidance to each MTF to support compliance with DOD policy requirements. This includes:
- Model the behaviors and beliefs as well as speak the language of patient safety through training / education forums, webinars, focused group teleconferences, and routine consultation with facility Patient Safety Managers (PSMs).
- Advocate for an environment of non-blame and reduction of the fear of retribution through recognizing and encouraging good catch, near miss, and event reporting, conducting leadership rounds, and encouraging proactive approaches to problem solving with the end goal of process improvement.
- Submit all MTF reviewable sentinel events through AFMS leadership to DoD Patient Safety Office.
- Root Cause Analysis (RCA) review team; guides facility RCA teams to conduct the analysis, review each RCA completed for credibility and thoroughness, track corrective action plan implementation.
- Developed and disseminated Patient Safety Handbook, which describes how to implement PSP requirements and other leading practices for patient safety.
- Promote compliance with National Patient Safety Goals and initiatives working closely with the facility PSM and goal champions.
- Focus on prospective and retrospective analysis of events, new and revised processes and systems to identify areas of high risk, high volume problem prone and high costs.
- Reinforce responses to alerts and Notice to Airmen through thorough assessment of impact to the facility.
- Monitor AFMS patient safety activities and performance improvement recommendations in regularly scheduled Performance Management Forums.

Facility PSMs serve as the local PS resource and confer with all levels of facility personnel to develop and manage the program at the MTF. PSMs collect, collate, analyze and display data from event reviews, near misses, good catches, RCAs, Proactive Risk Assessments, and other sources. PSMs disseminate information to appropriate MTF committees / functions, quality managers and other individuals for patient safety improvement purposes and awareness. Under the direction of the Chief of the Medical Staff, the MTF PSM notifies AFMOA/SGHQ of all sentinel events, and adverse incidents as required by DoD policy.

Army Governance

The Army SG has direct authority and responsibility for establishing policy and delegating broad oversight to the Deputy Surgeon General/Deputy Commanding General (Operations) (DA SG-ZB), who is directly responsible to the Army SG and has direct oversight over the Clinical Performance Assurance Directorate (CPAD). As illustrated in Figure 5.2-3, the CPAD has direct oversight over Quality Management, Risk Management, and the Library. Quality Management has direct oversight over Patient Safety, The Joint Commission/Performance Improvement, Evidence Based Practice, the USAR Liaison, Credentials & Privileging and Adverse Actions.

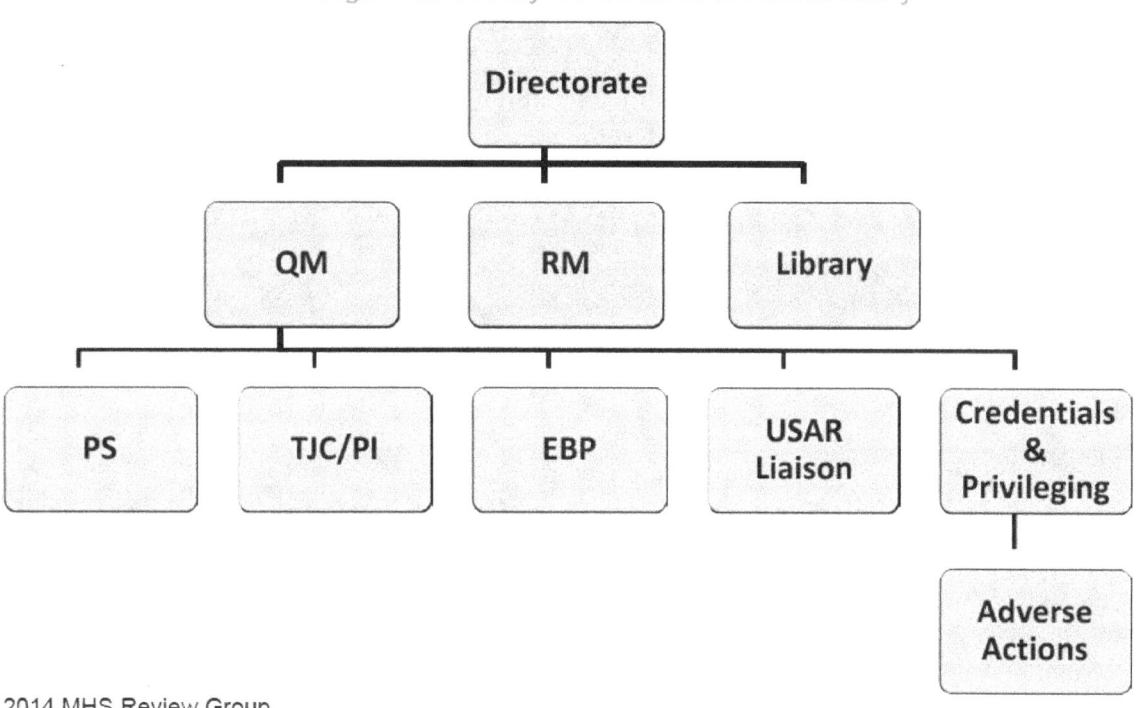

Figure 5.2-3 Army Governance of Patient Safety

2014 MHS Review Group
Source: COL. Karen T. Grace, USARMY MEDCOM HQ, July 2014

The CPAD Director is responsible for delegating management of the program to the Patient Safety Manager, CPAD who executes program requirements, which provides the manpower and expertise to operationalize the program within MEDCOM, the Regional Medical Commands (RMC), and at each MTF. SMEs within the MEDCOM PSP develop, implement, and evaluate policies at the MEDCOM level; provide mentoring, coaching, and training in collaboration with the Regional Medical Command (RMC) Leadership and RMC Quality Management cells to the Quality and Patient Safety Managers (PSMs) within the MTFs throughout the MEDCOM. In turn, each MTF Commander is responsible to ensure the program is implemented and in compliance with DoD and Army policy.

Facility PSMs serve as the local PS resource and confer with all levels of facility personnel to develop and manage the program at the MTF. PSMs collect, collate, analyze and display data from event reviews, near misses, good catches, RCAs, Proactive Risk Assessments, and other sources. PSMs disseminate information to appropriate MTF committees / functions, quality managers and other individuals for patient safety improvement purposes and awareness. Under the direction of the Chief, Quality Management Department, the MTF PSM notifies the RMC and MEDCOM of all sentinel events, and adverse incidents as required by MEDCOM policy. MEDCOM PSP in turn, notifies Health Affairs at the SGHQ of all sentinel events.

National Capital Region Medical Directorate

NCR MD headquarters develops policy and has direct authority and responsibility for PSPs within the Joint Facilities. The Quality Management Programs (Patient Safety, Quality, Risk Management, Credentials, and Performance Improvement) are located within NCR MD's Clinical Operations Division. As directed in the NCR MD Clinical Quality Manual (CQM), each inpatient MTF Director is responsible for establishing and implementing a PSP within their respective facilities. Facility level PSMs collaborate with staff to analyze and identify trends from adverse-event reports, support educational programs in patient safety, implement safety initiatives, and help extend best practices and "lessons learned" from adverse events to other units and departments.

Appendix 5.3
Patient Safety Policies

Navy Medicine Policies

1. Patient Safety and Quality are a strategic priority for Navy Medicine. The Chief Bureau of Medicine and Surgery issued a policy memorandum on January 3, 2014, SUB: Culture of Safety in Navy Medicine. The Chief outlined the measures Navy Medicine will take to begin the transition to a high reliability organization where staff feels safe in expressing concerns or asking questions of colleagues. The metrics that have been mandated include:
   - Leadership rounds
   - PS Recognition Programs
   - TeamSTEPPS® training and implementation
   - Monitoring the impact of the above
2. Effectively promoting patient safety focuses on creating strong incentives to disclose errors made/ observed, as well as building teamwork, communication and problem solving skills. On December 18, 2002, BUMED Instruction 6010.23 "Participation in the Military Health System Patient Safety Program (MHSPSP)" was established.
   The goal of the Patient Safety Program is to:
   - Prevent injuries to patients/visitors/personnel
   - Minimize negative consequences of injuries when they do occur
3. On October 9, 2013, BUMED Instruction 3100.1 "Commander's Critical Information Requirements" was established. The following patient safety events must be reported immediately via voice reports to the Chief, BUMED:
   - Sentinel events
   - Reporting medical-related events that may adversely affect mission accomplishment
4. On January 8, 2009, the Chief, Bureau of Medicine and Surgery issued a policy memorandum SUB: Reporting Infection Prevention and Control Data to the Centers for Disease Control and Prevention (CDC). This is in support of Health Affairs Policy Memo 08-020 of December 4, 2008.
5. On January 22, 2009, the Chief, Bureau of Medicine and Surgery issued a policy memorandum SUB: Application of the Joint Commission (TJC) Universal Protocol (UP) stating that Navy Medicine will effectively address its system and processes around effective implementation of The Joint Commission's Universal Protocol.
6. On April 14, 2011, BUMED Instruction 6620.9B, "Healthcare-Associated Infection Prevention and Control Program" was implemented. This policy establishes guidance for establishing infection control program. The policy applies to all MTFs, DTFs, branch health clinics, and shipboard and Marine Corps field medical units.
7. Medicine is very complex and even well-trained, well intentional dedicated professionals can make an error. Navy Medicine implemented BUMED 6010.28, "HealthCare Resolutions Program" on May 23, 2011. The policy promotes a culture of transparency and full disclosure following unanticipated or adverse outcomes of care. Commanders from MTFs will establish a Special Assistant for Healthcare Resolutions Position or ensure that services of a Special Assistant for Healthcare Resolutions are available. All Licensed Independent Practitioners (LIP) will receive disclosure training by health care resolutions specialists and

that full transparency is practiced when there are unanticipated or adverse outcomes of care, treatment or services.

Air Force Policies

The Air Force Medical Service's (AFMS) policy (AFI 44-119) for patient safety complies with DOD policy requirements, civilian accreditation standards, and aligns with current National Patient Safety standards. The policy clearly defines patient safety program roles and responsibilities for each health care team member rendering care and for the executive leadership. Additionally, the AFMS compliments this policy with a current patient safety guidebook, which further delineates process details to ensure uniform implementation of policy requirements. The Air Force Knowledge Exchange provides AFMS personnel easy online access to tools to enhance patient safety program effectiveness.

AFMS patient safety policy focuses on personal responsibility to identify and timely report near miss and actual adverse events. The Air Force analyzes each patient safety report to ensure lessons are learned from every event for performance improvement and to share lessons learned. The Air Force policy articulates our philosophy that building a culture of safety is leadership-driven and requires every team member value and commit to the principles and practices of safe care.

Army Policies

All programs have specified roles under AR 40-68 and as directed by the MHS. These roles include collaboration and input to DoD level Quality Meetings and policy development groups. CPAD serves as the Army representative to the Clinical Quality Forum, the Clinical Measures Steering Committee, Scientific Advisory Committee, Risk Management Committee, Patient Safety Planning and Coordination Committee, Evidence Based Practice Steering Committee, Various DoD Clinical Practice Guidelines (CPG) and Clinical Advisory Group (CAG) workgroups, DoD Pharmacy and Therapeutics Committee and various tri-service pharmacy working groups. Additionally, Army MEDCOM sends a representative to the National Guard Bureau Credentialing Board and the Army Reserve Component Credentialing board as a voting member and educational consultant.

The CPAD oversees MTF implementation of policies and procedures in collaboration with the Regional Medical Commands who have direct Command authority over the facilities. The ultimate aim is an operating company model where variation is minimized and accountability is recognized at the local and corporate level. Each region has a Quality Management cell. The manning varies somewhat, however the functions include overarching Quality management, The Joint Commission (TJC) accreditation, medical staff issues including credentialing and privileging, adverse practice and privilege actions, risk management, patient safety to include sentinel event reporting and root cause analysis, and performance improvement initiatives.

The CPAD Evidence Based Practice (EBP) section is the DoD lead with the Veterans Health Administration in the development of the DoD/VA Clinical Practice Guidelines (CPG). The

Director, CPAD serves as the Co-Chair of the Evidence Based Practice Workgroup. This work group is a direct report to the Health Executive Committee. EBP is an active member of the TRI-Service Workflow group working to develop AHLTA AIM forms for the CPGs streamlining documentation and putting the CPGs to work at the point of care. This encourages the use of evidence-based medicine and improves documentation of these practices across the AMEDD. CPGs are evidence based guidelines developed based on the needs of the beneficiary population. Each CPG has a toolkit that provides a variety of educational materials and guides for the clinicians and patient.

The CPAD provides corporate level oversight through tracking quality metrics and patient safety reports, reacting to trends, educating and training, measuring success against internal and external benchmarks and looking for future improvement projects in collaboration with Service and DHA representatives. The cornerstone is the education and engagement of leadership at all levels to apply lessons learned, anticipate the next issue and to hold providers and staff accountable for evidence based practices.

Appendix 5.4
Global Trigger Tool

The MHS performed a pilot implementation of the Institute of Healthcare Improvement (IHI) Global Trigger Tool (GTT) in inpatient MTFs to evaluate it in relation to other patient safety monitoring tools currently used within the MHS. The GTT method uses random sample inpatient medical record reviews to identify iatrogenic adverse events (AEs) leading to patient harms and to measure changes in harm rates over time. The DoD currently uses AHRQ Patient Safety Indicators (PSIs), derived from administrative data, and a voluntary Patient Safety Reporting system (PSR); however, previous studies found that GTT methods identify a greater number of harms than do PSI or voluntary reporting.

Two inpatient facilities participated in the pilot, a large tertiary care medical center with a varied patient population, delivering relatively more complicated health care services (Site #1) and a community hospital primarily serving an active duty and dependent population (Site #2). Three clinically experienced medical records reviewers and a physician adjudicator underwent training in GTT methods. A random sample of 120 adult, non-psychiatric, non-rehabilitative hospitalizations, occurring during the 6-month period of October 2011 through March 2012, was obtained from each MTF. Sampling was affected by choosing 10 records from each of the 12 semimonthly periods to assure consistent temporal representation over the six months. Pre-existing data from the DoD's voluntary PSR system, as well as DoD's implementation of AHRQ PSIs, were compared to the GTT results for the two participating MTFs.

During the six-month review period, overall harm rates at Site #1 were 286.8 harms/1,000 patient days, 90.8 harms/100 hospitalizations, and 47.5 percent of hospitalizations with an identified harm. At Site #2, there were 128.8 harms/1,000 patient days, 28.3 harms/100 hospitalizations, and 22.5 percent of hospitalizations with an identified harm. The majority of harms (65.0 percent) were classified as temporary harms that required medical intervention but had no long-term effects. For Site #1, 33 voluntary PSR reports were entered into the PSR system for the same six-month period, and for Site #2 it was only one report. The majority of the 17 individual PSI calculations revealed 0.0 percent six-month prevalence rates for both sites. Combining both sites, only three of the hospitalizations where harms were observed using GTT methods also had a corresponding AHRQ PSI identified.

Based on the literature, estimated harm rates were somewhat higher than anticipated at Site #1 but consistent with expectations at Site #2. The results of this pilot altogether support the GTT as potentially filling gaps in current patient safety monitoring that PSR and AHRQ PSI cannot.

Table 5.4-1 Adverse Events Reported Across Patient Safety Measures

	Hospitalizations With a Patient Safety Measure Event; n (Number of Hospitalizations With an Event / Total Number of Hospitalizations)					
	DoD PSR[a]		AHRQ PSI[b]		GTT Harm[c]	
Site #1	33	(1.07%)	0-6	(0.0 – 13.3%)	57	(47.5%)
Site #2	1	(0.08%)	0-5	(0.0 – 15.2%)	27	(22.5%)

a DoD PSR Totals and Rates.
b AHRQ PSI Totals and Rates.
c Percent of Hospitalizations With a Harm Event.

2014 MHS Review Group
Source: Pilot implementation of the Institute for Healthcare Improvement Global Trigger Tool at Two Military Treatment Inpatient Facilities

Appendix 5.5
Education and Training

The following section provides details on three components of the PSP that provide the field with the skills and knowledge needed to ensure patient safety: (1) Key PSP Initiatives, (2) PS Resources and Trainings, and (3) Recognition. The section concludes with a discussion on the education and training programs taking place at the Service level.

Key PSP Initiatives

Basic Patient Safety Manager Course

Results show that DoD PSP initiatives and integration efforts are making an impact. This is evident in the positive feedback from participants in the Basic Patient Safety Manager (BPSM) Course, targeting entry-level patient safety professionals in the DoD. BPSM learners reported "high confidence" in their attainment of skills through this important training, with average evaluation scores ranging between 90 and 100 percent.

Established in 2010, the DoD BPSM Course is a workforce development system designed to provide entry-level patient safety managers (PSMs) with the competencies they need to perform effectively during their first year on the job. PSMs manage patient safety programs in installations across the MHS, functioning as change agents at the frontlines of care to eliminate preventable patient harm. Given the PSM's critical role, the DoD PSP launched a multi-year effort in 2009 to build a state-of-the-art PSM ongoing learning program integrating leading-edge findings from the patient safety and workforce development sciences. The BPSM Program consists of three components: 1) Course Pre-work - three to four hours of preparatory learning activities to familiarize participants with the field of patient safety; 2) BPSM Course - five-day integrated classroom training focused on the practical application of a systems-based approach to patient safety; and 3) Coaching - follow-up sessions between course participants and trained BPSM coaches at 3, 6 and 12 months post-course to reinforce course content, provide performance support and facilitate learning transfer to the job.

The BPSM Program's comprehensive multi-level evaluation strategy assesses program effectiveness and identifies opportunities for improvements and future learning. Additionally, the course includes a lesson on the principles and tools of event reporting in the Patient Safety Reporting (PSR) system and PSMs have access to additional online PSR courses.

TeamSTEPPS

Developed by the DoD in collaboration with federal partners at the Agency for Healthcare Research and Quality (AHRQ), Team Strategies and Tools to Enhance Performance and Patient Safety (TeamSTEPPS®) includes a suite of evidence-based, ready-to-use materials and resources to integrate teamwork into any health care system. TeamSTEPPS® is designed to improve the quality, safety, and efficiency of health care to optimize patient outcomes by improving communication and other teamwork skills among health care professionals. It consists of customizable curricula necessary to successfully integrate teamwork principles into all areas of a health care system. Several customized versions of the training curriculum have been developed by AHRQ with DoD collaboration relative to Primary Care, Long Term Care, Enhancing Patient Safety for Patients with Limited English Proficiency, Dental Care, and Simulation. Many health care organizations and MTFs use simulation as an adjunct to training initiatives. Simulation is completed in designated centers and affords the opportunity for teams to practice team skills and behaviors in a controlled environment.

AHRQ began the National Implementation of TeamSTEPPS® in 2007 with DoD support. This program provides support and guidance for all TeamSTEPPS® users through an online user support network for implementation. It also provides training through six regional training centers and has trained approximately 5,000 Master Instructors from 1,500 civilian hospitals. Approximately 35 percent of U.S. hospitals are currently engaged with TeamSTEPPS®. As a result, DoD beneficiaries who use the purchased care component to receive care at civilian hospitals also benefit from patient care team that have integrated TeamSTEPPS® into daily practice.

Through award-winning TeamSTEPPS® (Team Strategies and Tools to Enhance Performance and Patient Safety), DoD has reached nearly 132,000 stakeholders[8] including 4,400 TeamSTEPPS® trainers through its Train the Staff and Train the Trainer courses since 2010. Course evaluation data shows strong evidence that TeamSTEPPS® trainings result in increased learner confidence in abilities surrounding the five TeamSTEPPS® competency areas. Before training, 45 to 65 percent of participants reported high confidence compared to 82 to 89 percent after training. At least 84 percent of participants intended to use the tools and strategies on the job. In addition, training empowered participants to speak up for patients' safety with 82 percent reporting high confidence after training compared to 55 percent without the training.

DoD emphasis has shifted from "awareness training" to sustainment and spread of positive TeamSTEPPS® changes, requiring an increasing focus on the organizational drivers of TeamSTEPPS® success. Key organizational drivers of TeamSTEPPS® success include supportive and involved learning environment, leadership engagement at all levels, rewards and accountability systems, frontline champions, peer support, impact measurement, on-site coaching, and training and alignment with strategic goals. During coaching sessions, MTFs report a heightened focus on training with difficulty in the implementation of the tools on the units, sustainment of trainer cadres, and lack of leadership engagement.

MTFs have reported broad TeamSTEPPS® impact/outcomes, including reduced patient harm events and improved communications, clinical processes, patient activation, staff and patient satisfaction and efficiency. Integrating teamwork efforts into a coherent Quality Improvement framework is essential. TeamSTEPPS® has been effectively integrated into efforts such as Partnership for Patients (PfP), Patient Centered Medical Home (PCMH), and the various

---

[8] The DoD PSP tracks TeamSTEPPS® training in the ORC, while the Army and Air Force track training numbers in Service-Specific systems. Due to lack of standardization around tracking of TeamSTEPPS® training, it is not possible to know if these additional Service numbers are duplicative of those tracked in the Online Registration Center.

perinatal safety initiatives. Emphasizing teamwork improvement as a separate stand-alone initiative was never the goal.

Partnership for Patients

In April 2011, the White House and the Department of Health and Human Services unveiled a new patient safety initiative, known as the Partnership for Patients (PfP), which focuses on decreasing hospital readmissions and hospital acquired conditions (HACs) by 20 percent and 40 percent, respectively by the end of 2013.

In June 2011, the ASD(HA) pledged to support the initiative, along with 3,700 other hospitals across the nation, and agreed to work toward making DoD hospital care safer, more reliable and less costly for every patient every time. As part of this initiative, HA and Services committed to implementing standardized evidence based safety practices for 10 specific areas of preventable harm (including Readmissions) across the DoD. The goals of the PfP support the DoD Quadruple Aim and have helped the DoD achieve improved population health, experience of care, overall military readiness and lower per capita cost. PfP also supports the Assistant Secretary of Defense for Health Affairs ASD(HA) strategic initiative to implement evidence-based practices across the MHS to improve the quality and safety of care provided to our beneficiaries. Implementation of PfP was the initial step in developing a 21st century Patient Safety and Quality Program across the DoD and moving the system toward becoming a high reliability organization.

In December 2011, the Surgeons General of the component Services discussed a model for a 21st century Patient Safety and Quality Program, as well as recommendations for meeting the aims of the PfP. In order to achieve the aims of the PfP, a three phased approach was discussed:

- Planning and Design: 1 January 2012 – 30 September 2012
- Implementation: 1 October 2012 – 31 December 2012
- Monitoring and Sustainment: 1 January 2013 – Present

The DoD continues to focus on ongoing, system-wide improvement activities in an effort to further decrease incidence of harm across the board. Based on the most current CY13 data, the MHS has achieved an overall harm reduction of 18 percent between CY13 and the baseline year (CY10). The DoD has also achieved an overall 11.1 percent reduction in readmissions from the baseline year (CY10) to CY13. DoD data will be incorporated into the national results. According to The Department of Health and Human Services report dated May 7, 2014, there was a national overall 8 percent reduction for readmissions.[9] Additionally, preliminary health care data for 2011 and 2012 indicated a 9 percent decrease in HACs nationally.[10]

---

[9] The Department of Health and Human Services Report. May 7, 2014. http://innovation.cms.gov/Files/reports/patient-safety-results.pdf.

[10] NASDAQ. (2014). http://m.nasdaq.com/press-release/lifepoint-achieves-significant-results-through-partnership-with-centers-for-medicare--medicaid-services-20140520-00345.

Patient Safety Portfolio of Resources

- *Annual Summaries:* The PSAC annually publishes two summaries of information submitted by the Services, an Annual Report that covers the entire Fiscal Year, and a Mid-year Report. These summaries provide an analysis of the patient safety reports (medication events, non-medication events, Root Cause Analyses, Proactive Risk Assessments, and other reports) submitted by the Services and MTF personnel during the respective reporting period. They identify trends, lessons learned, and other observations impacting the safety of patient care.
- *Focused Reviews:* In-depth, event driven analyses of specific topics based on what facilities are experiencing and reporting such as falls or unintended retained foreign objects. These analyses inform those directly engaged in providing health care of trends, notable causal factors, and useful lessons learned from events reported in MTFs and provide the latest research and innovations relative to the topic
- *Data Pulse:* The Data Pulse is published monthly and offers a Tri-Service snapshot of the PSR data, such as events by degree of harm, month and type, location type, and cumulative reporting for the DoD, as well as focus areas such as specific Partnership for Patients topics.
- *PSR SBAR:* The PSR SBAR highlights PSR-specific topics to enhance reporting and data quality, distribute knowledge, and increase learning across the DoD. Information is presented using the Situation, Background, Assessment, and Recommendation (SBAR) communication tool. The intent of the PSR SBAR product is to succinctly and quickly address issues and learning opportunities related to PSR, such as entering events, classifying events, generating reports, trending.
- *Sentinel Event Watch:* Sentinel Event Watch is a monthly publication provided to leadership with two overarching principles: near real-time distribution of Sentinel Event data and inter-service transparency of this information across the DoD. Includes a Sentinel Event Spotlight section which focuses on specific Sentinel Event category(s) and emerging trends seen at the Patient Safety Analysis Center (PSAC).
- *Alerts and Advisories:* Brief, often time-sensitive reports targeted at error-prone patient safety issues in which all targeted providers and staff should receive timely notification. The issues may involve anything used in or on patients (e.g., equipment, devices, etc.) that places them at increased risk. These notices provide background, general information, and recommendations for addressing the patient safety issue.
- *Learning Updates:* Since it was first launched in March 2011, approximately 27 issues of the Learning Update have been published and disseminated to 6,216 subscribers. Five Partnerships for Patients (PfP)-related Learning Circles have been held with an average of 49 attendees per month between October 2012 and August 2013.
- *Learning Circles:* DoD PSP hosts regular interactive webinars open to all MTFs, which focus on a variety of patient safety topics and feature subject matter experts (SMEs) who share the latest evidence, lessons learned, leading practices, and success stories from the DoD and civilian communities. Webinar materials are archived on the PSLC for users worldwide to access at a time that is convenient to their schedule and/or as "just-in-time" learning--when the topic may be particularly relevant.

- *eBulletin:* DoD PSP publishes and disseminates a monthly eBulletin to share activities, topics of interest, and PSP updates. Since September 2010 when it was first launched, 36 issues of the eBulletin have been published and disseminated to 7,253 subscribers.
- *Patient Safety Toolkits:* DoD PSP Toolkits offer just-in-time training, action steps and resource guides for specific patient safety issues targeted for health care providers, education specialists, and PSMs. Toolkit topics include: Briefs and Huddles, Debriefs, SBAR, Patient Falls Reduction, Patient Activation, and Professional Conduct.

In order to leverage national patient safety resources, the PSP also provides Military Treatment Facilities (MTFs) memberships to programs such as National Patient Safety Foundation (NPSF) Stand Up for Patient Safety and the Institute for Safe Medication Practice (ISMP). Stand Up for Patient Safety is designed to provide the tools, resources, and education necessary to launch, sustain and advance patient safety initiatives in inpatient and outpatient settings respectively. The resources help to embed patient safety principles into organizational practice, align with national patient safety goals and meet critical regulatory requirements. MTFs receive access to: professional learning series; online, self-paced, educational modules and patient safety curriculum; information updates to help staff stay current on emerging research and news; Ask Me 3 materials, a patient education/engagement program designed to promote communication between health care providers and patients; ready-to-use Patient Safety Awareness Week Toolkits; and discounted attendance at the NPSF Annual Patient Safety Congress. ISMP makes communication and education about medication errors a priority, publishing four electronic medication safety newsletters for health care professionals and consumers that collectively reach more than three million readers. ISMP's newsletters are widely recognized as some of the most timely and comprehensive medical alert systems in the world. All DoD facilities receive the following Medication Safety Alert newsletters: ISMP Medication Safety Alert! Acute Care edition; ISMP Medication Safety Alert! Community/Ambulatory Care Edition; and the ISMP Medication Safety Alert.

Publications

Significant contributions have been made to the field of Patient Safety, including 35 peer review journal articles and 7 book chapters since 2005. International and domestic leaders, including the DoD, have co-authored health care team training publications that include topics such as: TeamSTEPPS®, Teamwork, Team Training Evaluation and Simulation.

Recognition

The Quality and Patient Safety Awards, first presented in 2004, were conceived as a way to encourage and inspire organizations, raise awareness, reward successful efforts, and to communicate successes and lessons learned throughout the MHS. The award provides Senior MHS Leadership an opportunity to recognize efforts designed to improve the care delivered within the MHS. The award helps to identify those who have shown innovation and commitment to the development of systems and processes that are tightly organized around the needs of the patient. DoD seeks to promote efforts that create an environment where safe, quality care is provided and is the responsibility of all members of the team. Quality and Patient safety initiatives submitted were focused on eliminating preventable harm, keeping patients from getting injured or sicker and helping patients heal without complications. Award submissions were evaluated through an internal board review process with evaluators familiar with expertise in education, data analysis, quality improvement, and patient safety. DoD has presented 44 awards since the inception of the award.

The DoD encourages a systems approach to creating a safer patient environment; engaging leadership; promoting collaboration across all three Services; and fostering trust, transparency, teamwork and communication. To promote a culture of safety and eliminate preventable patient harm, the PSP engages with stakeholders across the health care system – leadership, health care professionals, and beneficiaries – to provide education to ensure positive patient safety practices and safe patients.

Service Patient Safety Initiatives

In addition to the comprehensive patient safety resources made available at the DHA level, each Service also has other patient safety educational initiatives led at the headquarters level.

Navy

Navy Medicine offers the following education and training to its medical personnel:
- All new patient safety managers attend the DHA Basic Patient Safety Manager Course. This is a five day integrated classroom training focused on patient safety and root cause analysis and TapRooT® methodology. BUMED follows up with the new patient safety manager one month after the course to address questions or concerns.
- Advanced TapRooT® training is offered for patient safety/quality management staff that performs root cause analyses on a frequent basis.
- Annual The Joint Commission/Navy training for patient safety, quality improvement and risk management staff as well as the Chairperson of the Executive Committee of the Medical Staff of each MTF. This training is held at The Joint Commission (TJC) headquarters.
- AHRQ TeamSTEPPS® training (initial training and train the trainer) is implemented and attendance at the AHRQ TeamSTEPPS® conference is facilitated by BUMED.
- Membership in the American Society for Healthcare Risk Managers –the leading organization for health care risk managers is provided to each MTF Risk Manager. This organization provides current information on risk management so Navy risk managers can be cognizant of national trends and the latest approaches, innovations and resources.
- Subscription Membership in the Emergency Care Research Institute (ECRI) is provided to each MTF Risk Manager. ECRI is an independent, nonprofit organization that researches the best approaches to improving the safety, quality, and cost-effectiveness of patient care. They provide tools and references for problem solving and ongoing assessment.
- Training on the Systems Engineering Initiative for Patient Safety (SEIPS) provides a model that addresses work systems and patient safety, it provides a framework for

understanding the structures, processes and outcome in health care (hospital) related to human factors.
- Active Duty Middle managers attend the Advanced Medical Department Officer Course (AMDOC) where instruction on patient safety and risk management is taught.
- Navy Infection Preventionists are encouraged to be familiar with the products of the Association for Professionals in Infection Control and Epidemiology (APIC). They also attend epidemiology courses.
- Educational materials on patient safety are provided to facilities during National Patient Safety Week.
- Scenarios based upon content from real situations are provided to MTFs for use in simulation centers and in drills.

In addition, Navy Medicine Patient Safety/Quality Management/Risk Management Department provides formal communication sessions to discuss current progress on initiatives through:
- Monthly infection prevention video teleconferences (VTCs)
- Bi-monthly patient safety/risk/quality management VTCs
- Quarterly VTCs for the Executive Committee of the Medical Staff and medical staff services professionals.
- Annual update to BUMED leadership on the patient safety program and status of initiatives.
- Status of key patient safety program initiatives provided to BUMED Strategic Planning Group.
- Updates upon request to BUMED Advisory Boards, e.g. Women's Health-Perinatal group and key specialty leaders.
- Updates to Regional Commanding Officers on a semi-annual basis on status of the patient safety program and areas of MTF specific successes or challenges.
- Routine communications including results of data analysis, alerts, and advisories are provided on a regular basis to the MTF and Regional PS/RM/QA managers through emails and consultations.

Air Force

To support and maintain a culture of safe patient care, the Air Force has established numerous educational and training forums for health care teams and leadership. These forums focus on the importance of imbedding safe principles and practices into every patient encounter and in the systems of care overall. Germane to each educational forum are the key components to building a safe patient culture in each AFMS facility. AFMS courses are of various levels of detail dependent on the individuals' role and responsibilities. The courses vary from one hour instruction periods to five day formal courses. Patient safety topics are disseminated in non-formal means such as Annual Patient Safety reporting, AFMOA newsletters, Patient Safety Awareness Week celebrations, commanders' calls, and safety briefings. Below are examples of patient safety training within the AFMS.

Individuals (AFMS medics)

- Patient Safety Training at Newcomers Orientation
- Annual PS refresher (CBT or face to face offered)
- TeamSTEPPS® four hour initial training
- TeamSTEPPS® annual face to face re-dosing
- PSR Tool User CBT
- Commanders Calls, Just in Time training
- DoD Patient Safety Learning Center documents (SE watches, Focused Reviews, etc.) are shared with all Medics
- PS briefing at Nurse Residency Program
- AFMOA eBLAST sent to the field with PS topics
- MTFs participate in National PS week seminars
- Tailored education when required/desired
- Simulation training is conducted in multiple clinical areas for team training to enhance communication as well as improve individual currency for skills maintenance.

Patient Safety Staff

- All Patient Safety Managers (PSMs) attend five day Basic Patient Safety Managers Course
- All PSMs spend 1 day orientation at Air Force Medical Operations Agency PS/Quality Division
- IHI open school training available to all PSMs
- Duke University PS leadership course, John Hopkins PS Leadership course – attended by 37 PSMs in last three years
- AHRQ Annual TeamSTEPPS® collaborative available for some PSMs
- AF Annual five day QSPAR conference, (Quality Systems Program Assessment Review) attended by Chief of Medical Staff, Patient Safety, Quality and Risk Managers and Credentials Staff
- Aerovac and Deployed PSM courses available for JIT training
- DoD PSP offers frequent video/teleconferences for hot topics for PSMs and field
- AFMOA PS staff attend annual training for TapRooT®
- PS concepts incorporated into Medical School and GME resident education
- AF requested conference approval for attendance for The Quality and Patient Safety Educators Academy (QPSEA) – Train resident and Faculty of GME programs
- Staff Education Visits provided to MTF PS/Quality Team by AFMOA experts
- Formal Fellowship training opportunities in Patient Safety, Program offered annually
- Monthly Teleconferences offered by AFMOA SMEs with field functional managers on the Quality Team.

Leaders
- PS/Quality and Performance Management key topics addressed in MDG Commanders Course, Joint Services Intermediate Executive Skill, AF Intermediate Executive Skills, and the Annual AF Senior Leader Workshop.
- Key AF General Officers participate as mentors within the training noted here.
- DoD published Annual PS Report and DoD PS Culture Survey area shared across the AF.

Army

CPAD provides multiple training opportunities and educational resources across the AMEDD for leaders, SMEs and support staff. Alerts, information on products and best practices and opportunities for education are shared with the MTFs through their regional leads.

The baseline training and educational opportunities include:
- Monthly QM VTCs (prepared and presented by CPAD staff and including TJC education webinars).
- Data shared to date includes sentinel event data drill down by category and facility (result is sharing across the organizations; discussion of lesson learned).
- TJC findings have data for findings from 2011-2013 that shows areas to look for in preparation and is guiding policy development for the enterprise.
- Quarterly Patient Safety DCO sessions with facility and region PSMs, and bi-monthly regional patient safety manger collaborative calls.
- Bi-monthly Risk Management DCO sessions with facility and region Risk Managers.
- Scheduled and on demand DCO instruction in CCQAS and PSR.
- Patient Safety and Risk Management have milSuite sites with regular updates and discussions.
- Patient Safety Program "Root Cause" - newsletter highlighting Sentinel event lessons learned.
- DHA PSAC Focused reviews and Sentinel Event Watch, Patient Safety Annual report, Partnership for Patients (PfP) newsletters and the Data pulse highlighting patient safety metrics across the DoD.
- Blocks of instruction at AMEDD C&S courses. All of these leaders get a block of instruction on quality, patient safety and risk management and how they are to operationalize it at their MTF.
    - Pre-Command Course
    - Executive Skills Course
    - Captain's Career Course
    - Basic Officer Leader Course
    - Nurse Case Manager Course
    - Baylor Master's Program
    - Patient Administration Division Course
    - Clinical Nurse OIC Course
- Traveling team training opportunities
    - Surgical Services TeamSTEPPS® Training

- TapRooT® Methodology and Software training
- Team and Organizational Development Directorate (Organizational Coaching, Development, and Resilience; Self-awareness, Team Building, Change Management, Interpersonal Communication, Leader Development, and Service Excellence)
- Basic Patient Safety Manager Course in collaboration with AF, Navy and DHA.

Sharing of enterprise wide lessons learned:
- Newsletters, email notifications, phone calls, DCO, VTC, PSAC educational products are shared directly with regional and MTF leads.
- MTFs present to the AMEDD on sentinel event lessons learned, best practices in communities of practice and serve as mentors to the other facilities.
- Data from DHA and MEDCOM sources on a variety of metrics is shared as quickly as it becomes available.

National Capital Region Medical Directorate

NCR MD Patient Safety staff is required to attend the DHA sponsored Basic Patient Safety Manager Course, TapRooT®, PSR, TeamSTEPPS® trainings. Additionally, Patient Safety staff is encouraged to participate in monthly MEDCOM Quality VTCs (as per formal agreement with the Army).

Appendix 5.6
Hospital Survey on Patient Safety Culture

Table 5.6-1 Direct Care Comparison to the National Average – Safety

Hospital Survey on Patient Safety Culture 2005, 2008, and 2011: AHRQ comparison culture survey dimensions	DC Actual 2005	DC Actual 2008	DC Actual 2011	AHRQ 2012 Average
D1: Management Support for Patient Safety	71%	72%	72%	72%
D2: Supervisor/Manager Expectations and Actions Promoting Patient Safety	72%	73%	73%	75%
D3: Organizational Learning – Continuous Improvement	68%	69%	67%	72%
D4: Non-punitive Response to Error/Mistakes	44%	44%	42%	44%
D5: Feedback and Communication about Error	64%	64%	62%	64%
D6: Frequency of Events Reported	60%	60%	64%	63%
D7: Communication Openness	61%	61%	61%	62%
D8: Teamwork within Units	75%	75%	75%	80%
D9: Teamwork across Units	59%	59%	59%	58%
D10: Handoffs and Transitions	47%	47%	49%	45%
D11: Staffing	45%	45%	48%	56%
D12: Overall Perception of Patient Safety	66%	66%	66%	66%
Response Rate	54%	58%	43%	53%

2014 MHS Review Group
Source: Final MHS Overall Culture Survey Final Report, January 2013

Table 5.6-2 Direct Care Comparison to a National System – Safety

Hospital Survey on Patient Safety Culture 2011: AHRQ comparison culture survey dimensions	Direct Care Compared to HS3	
	DC Actual	HS3
D1: Management Support for Patient Safety	72.0%	76.7%
D2: Supervisor/Manager Expectations and Actions Promoting Patient Safety	73.0%	77.8%
D3: Organizational Learning – Continuous Improvement	67.0%	78.8%
D4: Non-punitive Response to Error/Mistakes	42.0%	45.3%
D5: Feedback and Communication about Error	62.0%	68.2%
D6: Frequency of Events Reported	64.0%	62.3%
D7: Communication Openness	61.0%	63.0%
D8: Teamwork within Units	75.0%	86.8%
D9: Teamwork across Units	59.0%	69.0%
D10: Handoffs and Transitions	49.0%	56.4%
D11: Staffing	48.0%	59.5%
D12: Overall Perception of Patient Safety	66.0%	74.5%
Response Rate	N/A	N/A

2014 MHS Review Group
Source: Final MHS Overall Culture Survey Final Report, January 2013

Appendix 5.7
PSI #90 Composite

Table 5.7-1 National PSI and IQI Results for the Medicare Population – Supplementary Information (2010 – 2013)

Metric Name	Benchmark	DC Actual
PSI #90 Composite (% of MTFs Performing as well as Benchmark)	CMS .68(2010, 2011) .61(2012) and .62(2013)	2010-63% 2011-75% 2012-75% 2013-73%
	AHRQ Reference Population*	2010-81% 2011-85% 2012-93% 2013-88%

*CMS National Achievement Threshold
2014 MHS Review Group
Source: Agency for Healthcare Research and Quality (AHRQ) and Centers for Medicare & Medicaid Services (CMS), July 2014

Appendix 5.8
National Health Safety Network

Figure 5.8-1 CAUTI Med/Surg: Major Teaching CY10 – CY13

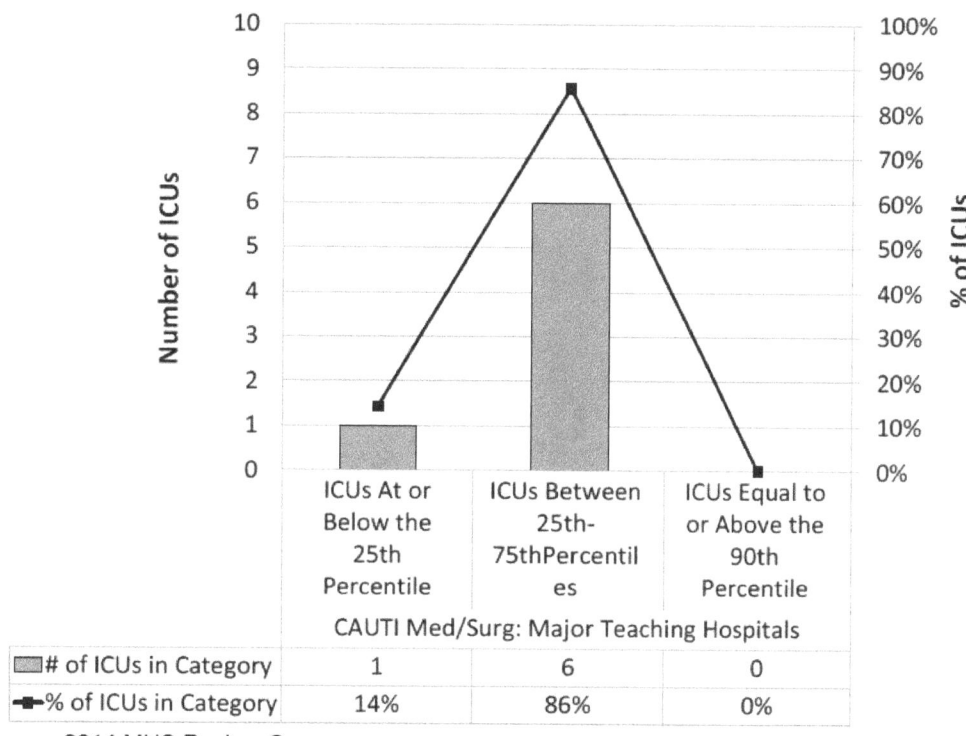

2014 MHS Review Group
Source: National Health Safety Network, July 2014

Figure 5.8-2 CAUTI Med/Surg: Other Hospitals Less Than 15 ICU Beds CY10 – CY13

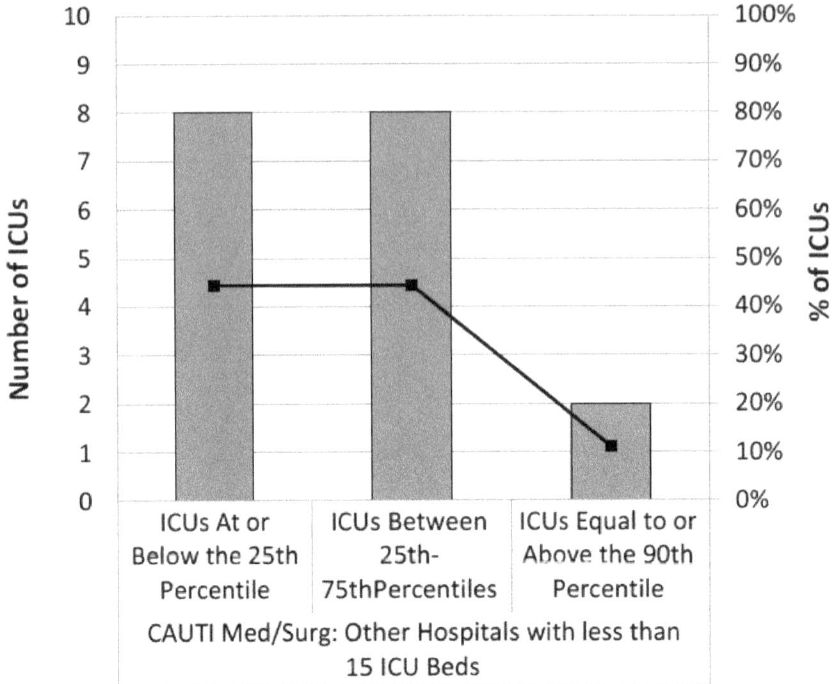

CAUTI Med/Surg: Other Hospitals with less than 15 ICU Beds	ICUs At or Below the 25th Percentile	ICUs Between 25th-75th Percentiles	ICUs Equal to or Above the 90th Percentile
# of ICUs in Category	8	8	2
% of ICUs in Category	44%	44%	11%

2014 MHS Review Group
Source: National Health Safety Network, July 2014

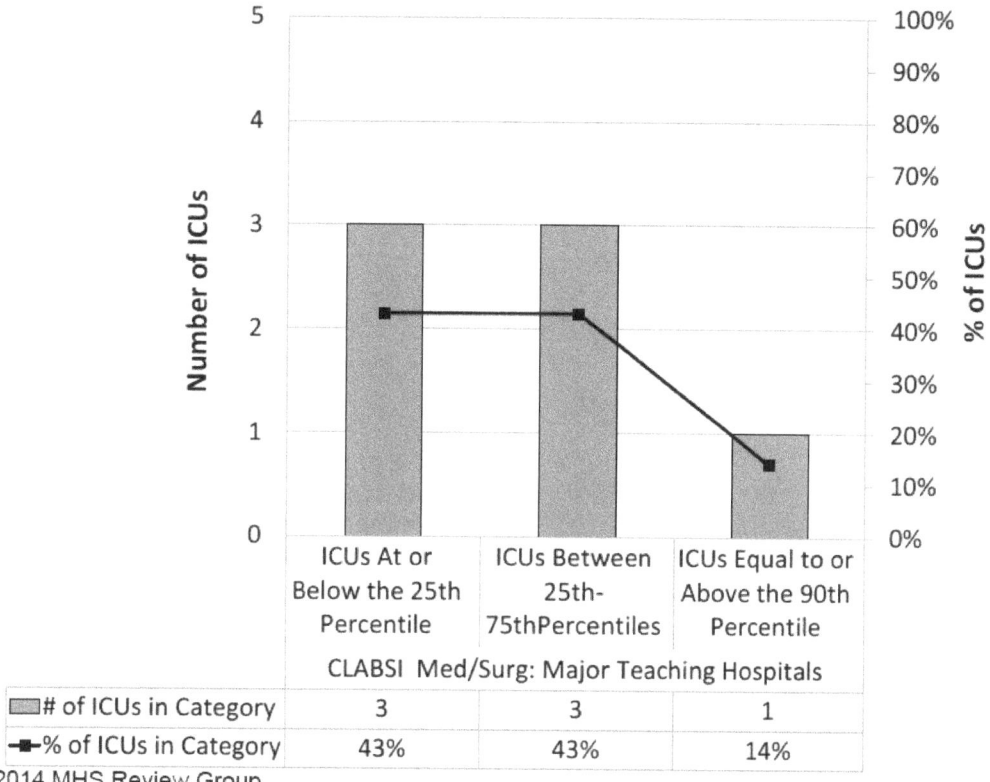

Figure 5.8-3 CLABSI Med/Surg: Major Teaching CY10 – CY13

2014 MHS Review Group
Source: National Health Safety Network, July 2014

Figure 5.8-4 CLABSI Med/Surg: Other Hospitals with Less Than 15 ICU Beds CY10 – CY13

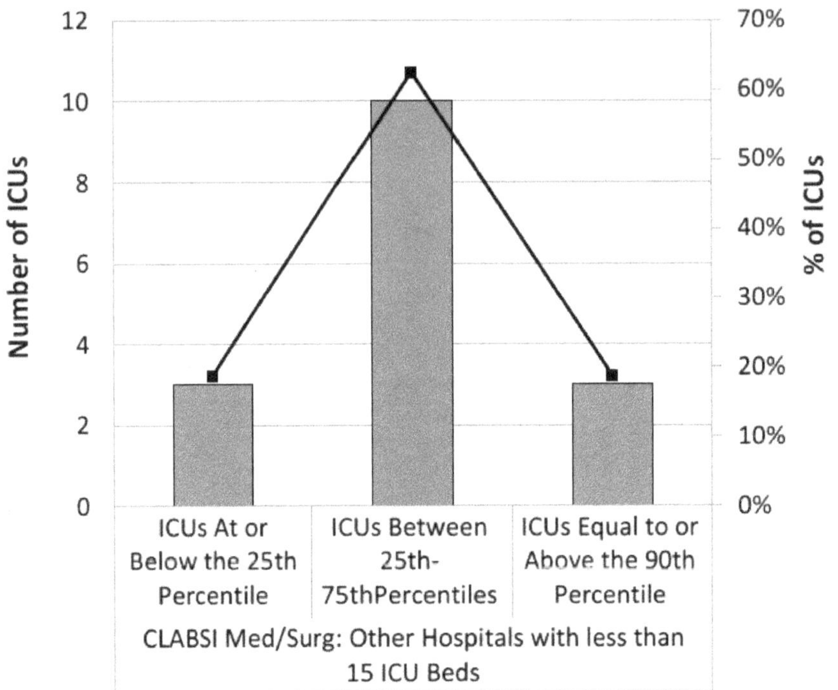

CLABSI Med/Surg: Other Hospitals with less than 15 ICU Beds	ICUs At or Below the 25th Percentile	ICUs Between 25th-75th Percentiles	ICUs Equal to or Above the 90th Percentile
# of ICUs in Category	3	10	3
% of ICUs in Category	19%	63%	19%

2014 MHS Review Group
Source: National Health Safety Network, July 2014

Figure 5.8-5 VAP Med/Surg: Major Teaching Hospitals CY10 – CY13

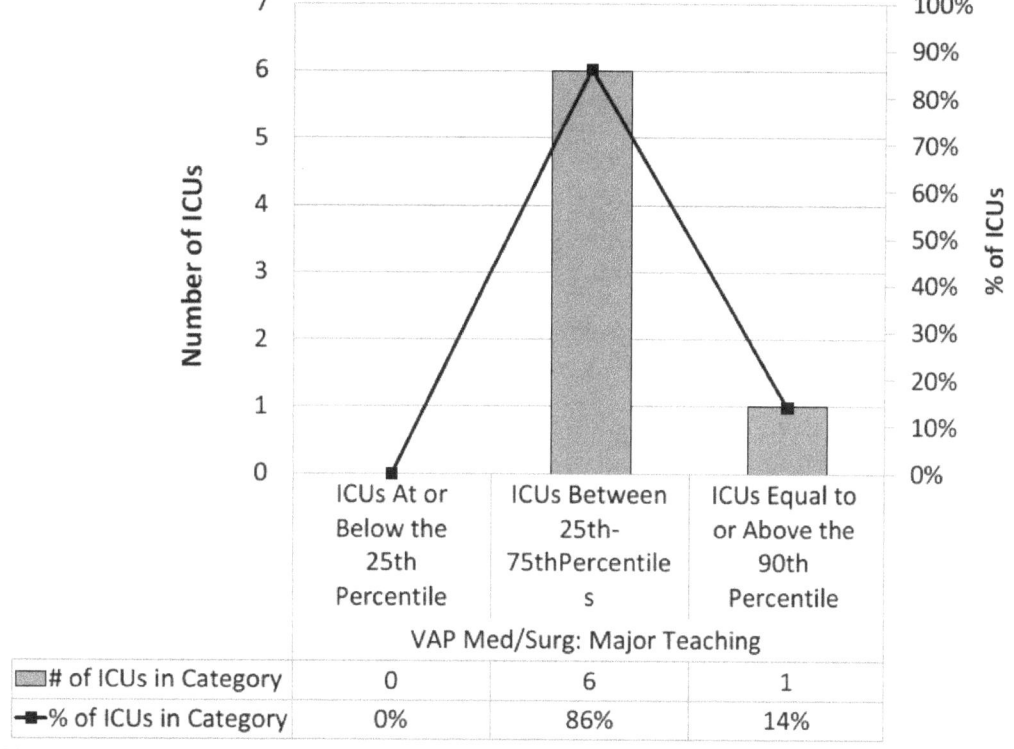

2014 MHS Review Group
Source: National Health Safety Network, July 2014

Figure 5.8-6 VAP Med/Surg: Other Hospitals with Less Than 15 ICU Beds CY10 – CY13

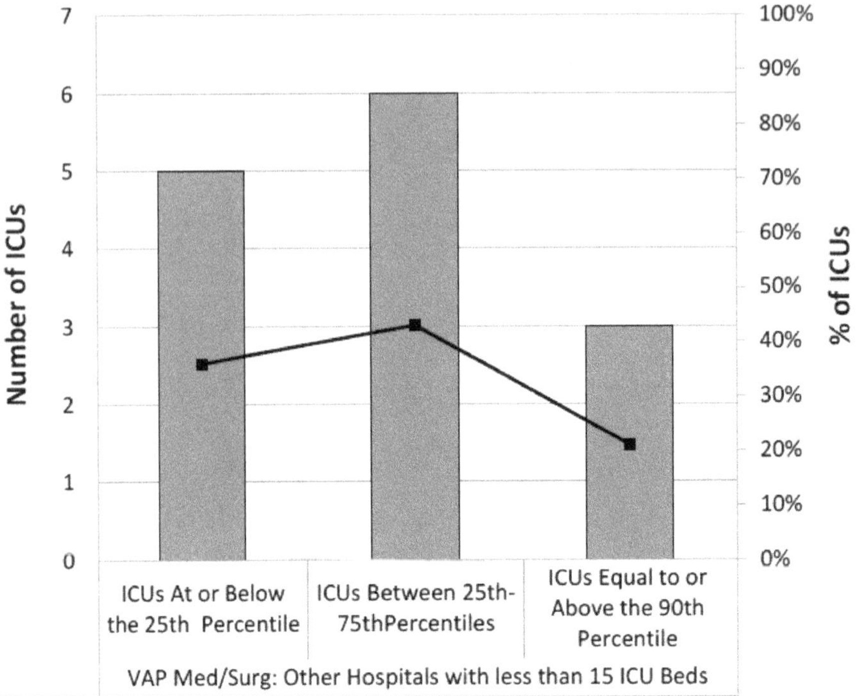

	ICUs At or Below the 25th Percentile	ICUs Between 25th-75th Percentiles	ICUs Equal to or Above the 90th Percentile
# of ICUs in Category	5	6	3
% of ICUs in Category	36%	43%	21%

2014 MHS Review Group
Source: National Health Safety Network, July 2014

Appendix 5.9
Reviewable Sentinel Events

The definition of a reviewable sentinel event takes into account a wide array of occurrences applicable to a wide variety of health care organizations. Any or all occurrences may apply to a particular type of hospital. Thus, not all of the following occurrences may apply to your particular hospital. The subset of sentinel events that is subject to review by The Joint Commission includes any occurrence that meets any of the following criteria:

- The event has resulted in an unanticipated death or major permanent loss of function not related to the natural course of the patient's illness or underlying condition, or
- The event is one of the following (even if the outcome was not death or major permanent loss of function not related to the natural course of the patient's illness or underlying condition):
  - Suicide of any patient receiving care, treatment and services in a staffed around-the-clock care setting or within 72 hours of discharge.
  - Unanticipated death of a full-term infant.
  - Abduction of any patient receiving care, treatment, and services.
  - Discharge of an infant to the wrong family.
  - Rape, assault (leading to death or permanent loss of function), or homicide of any patient receiving care, treatment, and services.
  - Rape, assault (leading to death or permanent loss of function), or homicide of a staff member, licensed independent practitioner, visitor, or vendor while on site at the health care organization.
  - Hemolytic transfusion reaction involving administration of blood or blood products having major blood group incompatibilities (ABO, Rh, other blood groups)
  - Invasive procedure, including surgery, on the wrong patient, wrong site, or wrong procedure.
  - Unintended retention of a foreign object in a patient after surgery or other invasive procedures.
  - Severe neonatal hyperbilirubinemia (bilirubin >30 milligrams/deciliter).
  - Prolonged fluoroscopy with cumulative dose >1,500 rads to a single field or any delivery of radiotherapy to the wrong body region or >25% above the planned radiotherapy dose.

Appendix 5.10
Site Visit Patient Safety Questions Analyzed

MTF Leadership Questions

1. What are you doing to improve patient safety?
2. Give examples of safety measures currently in place to reduce patient harm?
3. Describe how you create an environment where staff feels safe reporting errors and failures?
4. What areas did you focus on and what improvements have been made from the results of the cultural surveys?

Functional Staff & Staff Questions

1. Describe how your organization creates an environment where staff feels safe reporting errors? GIVE AN EXAMPLE
    a. How likely are you to report errors and related concerns?
2. Describe how your organization creates an environment where staff feels safe reporting near misses? GIVE AN EXAMPLE.
    a. How likely are you to report near misses?
3. Were the results of the 2011 CULTURE SURVEY communicated to you as a priority?
4. How effectively has leadership fostered a culture of safety?

Patient Questions

1. Do you feel comfortable asking questions to your care providers and MTF staff?

Town Hall Staff Questions

1. How do you report a safety issue or concern?
2. When concerned, how does the process work?
3. If you don't report, describe what steps you take to address the concern?

Town Hall Patient Questions

1. Do you feel you receive safe care here?
2. Do you feel comfortable asking questions to your care providers and MTF staff?
3. How do you report a safety issue or concern?
    a. If you don't, what steps do you take? (Subjective Response)
4. Have you been referred for care in the civilian sector? (yes/no)
    a. Did you feel like you received safe care?

Appendix 5.11
Site Visit Data

Table 5.11-1 Number of Respondent Types

Survey Site	Leadership	Subject Matter Expert (SME)*	Staff	Patient	Total
Site 1	7	5	16	10	**38**
Site 2	4	3	37	28	**72**
Site 3	4	3	16	6	**29**
Site 4	5	2	22	10	**39**
Site 5	6	3	24	11	**44**
Site 6	5	1	10	14	**30**
Site 7	5	5	13	16	**39**

*The Focus Group SMEs at Site 1 were present during the Executive Leadership session.
2014 MHS Review Group
Source: 2014 MHS Review Site Visit Survey, July 2014

Appendix 5. Patient Safety

Table 5.11-2 Associated Comments from Site Visits

Theme Concept	Associated Comments from Site Visits
Staff training	Initial and annual culture of [patient] safety training, orientation and ongoing training, lots of diversity and training, culture and safety training
Communication	have good communication throughout the facility, there is two way communication, increased communication on [patient] safety, working to improve communication between disciplines
Feedback	encouraged to report incidents, non-punitive
Patient Centered Practices	Protocol for Radio tag sponges, Sharp container - moved away from duty area, Security doors, check bands on patients, hourly rounds
Patient Focus	speaking up for patient care, Patient safety is one of CMD goals, I care about my patients
Open Door Policy	Open door policy is great, CO- encourages open door policy
TeamSTEPPS®	TeamSTEPPS® training, team huddles, rewards for speaking up, mustering, sharing lessons learned, SBAR
Staff Recognition	rewards for speaking up, good catch awards, Commander Coins
2011 Patient Safety Culture Survey	I do not recall, probably happened but do not recall it, they were communicated
Event tracking	report in PSR, QA logs, leadership fixed it, patient procedure held off until more X-ray were complete
Report Errors and Related Concerns	definitely, 100%, Not supported in the past; culture is not here, Not often. No finger pointing, Advocate PSR as non punitive, staff free to report
Report Near Miss	Always, Neutral - depends on the severity, If it is something that can be improved
Comfortable Inquiring Staff about Care*	Yes, would talk with provider and RN, I've asked questions of both staff and provider

*Theme concepts from only Patient respondents
2014 MHS Review Group
Source: MHS Review Site Visit Survey, July 2014

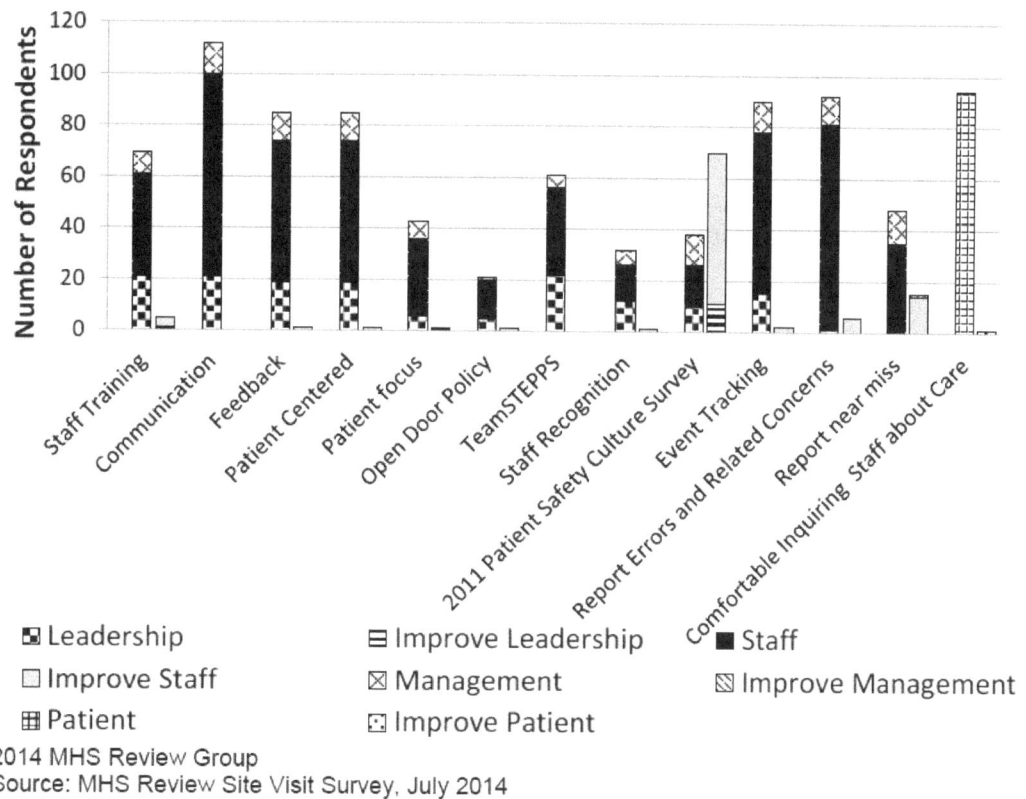

Figure 5.11-1 Number of Themed Concepts from Patient Safety Site Visit Rollup, CY14

2014 MHS Review Group
Source: MHS Review Site Visit Survey, July 2014

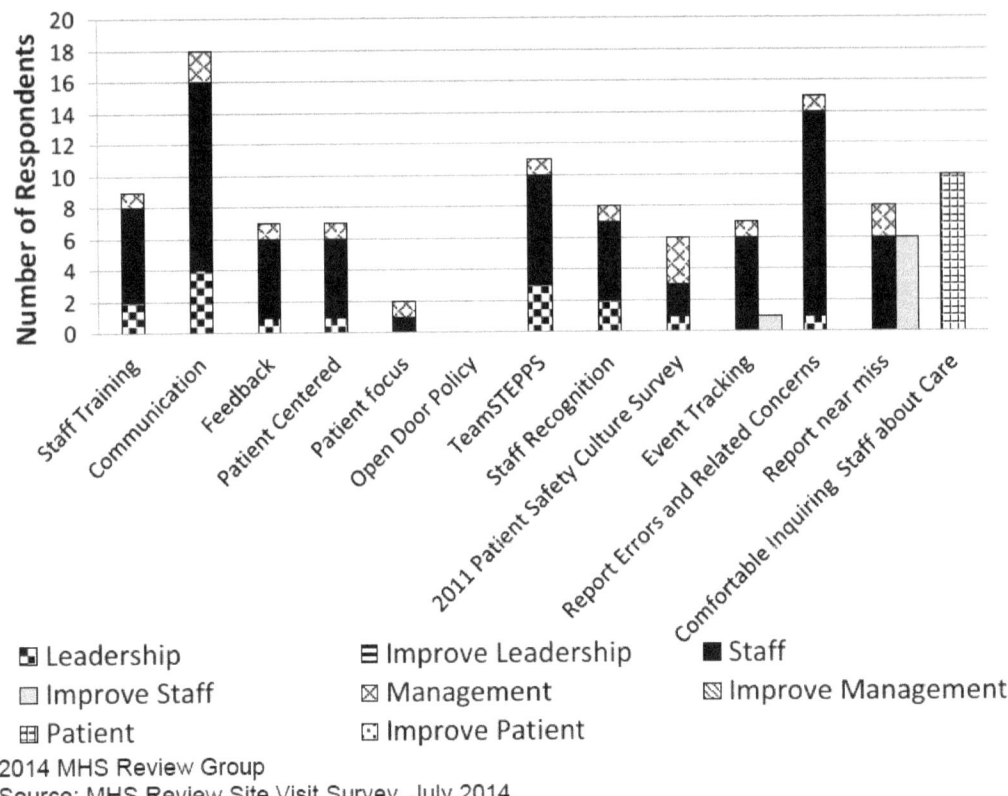

Figure 5.11-2 Number of Themed Concepts by Site: Site 1, CY14

2014 MHS Review Group
Source: MHS Review Site Visit Survey, July 2014

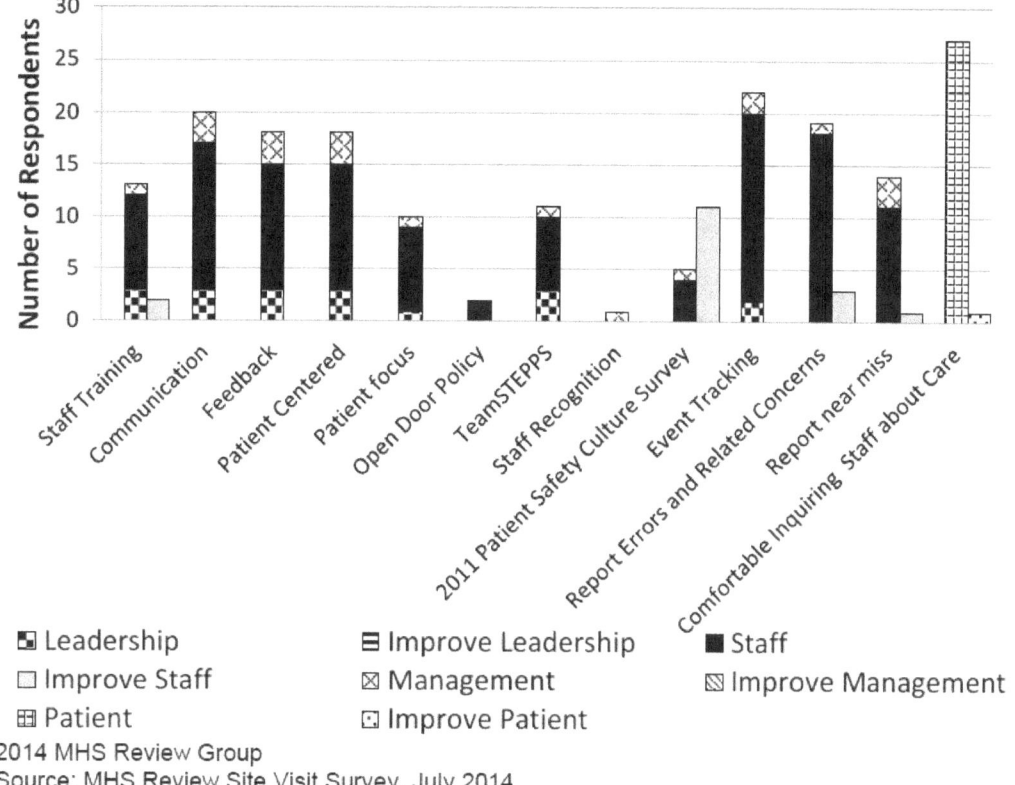

Figure 5.11-3 Number of Themed Concepts by Site: Site 2, CY14

2014 MHS Review Group
Source: MHS Review Site Visit Survey, July 2014

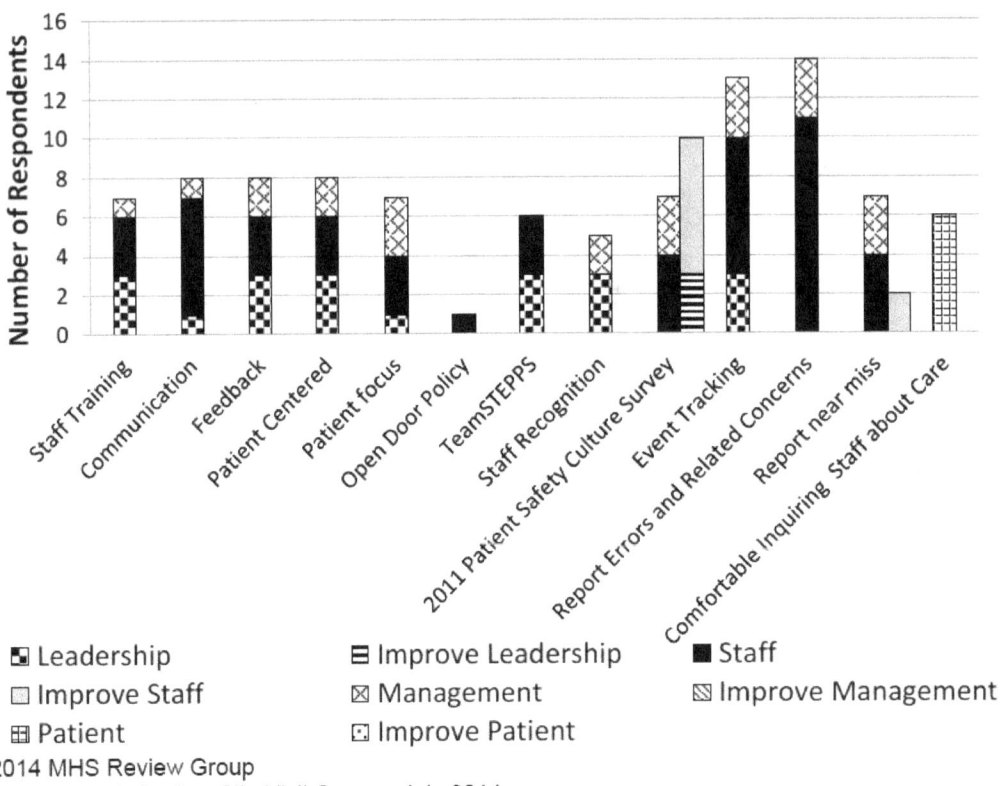

Figure 5.11-4 Number of Themed Concepts by Site: Site 3, CY14

2014 MHS Review Group
Source: MHS Review Site Visit Survey, July 2014

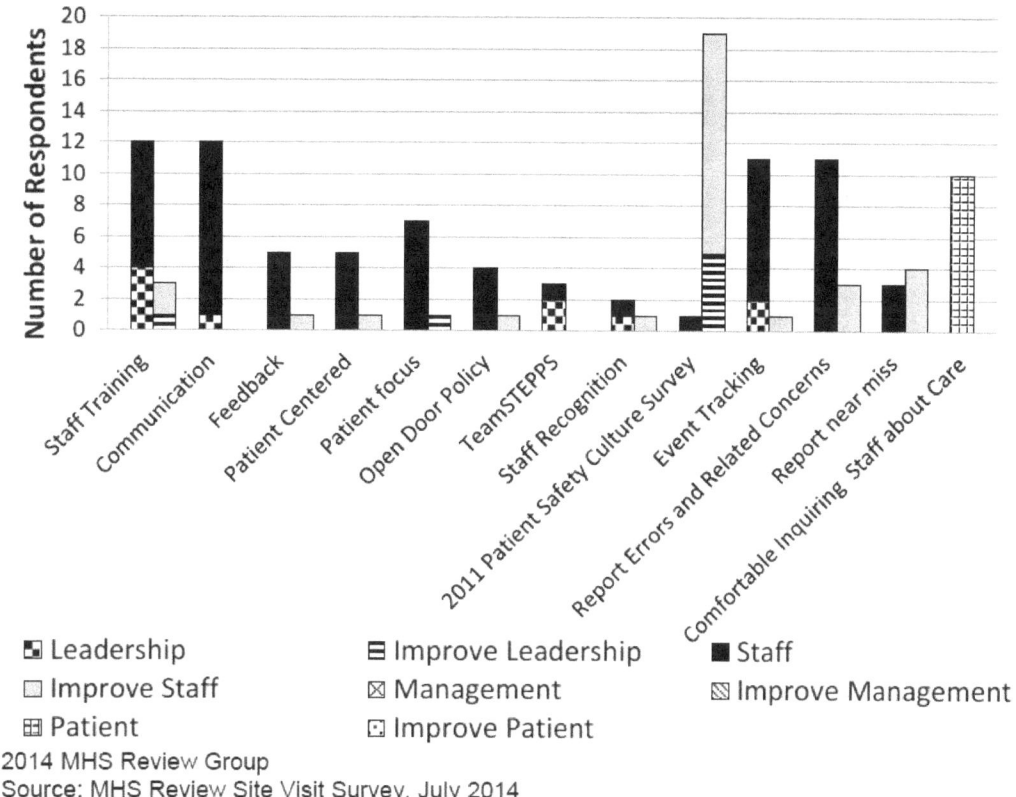

Figure 5.11-5 Number of Themed Concepts by Site: Site 4, CY14

2014 MHS Review Group
Source: MHS Review Site Visit Survey, July 2014

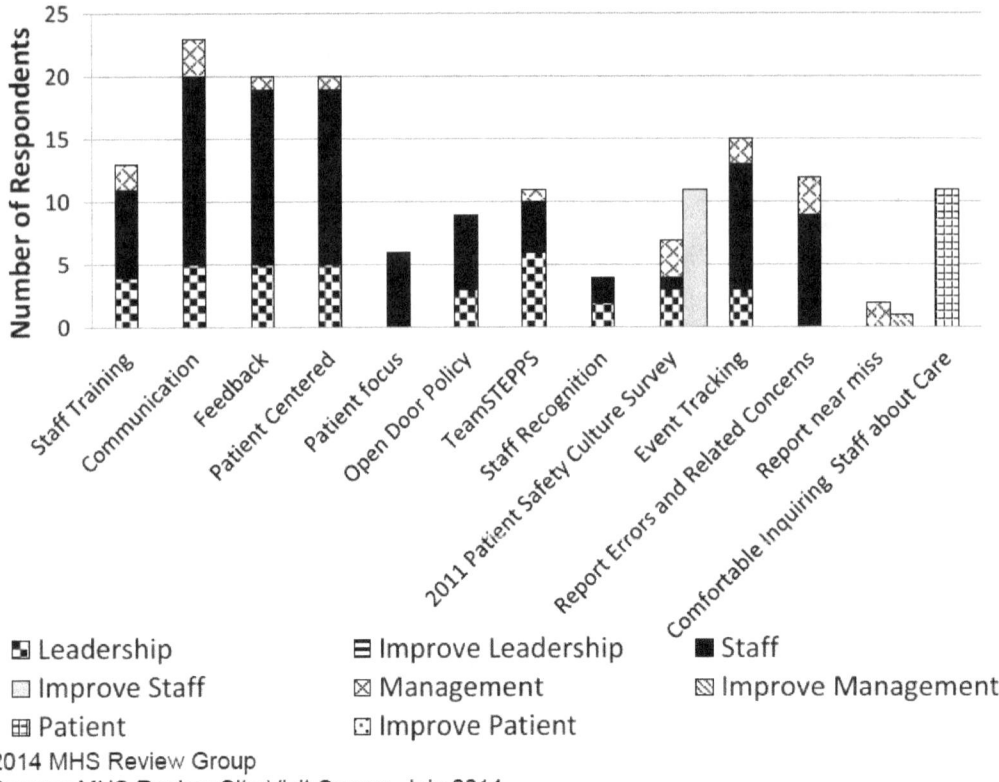

Figure 5.11-6 Number of Themed Concepts by Site: Site 5, CY14

2014 MHS Review Group
Source: MHS Review Site Visit Survey, July 2014

Figure 5.11-7 Number of Themed Concepts by Site: Site 6, CY14

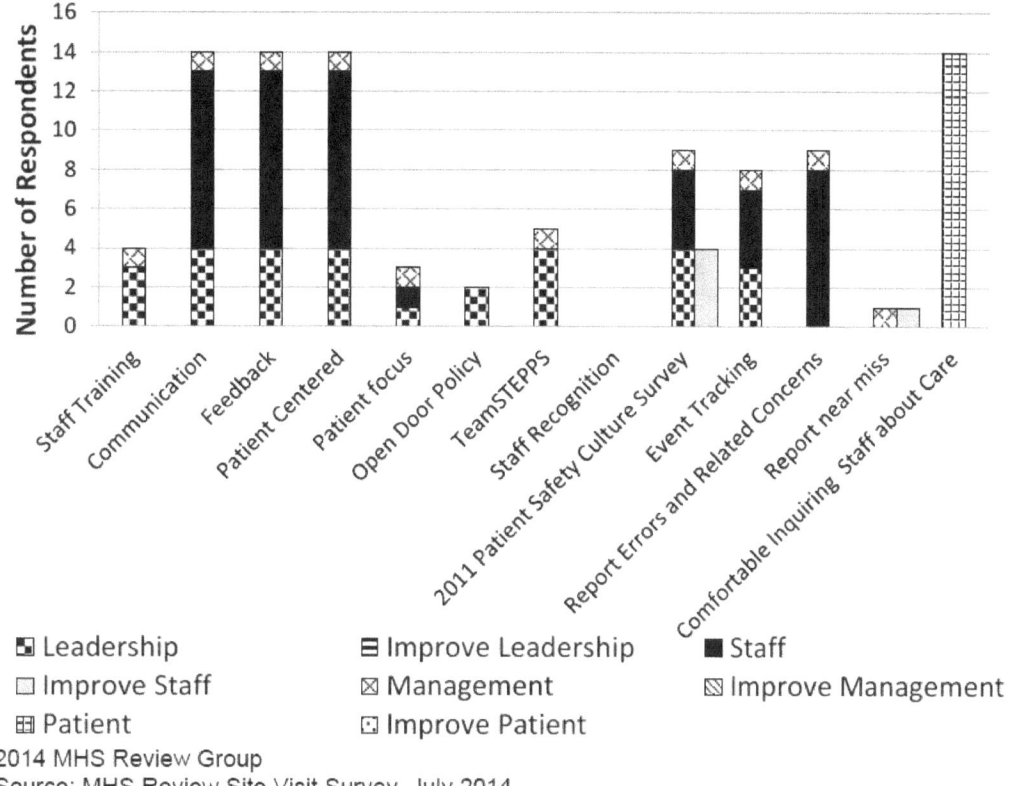

2014 MHS Review Group
Source: MHS Review Site Visit Survey, July 2014

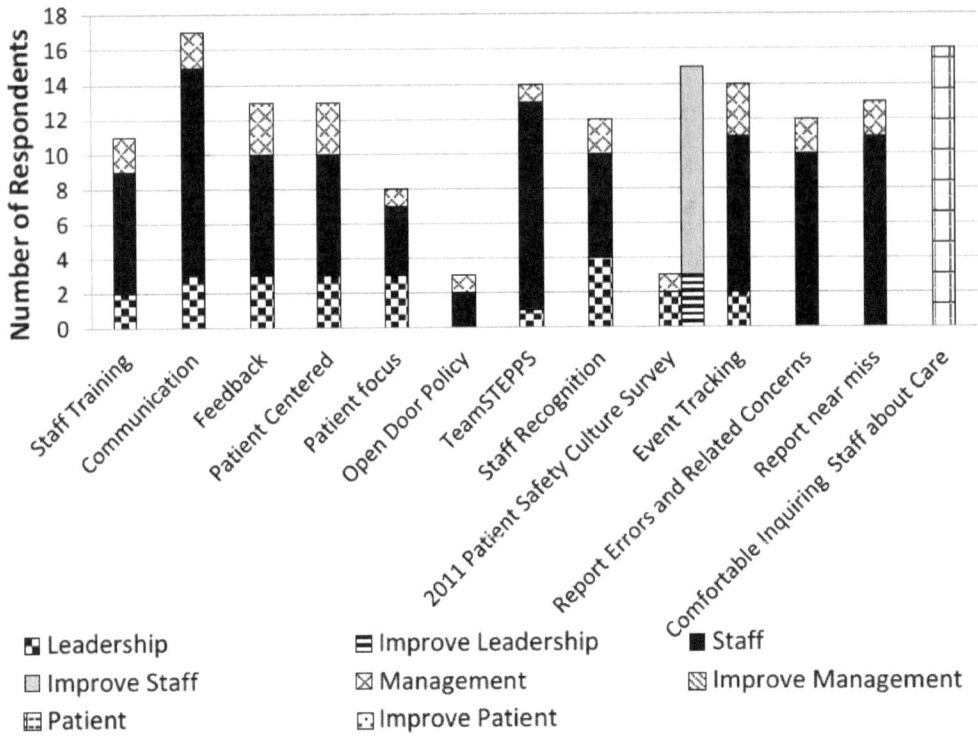

Figure 5.11-8 Number of Themed Concepts by Site: Site 7, CY14

2014 MHS Review Group
Source: MHS Review Site Visit Survey, July 2014

Appendix 5.12
Performance Improvement Initiatives

DHA and Service-level Performance Improvement Initiatives

Patient Safety has been a focus of the MHS direct care component for many years; service-wide performance improvement initiatives are described below:

Defense Health Agency (DHA) – Partnership for Patients

Partnership for Patients (PfP) was the first ever enterprise-wide approach to improving the safety and quality of care across the MHS for every patient every time and a key step in becoming a HRO. It is focused on making hospital care safer, more reliable, and less costly through the achievement of two goals:

- Making Care Safer: By the end of 2013, preventable hospital-acquired conditions would decrease by 40 percent compared to 2010.
- Improving Care Transitions: By the end of 2013, preventable complications during transition from one care setting to another would be decreased so that all hospital readmissions would be reduced by 20 percent compared to 2010.

PfP implemented Evidence-Based Practices (EBPs) around ten core patient safety areas of focus that included nine hospital-acquired conditions. These areas are: Adverse Drug Events; Catheter-Associated Urinary Tract Infections; Central Line Associated Blood Stream Infections; Injuries from Falls and Immobility; Obstetrical Adverse Events; Pressure Ulcers; Surgical Site Infections; Venous Thromboembolism; Ventilator-Associated Pneumonia/Ventilator Associated Events; and Readmissions. The EBPs are outlined in a series of Implementation Guides and developed for each harm condition and readmissions.

Process and outcome measures for each harm condition and readmissions were tracked and monitored by the PfP Working Group. Analysis of the Outcome data continues to occur on a quarterly basis; the Services report MTF-level harm data on a monthly basis for more real-time opportunities for performance improvement. The Services have established systems for tracking compliance with using the relevant EBP with every patient every time, which include tracers, compliance metrics, and checklist.

The Learning Action Network (LAN) structure allowed the MHS to move toward its goal of becoming a learning organization. The LAN consisted of Learning Circles focused on performance improvement and Communities of Practice (CoPs). The CoPs are harm condition-specific champions and teams allowing all MTFs to share best practices and lessons learned surrounding PfP implementation and data tracking, and external subject matter experts to present leading practices. MTF representatives used both of these learning opportunities to help their own MTF and others fully implement standard practices and achieve PfP aims. As part of the PfP initiative, there were five Learning Circles and 171 CoP sessions with nearly 370 participants each month.

MHS has made significant impact to patient safety through the collaborative efforts with Services and DHA. Through PfP, MHS reduced overall harm by 18 percent from CY2010 (baseline) to CY2013. Comparing the current rate (CY2013Q4) to when implementation began (October 1, 2012), there has been an 18 percent reduction. MHS readmissions decreased by 11.1 percent between CY2010 (baseline) and CY2013. Since the implementation of PfP, approximately 527 total fewer harms affected patients (averaging 105 harms per quarter) and $14 million in HAC associated costs (averaging $2.8M per quarter) were avoided. Areas of opportunity for improvement include, adverse drug event (ADE) and falls, which are self-reported harms. The Services and DHA continue to collaboratively focus on PfP sustainment and ongoing patient safety and quality improvement efforts via PSIC discussions and centrally reported outcome data.

Some of the key accomplishments of PfP throughout the MHS include establishing a framework for Transformative Performance Improvement; engaging front line clinical staff and leadership; promoting data-driven decision-making; creating an effective learning organization model; and reducing overall incidence of preventable harm and readmissions since PfP implementation (CY2012 Q4).

Army – Patient CaringTouch System

The Patient CaringTouch System (PCTS) is a strategic, patient-centered comprehensive nursing framework. It was first implemented across the Army Medical Department in 2011. The PCTS is an evidence-based framework developed to reduce unwanted variance, improve care, and reduce nursing turnover.

The PCTS is based on five core elements: 1) patient advocacy, 2) enhanced communication, 3) capability building, 4) evidence-based practices, and 5) healthy work environments. These elements are supported by six standards that are implemented at the clinic and unit level: 1) care teams (a care delivery model), 2) peer feedback (review and reflection on practice), 3) shared accountability (shared governance), 4) core values (guiding tenants), 5) skill building (improving knowledge), and 6) optimized performance (nurse-sensitive metrics). Four additional components reside at the regional or higher level including the Centers for Nursing Science and Clinical Inquiry, standardized documentation, leader development, and talent management.

Initial trends demonstrate improvement in several of the 10 nurse sensitive metrics such as voluntary nursing turnover, falls, falls with injury, patient satisfaction, and the practice environment. These metrics are reviewed and analyzed from the unit/clinic level to the Corps Chief. An early analysis revealed a cost avoidance of more than $9 million in nursing staff voluntary turnover and falls with injury. In 2013 Practice Environment Scale of Nursing Work Index, Army Facilities scored higher than Magnet facilities in three out of five subscales and in the overall composite scale (See Figure 5.12-1). In evaluation with the comparable health systems 2013 data, Army Hospitals had the same PES composite score (2.95) as the Magnet designated medical centers. Hospitals with Magnet designation are recognized for nursing excellence, better patient outcomes, and reduce mortality rates[11].

Although initially an Army program, other MTFs such as Walter Reed National Military Medical Center and Ft. Belvoir adopted some of the standards of PCTS and continue towards full implementation. This program is in its fourth year and research validates the difficulty of sustaining innovations in health care. The degree to which PCTS is embedded into the organizational culture is varied. The Army, Air Force, and Navy Nurse Corps Chiefs approved a grant to formally study the degree of sustainment, patient outcomes, practice environment and make program recommendations. The results of the study are expected in early 2015.

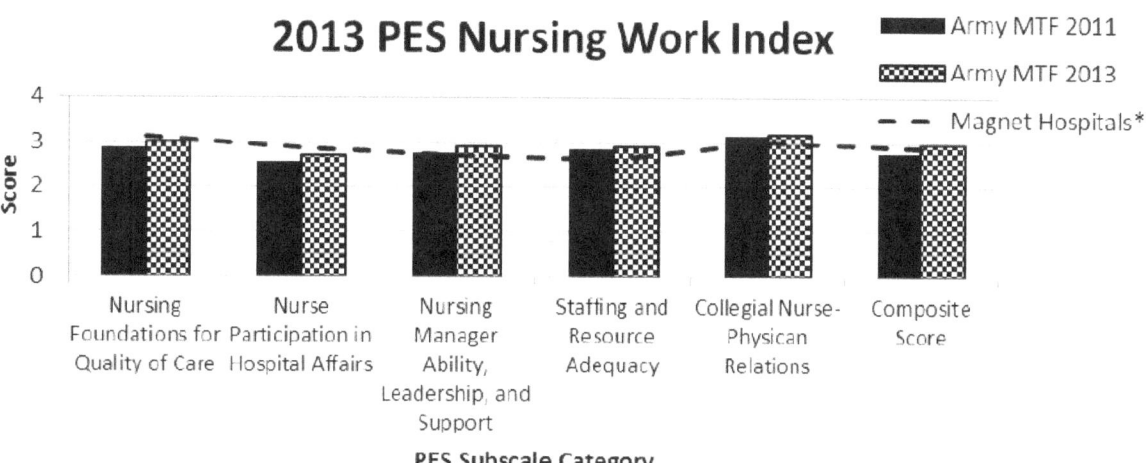

Figure 5.12-1 PES Nursing Work Index, CY13

*McHugh, Matthew, PhD, JD, MPH, RN, "PES scores-comparisons" email to D. Patricia Patrician, 27 August 2013.
2014 MHS Review Group
Source: Patient CaringTouch System, 2013

Navy – Culture of Safety

In January 2014 after analysis of data obtained using the AHRQ patient safety culture tool, the Navy Surgeon General initiated the PS Culture Initiative. The goal of the initiative is making sure that every staff member feels empowered to speak up to protect patients, and to feel safe in expressing concerns or asking questions of colleagues regarding care provided to a patient. The Surgeon General set the following expectations of leadership:

- Participation in weekly rounds and findings/actions resulting from the rounds are shared with staff
- Establishment or enhancement of PS Recognition Programs to focus on identification of process and system issues with subsequent recognition of staff in key forums

---

[11] McHugh, M.D. Kelly, L.A. Smith, H.L. Wu, E.S. (2012) Lower Mortality in Magnet Hospitals. Medical Care 51(5), 382-388.

- Implementation of TeamSTEPPS® training principles and tools such as huddles, briefings, debriefs and two challenges rule
- Include TeamSTEPPS® training in the Command Orientation Program
- Five staff per week are interviewed using the communication openness and non-punitive response to error questions

Four months of data show progress in staff awareness and willingness to share concerns. The command managers and leadership find the rounds informative. Staff are asking questions and receiving feedback. This is expected to be an ongoing evolution with increasing staff involvement and empowerment.

Air Force – Surgical Site Consultant

The Air Force Medical Service (AFMS) Clinical Consultant for Surgery in collaboration with the Patient Safety Program (PSP) initiated a Lean event to reduce wrong-site/wrong person surgical events. Surgical team members participated in this Lean event as essential stakeholders in this process. The documentation of compliance is automated and sent to the Air Force Medical Operations Agency for analysis. The final data sets are being evaluated and results are pending. This initiative resulted with a team-focused process and associated checklist to assure all critical Time-Out steps are followed and documented. The intent of this new safety initiative is to reduce wrong site surgical events.

APPENDIX 6. RECOMMENDATIONS AND COMMENTS

Appendix 6.1
Compiled Recommendations and Proposed Action Items and Associated Timelines

Compiled Recommendations

Overarching Recommendations

I. The MHS should identify the cause of variance for MTFs that are outliers for one or more measures and, when due to poor performance, develop corrective action plans to bring those MTFs within compliance.

II. The Military Health System (MHS) should develop a performance management system adopting a core set of metrics regarding access, quality, and patient safety; further develop MHS dashboards with systemwide performance measures; and conduct regular, formal performance reviews of the entire MHS, with the Defense Health Agency (DHA) monitoring performance and supporting MHS governance bodies in those reviews.

III. The MHS should develop an enterprise-wide quality and patient safety data analytics infrastructure, to include health information technology systems, data management tools, and appropriately trained personnel. There should be clear collaboration between the DHA's analytic capabilities, which monitor the MHS overall, and the Service-level analytic assets.

IV. The MHS should emphasize transparency of information, including both the direct and purchased care components, with visibility internally, externally, and to Department of Defense (DoD) beneficiaries. Greater alignment of measures for the purchased care component with those of the direct care component should be incorporated in TRICARE regional contracts.

V. Through MHS governance, policy guidance can be developed to provide the Services with common executable goals. While respecting the Services' individual cultures, this effort would advance an understanding of the culture of safety and patient-centered care across the MHS.

VI. The MHS should continue to develop common standards and processes designed to improve outcomes across the enterprise in the areas of access, quality, and patient safety where this will improve quality, or deliver the same level of quality at decreased cost (i.e., better value).

Access to Care

1. MHS governance should increase the focus on the standardization of specialty care for the direct care component through the following: a) create the Tri-Service

Specialty Care Advisory Board, b) fund requirements to standardize specialty product lines, c) establish business rules for access, and d) define performance review metrics for specialty care product lines.

2. MHS governance should standardize MHS direct care component access to care business practices by replacing the MHS Guide to Access Success with a MHS policy memorandum and subsequent DoD Instruction.

3. MHS governance should commission an external study to evaluate purchased care access for TRICARE Prime enrollees as it relates to 32 C.F.R. § 199.17. This study should include a review of all data available and recommend metrics to be incorporated into the current and future TRICARE contracts.

4. MHS governance should continue implementation of the Joint Service survey tool, refining access satisfaction questions to include satisfaction with office wait times.

5. MHS governance should standardize reporting on access from the TRICARE Regional Offices to the Services.

6. MHS governance should promote Secure Messaging and TRICARE On-Line through direct care component standardized business processes and a strategic marketing approach.

7. MHS governance should standardize both access to care and customer service training across the direct care component.

Quality of Care

8. It is clear that the MHS is dedicated to quality health care and performance improvement. In several areas, the MHS outperforms or is equal to national benchmarks. Other areas were identified for focused improvement in performance and to reduce variation in performance. It will be necessary to refocus the organization's quality culture for more rapid and continued improvement in quality of care. The MHS Review Group recommends that MHS governance research and implement health care industry best practices of a high reliability organization to revitalize and sustain the needed cultural changes throughout the MHS.

9. While comparison to national benchmarks is helpful, because of the variances inherent among health care systems, direct comparison between the MHS and civilian health systems proved challenging, with limitations in the comparative portion of the analysis. The MHS Review Group recommends that the MHS continue building relationships with civilian health systems to participate in collaboration and data sharing in order to facilitate more complete comparisons.

10. Under-developed MHS-level enterprise processes currently limit data standardization, collection, and analysis to drive system-wide improvement (e.g., governance, standard business and clinical processes, shared services). Variation exists in the use of existing data to identify and prioritize objectives. The MHS Review Group recommends that the MHS develop and implement a performance management system that links to MHS and Service strategies with MHS dashboards and common system-wide performance measures to support visibility of those measures across the enterprise. The MHS should also create and use a MHS data analytics capability to provide analysis and actionable information to the Services and DHA.

11. DOD quality policy (DODI/DODM 6025.13) lacks specificity with regard to quality measurement and performance improvement. The MHS should update or supplement DoDI and DoDM 6025.13 with specific guidance on quality measurement, performance improvement, and requirements necessary for assessing and improving quality education and training.

12. While there is a significant amount of quality training occurring in the Services, there is no clearly prescribed quality-specific training and education by MHS policy. The DHA Education and Training Directorate should conduct a more in-depth review and needs assessment of quality training to adequately assess the efficacy of training being accomplished.

13. There are gaps in the enterprise processes to validate Service compliance with policies and directives disseminated from ASD(HA). The MHS Review team recommends ASD (HA) develop and implement a process to manage and track compliance of Services and DHA with applicable DoD policies and directives.

14. The Assistant Secretary for Health Affairs ASD(HA) and DHA should develop policy guidance in support of DoDI and DoDM 6025.13 with specific direction on quality measurement, performance improvement, and requirements for education and training.

15. ASD (HA) should develop policy guidance to manage and track compliance of the Services and DHA with applicable DoD policies and directives.

16. The DHA Education and Training Directorate should conduct an in-depth review and needs assessment of quality training to adequately assess the efficacy of training.

17. DHA should integrate requirements for purchased care clinical quality data on TRICARE beneficiaries into the TRICARE Operations Manual and future TRICARE regional contracts.

18. MHS governance should determine the requirements to guide the development and implementation of a quality expert career path.

19. MHS governance should establish a mechanism to aggregate and communicate accreditation findings across the MHS.

20. MHS governance should evaluate the value of adding additional fellowship opportunities with The Joint Commission (TJC) or other nationally recognized programs, and the Services should explore optimizing and standardizing Service fellow utilization by aligning training with follow-on assignment after fellowship completion.

21. DHA Health Plans should give purchased care contractors the authority to use supplemental databases to improve the capture of clinical information for purchased care enrollees.

22. DHA Health Plans should evaluate alternative methods of incentivizing contractors and/or providers to improve the provision of clinical preventive services and Healthcare Effectiveness Data and Information Set (HEDIS®) performance. This may require statutory or regulatory changes, since new, innovative payment mechanisms may have to be developed to encourage compliance.

23. MHS governance should assess the value of expanding the number of HEDIS® measures monitored to evaluate care provided to enrolled beneficiaries.

24. MHS governance should establish policy to guide processes for verification of clinical data and capture in AHLTA (DoD Outpatient Electronic Health Record) regarding preventive services that are obtained outside of the direct care component.

25. DHA should develop plans to improve Other Health Insurance documentation in Defense Enrollment Eligibility Reporting System (DEERS) for all beneficiaries to ensure those with Other Health Insurance are not included in HEDIS® calculations.

26. MHS governance should develop a strategy for military treatment facilities (MTFs) to maximize the use of "action lists" generated by the MHS Population Health Portal to ensure beneficiaries receive clinical preventive services in a timely manner.

27. MHS governance should implement provider level Prevention Quality Indicators (PQI) education followed by an evaluation of MTF utilization of Agency for Healthcare Quality and Research PQI measures and implementation of a monitoring program requiring improvement plans as indicated.

28. MHS governance should establish an implementation plan for the MHS Population Health Portal readmissions site to ensure maximum utilization so as to reduce avoidable readmissions.

29. The DHA Healthcare Operations Directorate should complete transition to the HEDIS® All-Cause Readmission standardized measure, which is risk-adjusted and has national benchmarks.

30. DHA Health Information Technology should prioritize electronic health record upgrades by aligning needed data elements into Essentris® (the inpatient electronic health record). All inpatient MTFs should have the capability to remotely access health records to facilitate expeditious and timely data extraction for clinical measure calculation.

31. MHS governance should establish goals and processes for increasing the number of MTFs achieving The Joint Commission Top Performer status annually.

32. MHS governance should explore expanding National Surgical Quality Improvement Program (NSQIP®) participation to all remaining direct care inpatient facilities performing surgery. In addition, it should ensure ambulatory surgery platforms all participate in a similar surgical quality improvement program.

33. The DHA Healthcare Operations Directorate should partner with the American College of Surgeons NSQIP® staff to improve MTF collaboration and the sharing of best practices of top performing facilities, thereby decreasing overall direct care surgical morbidity and improving clinical outcomes.

34. MHS governance should task the NSQIP® working group to assess surgical morbidity shortfalls to the Medical Operations Group for Tri-Service/DHA engagement, collaborative support, and facility action.

35. The Perinatal Advisory Group should conduct a comprehensive review of clinical practices related to metrics where MHS is underperforming. Through a dashboard and standardized metric reporting requirements, intervention plans should be developed and actions prioritized.

36. Health Affairs policy is needed to standardize annual and interval training requirements related to perinatal team care.

37. MHS governance should require a review of perinatal provider documentation and coding practices at MTFs to validate data integrity.

38. MHS governance should ensure that standardization of accurate perinatal coding practices is implemented across direct care.

39. MHS governance should investigate readmissions of mothers and infants. This clinical review of diagnostic codes at readmission will identify the medical conditions that drive these rates and determine if lagging performance is a quality issue or related to military-unique issues and flexibility.

40. MHS governance should integrate measures of mortality into its quality monitoring and performance improvement programs.

41. MHS governance should require Service facilities with higher-than-expected mortality on an Inpatient Quality Indicators measure for more than one quarter to perform an investigation and implement improvement activities as indicated.

42. MHS governance should evaluate the use of the risk-adjusted standardized mortality ratio (SMR) model in direct care. Facilities with higher than expected mortality should validate the risk-adjusted SMR model data and perform a root cause analysis as indicated.

43. MHS governance should continue to study determinants of patient satisfaction and develop strategies to meet or exceed civilian benchmarks in satisfaction with primary care and obstetrics for every MTF.

44. MHS governance should continue to guide MTFs in implementation of strategies to optimize patient centered medical home (PCMH) operations and use of secure messaging, Nurse Advice Line, and other customer service tools.

45. Services and DHA should continue to evaluate determinants of satisfaction with primary care and ensure ongoing maturation of PCMH in all MTFs.

46. The PCMH Advisory Board should assess processes that affect Primary Care Manager (PCM) continuity at high-performing PCMH sites and promulgate best practices across the MHS to support improvement initiatives.

47. DHA should establish clear and consistent guidelines for the CONUS TRICARE Regions and the OCONUS Area Offices on reporting and processing quality and patient safety issues identified in the purchased care component.

48. MHS governance should work with the Services to increase the use of Clinical Practice Guidelines in the direct care component.

49. MHS governance should evaluate the feasibility of DoD and TRICARE regional contractor collaborations/MOUs with local purchased care organizations to support electronic health record accessibility.

50. MHS governance should develop processes to ensure standardized patient notification requirements for laboratory and radiology services.

Patient Safety

51. Implement principles of a high reliability organization with focus on leadership, culture of safety, and robust process improvement. This must be a strategic priority for executive leadership and will require revision of current policy and re-evaluation of Patient Safety Program.

52. Reevaluate the charter and membership of the Quality Patient Safety Risk Management Task Force and determine whether to use it to develop a framework for a high reliability organization for submission through existing governance structure.

53. DoD should develop a formal partnership plan with external health care organizations, TRICARE contractors, and national governing bodies to improve as a learning organization and be at the forefront of national benchmark development and initiatives for patient safety.

54. Refine DoDM 6025.13 policy to establish more than one mechanism for capturing harm events.

55. Health Affairs, through the DHA Clinical Support Division, with Service representation, should assess the revised TJC definition of "sentinel event" and determine if additional guidance in the DoDM 6025.13 policy is required.

56. Health Affairs, through the DHA Clinical Support Division and Office of General Counsel, with Service representation, should incorporate and define appropriate policy for patient/family engagement to proactively include patient/family perspectives in MTF decision-making.

57. Establish clear expectations in DoDM 6025.13 for the root cause analysis (RCA) process.

58. Establish a system-wide closed loop mechanism for documentation and disposition of a patient safety alert or advisory.

59. Ensure that the policy establishes attainable goals for "near miss" reporting.

60. Establish a system-wide structure to fully expand internal transparency of patient safety information in compliance with 10 U.S. Code 1102.

61. DHA should conduct a business case analysis that identifies the most effective method for staffing the Patient Safety Program.

62. The Services and DHA should evaluate their organizational structure to better align patient safety functions within their organizations to maximize leadership visibility.

63. Further define and standardize minimal patient safety training requirements as outlined in DoDM 6025.13 policy.

64. Develop an executive leadership toolkit; this best practice guide will address integral areas of patient safety.

65. MHS Governance must determine safety culture expectations and set targets based on opportunities.

66. Consider PSI #90 composite utilization as a component of a comprehensive safety measure set and develop an educational plan to support its implementation.

67. The Infection Prevention and Control Panel should review variance in performance in accordance with the Partnership for Patients Implementation Guides for Central Line-Associated Bloodstream Infection (CLABSI), and Ventilator Associated Pneumonia/Ventilator Associated Events (VAP/VAE).

68. The Infection Prevention and Control Panel should develop a comprehensive plan to standardize requirements for monitoring device-related infections.

69. Clarify policy and educate health care staff on the sentinel event definition and event types to reduce variation in interpretation.

70. MHS governance should pursue an enterprise-wide improvement process addressing the top five reported SEs, improve distinction between SEs occurring within ambulatory versus hospital settings, and monitor SE occurrence by rates using appropriate denominator estimates.

71. Establish clear expectations for the root cause analysis process and the follow up that will occur.

72. Standardize the performance improvement root cause analysis process with a focus on event type classification, a centralized repository, and dissemination of lessons learned.

73. Standardize the event type components of the event reporting process.

74. Standardize leadership activities to drive a culture of safety (i.e., Executive toolkit).

75. Adopt a chart audit based methodology such as the Institute for Healthcare Improvement Global Trigger Tool (GTT) to determine harm rate.

76. Incorporate best practices from all three contractors to develop a more standardized process that enhances transparency, minimizes variation, and incentivizes reporting for process improvement.

77. DoD direct care systems should pursue tracking infection rates at the unit level beyond intensive care units.

MHS Review Proposed Action Items and Associated Timelines

Action Items for Immediate Action (within 90 days)	Mapping to Overarching Recommendations / Timeline / Governance
ACCESS: MHS should further evaluate specialty care access data by individual product lines.	Global Recommendation VI Immediate Action MHS Governance
ACCESS: MHS should further evaluate the challenges of measuring access to care in the purchased care component by commissioning an external study to evaluate purchased care access for TRICARE Prime enrollees as it relates to 32 C.F.R. § 199.17.	Global Recommendation IV Immediate Action MHS Governance
ACCESS: MHS governance should continue implementation of the Joint Service survey tool, refining access satisfaction questions to include the addition of satisfaction with office wait times.	Global Recommendation VI Immediate Action MHS Governance
QUALITY: MHS governance should task the National Surgical Quality Improvement Program (NSQIP®) working group to assess surgical morbidity shortfalls to the Medical Operations Group for Tri-Service/Defense Health Agency (DHA) engagement, collaborative support, and facility action.	Global Recommendation II Immediate Action MHS Governance
QUALITY: DHA Healthcare Operations Directorate should partner with the American College of Surgeons NSQIP® staff to improve military treatment facility (MTF) collaboration and the sharing of best practices from the top performing facilities, thereby decreasing overall direct care surgical morbidity and improving clinical outcomes.	Global Recommendation II Immediate Action DHA
QUALITY: MHS governance should require a review of perinatal provider documentation and coding practices at MTFs to validate data integrity.	Global Recommendations II & III Immediate Action MHS Governance
QUALITY: MHS governance should develop strategy for MTFs to maximize the use of "action lists" generated by the MHS Population Health Portal to ensure beneficiaries receive clinical preventive services in a timely manner.	Global Recommendation III Immediate Action MHS Governance

Action Items for Immediate Action (within 90 days)	Mapping to Overarching Recommendations ---------- Timeline ---------- **Governance**
SAFETY: Revaluate charter and membership of Quality Patient Safety Risk Management Task Force and determine whether to use Task Force to develop framework for a high reliability organization (HRO) and submit through existing governance structure.	Global Recommendation V Immediate Action MHS Governance
SAFETY: Services and DHA evaluate their organizational structure to better align patient safety functions within their organizations to maximize leadership visibility.	Global Recommendation IV Immediate Action Services and DHA

Action Items for Campaign Plan Summit* POLICY	Mapping to Overarching Recommendations ---------- Timeline ---------- Governance
ACCESS: Health Affairs (HA) with support from MHS governance should standardize MHS direct care component access to care business practices by replacing the MHS Guide to Access Success with an MHS policy memorandum and subsequent DoD Instruction.	Global Recommendation VI Campaign Plan Summit HA (w/ MHS Governance support)
QUALITY: The Assistant Secretary of Defense for Health Affairs (ASD (HA)) and DHA should develop policy guidance in support of DoDI and DoDM 6025.13 with specific direction on quality measurement, performance improvement, and requirements for education and training.	Global Recommendation V Campaign Plan Summit HA (w/ MHS Governance support)
QUALITY: ASD (HA) should develop policy guidance to manage and track compliance of Services and DHA with applicable DoD policies and directives.	Global Recommendation V Campaign Plan Summit HA (w/ MHS Governance support)
QUALITY: HA policy is needed to standardize annual and interval training requirements related to perinatal team care.	Global Recommendations II & V Campaign Plan Summit HA (w/ MHS Governance support)
SAFETY: Refine DoDM 6025.13 policy to establish more than one mechanism for capturing harm events.	Global Recommendation V Campaign Plan Summit HA (w/ MHS Governance support)
SAFETY: Assess the revised The Joint Commission (TJC) definition of "sentinel event" and determine if additional guidance in the DoDM 6025.13 policy is required.	Global Recommendation V Campaign Plan Summit HA (w/ MHS Governance support)

Action Items for Campaign Plan Summit* **POLICY**	Mapping to Overarching Recommendations Timeline Governance
SAFETY: HA, through the DHA Clinical Support Division and Office of General Counsel, with Service representation, should incorporate and define appropriate policy for patient/family engagement to proactively embed patient/family perspectives in MTF decision-making.	Global Recommendations IV & V Campaign Plan Summit HA (w/ MHS Governance support)
SAFETY: Establish clear expectations in DoDM 6025.13 for the root cause analysis (RCA) process.	Global Recommendation V Campaign Plan Summit HA (w/ MHS Governance support)
SAFETY: Ensure that the policy establishes attainable goals for "near miss" reporting.	Global Recommendation V Campaign Plan Summit HA (w/ MHS Governance support)

Action Items for Campaign Plan Summit* **INFRASTRUCTURE, PROGRAMS, AND PROCESSES**	Mapping to Overarching Recommendations Timeline Governance
ACCESS: MHS governance should increase the focus on the standardization of specialty care for the direct care component through the following: creating the Tri-Service Specialty Care Advisory Board, funding requirements to standardize `specialty product lines, establishing business rules to support enhanced access, and defining performance review metrics for specialty care product lines.	Global Recommendation VI Campaign Plan Summit MHS Governance
ACCESS: MHS governance should standardize reporting from the TRICARE Regional Offices to the Services.	Global Recommendations IV & VI Campaign Plan Summit MHS Governance

Action Items for Campaign Plan Summit* INFRASTRUCTURE, PROGRAMS, AND PROCESSES	Mapping to Overarching Recommendations ---------- Timeline ---------- Governance
QUALITY: DHA Health Plans should evaluate alternative methods of incentivizing contractors and/or providers to improve the provision of clinical preventive services and Healthcare Effectiveness Data and Information Set (HEDIS®) performance. This may require statutory or regulatory changes, since new, innovative payment mechanisms may have to be developed to encourage compliance.	Global Recommendation II Campaign Plan Summit DHA
QUALITY: DHA should establish clear and consistent guidelines for the CONUS TRICARE Regions and the OCONUS Area Offices on reporting and processing quality and patient safety issues identified from the purchased care.	Global Recommendation VI Campaign Plan Summit DHA
QUALITY: MHS governance should establish goals and processes for increasing the number of MTFs achieving TJC Top Performer status annually.	Global Recommendations V & VI Campaign Plan Summit MHS Governance
QUALITY: MHS governance should explore expanding NSQIP® participation to all remaining direct care inpatient facilities performing surgery. In addition, ensure ambulatory surgery platforms all participate in a similar surgical quality improvement program.	Global Recommendation II Campaign Plan Summit MHS Governance
QUALITY: MHS governance should require Service facilities with higher-than-expected mortality on an Inpatient Quality Indicators (IQI) measure for more than one quarter to perform an investigation and implement improvement activities as indicated.	Global Recommendation II Campaign Plan Summit MHS Governance
ACCESS: MHS governance should promote Secure Messaging and TRICARE On-Line through direct care component standardized business processes and a strategic marketing approach.	Global Recommendation VI Campaign Plan Summit MHS Governance
QUALITY: MHS governance should continue to guide MTFs in implementation of strategies to optimize patient centered medical home (PCMH) operations and use of secure messaging, Nurse Advice Line, and other customer service tools.	Global Recommendations V & VI Campaign Plan Summit MHS Governance

Action Items for Campaign Plan Summit* INFRASTRUCTURE, PROGRAMS, AND PROCESSES	Mapping to Overarching Recommendations ---------- Timeline ---------- Governance
QUALITY: PCMH Advisory Board should assess processes that affect Primary Care Manager continuity at high performing PCMH sites and promulgate across the MHS to support improvement initiatives.	Global Recommendation VI Campaign Plan Summit MHS Governance
QUALITY: MHS governance should work with the Services to increase utilization of Clinical Practice Guidelines in the direct care component.	Global Recommendation VI Campaign Plan Summit MHS Governance
QUALITY: MHS governance should develop processes to ensure standardized patient notification requirements for laboratory and radiology.	Global Recommendation VI Campaign Plan Summit MHS Governance
QUALITY: MHS governance should establish a mechanism to aggregate and communicate accreditation findings across the MHS.	Global Recommendation IV Campaign Plan Summit MHS Governance
SAFETY: Implement principles of HRO with focus on leadership, culture of safety, and robust process improvement. Must be strategic priority for executive leadership and will require revision of current policy and re-evaluation of Patient Safety Program	Global Recommendation V Campaign Plan Summit MHS Governance
SAFETY: Establish a system-wide closed loop mechanism for documentation and disposition of a patient safety alert or advisory.	Global Recommendation III Campaign Plan Summit MHS Governance
SAFETY: Establish a system-wide structure to fully expand internal transparency of patient safety information in compliance with 10 US Code 1102.	Global Recommendations II, IV, & V Campaign Plan Summit MHS Governance

Appendix 6. Recommendations and Comments

Action Items for Campaign Plan Summit* INFRASTRUCTURE, PROGRAMS, AND PROCESSES	Mapping to Overarching Recommendations Timeline Governance
SAFETY: MHS Governance must determine safety culture expectations, set targets based on opportunities.	Global Recommendations II, V, & VI Campaign Plan Summit MHS Governance
SAFETY: MHS governance should pursue an enterprise-wide improvement process addressing top five reported sentinel events (SEs) and improve distinction between SEs occurring within ambulatory versus hospital settings, and monitor SE occurrence by rates using appropriate denominator estimates.	Global Recommendations II & III Campaign Plan Summit MHS Governance
SAFETY: Establish clear expectations for the RCA process and the follow up that will occur.	Global Recommendations II & V Campaign Plan Summit MHS Governance
SAFETY: Standardize performance improvement RCA process with focus on event type classification, centralized repository and dissemination of lessons learned.	Global Recommendations II, IV & V Campaign Plan Summit MHS Governance
SAFETY: Standardize event type components of the event reporting process.	Global Recommendations V & VI Campaign Plan Summit MHS Governance
SAFETY: Adopt a chart audit based methodology such as the Institute for Healthcare Improvement (IHI) Global Trigger Tool (GTT) to determine harm rate.	Global Recommendations II & III Campaign Plan Summit MHS Governance

Action Items for Campaign Plan Summit* **INFRASTRUCTURE, PROGRAMS, AND PROCESSES**	Mapping to Overarching Recommendations ---------- Timeline ---------- Governance
SAFETY: Incorporate best practices from all three contractors to develop a more standardized process that enhances transparency, minimizes variation, and incentivizes reporting for process improvement.	Global Recommendations IV & VI Campaign Plan Summit MHS Governance

Action Items for Campaign Plan Summit* **DATA COLLECTION, MONITORING, AND ANALYSIS**	Mapping to Overarching Recommendations ---------- Timeline ---------- Governance
ACCESS: MHS governance should commission an external study to evaluate purchased care access for TRICARE Prime enrollees as it relates to 32 C.F.R. § 199.17. This study should include a review of all data available and a recommendation for metrics to be incorporated into the current and future TRICARE contracts.	Global Recommendation IV Campaign Plan Summit MHS Governance
QUALITY: DHA should integrate requirements for Purchased Care clinical quality data on TRICARE beneficiaries into the TRICARE Operations Manual and future TRICARE regional contracts.	Global Recommendation IV Campaign Plan Summit DHA
QUALITY: DHA Health Plans should give purchased care contractors the authority to utilize supplemental databases to improve the capture of clinical information for purchased care enrollees.	Global Recommendation III Campaign Plan Summit DHA
ACCESS: MHS governance should continue implementation of the Joint Service survey tool, refining access satisfaction questions to include the addition of satisfaction with office wait times.	Global Recommendation VI Campaign Plan Summit MHS Governance

Action Items for Campaign Plan Summit* DATA COLLECTION, MONITORING, AND ANALYSIS	Mapping to Overarching Recommendations ---------- Timeline ---------- Governance
QUALITY: MHS governance should continue to study determinants and develop strategy to meet or exceed civilian benchmarks in satisfaction with primary care and OB for every MTF.	Global Recommendation V Campaign Plan Summit MHS Governance
QUALITY: Services and DHA should continue to evaluate determinants of satisfaction with primary care and ensure ongoing maturation of PCMH in all MTFs.	Global Recommendations II & VI Campaign Plan Summit MHS Governance
QUALITY: MHS governance should develop and implement an enterprise performance management system that links to MHS and Service strategy with dashboards and common performance measures to support visibility of those measures across the enterprise.	Global Recommendation II Campaign Plan Summit MHS Governance
QUALITY: MHS governance should create and task an MHS data analytics cell to provide actionable information to the Services and DHA at the enterprise level.	Global Recommendation III Campaign Plan Summit MHS Governance
QUALITY: MHS governance should establish policy to guide processes for verification of clinical data and capture in AHLTA (DoD Outpatient Electronic Health Record) regarding preventive services that are obtained outside of the direct care component.	Global Recommendation III Campaign Plan Summit MHS Governance
QUALITY: DHA should develop plans to improve Other Health Insurance documentation in Defense Enrollment Eligibility Reporting System (DEERS) for all beneficiaries to ensure those with Other Health Insurance are not included in HEDIS® calculations.	Global Recommendation III Campaign Plan Summit DHA
QUALITY: MHS governance should implement provider-level PQI education, followed by an evaluation of MTF utilization of Agency for Healthcare Quality and Research (AHRQ) Prevention Quality Indicators (PQI) measures and implementation of a monitoring program requiring improvement plans as indicated.	Global Recommendation II Campaign Plan Summit MHS Governance

Action Items for Campaign Plan Summit* DATA COLLECTION, MONITORING, AND ANALYSIS	Mapping to Overarching Recommendations ---------- Timeline ---------- Governance
QUALITY: MHS governance should establish an implementation plan for MHS Population Health Portal readmissions site to ensure maximum utilization to reduce avoidable readmissions.	Global Recommendation II Campaign Plan Summit MHS Governance
QUALITY: DHA Healthcare Operations Directorate should complete transition to the HEDIS® All-Cause Readmission standardized measure, which is risk-adjusted and has national benchmarks.	Global Recommendation II Campaign Plan Summit DHA
QUALITY: DHA Health Information Technology should prioritize electronic medical record upgrades by aligning needed data elements into Essentris®. All inpatient MTFs should have the capability to remotely access medical records to facilitate expeditious and timely data extraction for clinical measure calculation.	Global Recommendation III Campaign Plan Summit DHA
QUALITY: MHS governance should ensure that standardization of accurate perinatal coding practices is implemented across direct care.	Global Recommendation VI Campaign Plan Summit MHS Governance
QUALITY: MHS governance should integrate measures of mortality into their quality monitoring and performance improvement programs.	Global Recommendation II Campaign Plan Summit MHS Governance
SAFETY: The Infection Prevention and Control Panel will develop a comprehensive plan to standardize requirements for monitoring device-related infections as a component of a comprehensive safety measure set^.	Global Recommendation II Campaign Plan Summit MHS Governance
SAFETY: DoD direct care systems should pursue tracking infection rates at the unit level beyond intensive care units as a component of a comprehensive safety measure set^.	Global Recommendations II & III Campaign Plan Summit MHS Governance

Appendix 6. Recommendations and Comments

Action Items for Campaign Plan Summit* DATA COLLECTION, MONITORING, AND ANALYSIS	Mapping to Overarching Recommendations ---------- Timeline ---------- Governance
SAFETY: Establish rate-based SE reporting for DoD or other recognized frequency tracking as a component of a comprehensive safety measure set^.	Global Recommendation III Campaign Plan Summit MHS Governance
SAFETY: Consider PSI #90 composite utilization as a component of a comprehensive safety measure set^ and develop an educational plan to support implementation.	Global Recommendations II & VI Campaign Plan Summit MHS Governance

^ *Reference to "a comprehensive safety measure set" implies future development of such a set.*

Action Items for Campaign Plan Summit* EDUCATION AND TRAINING	Mapping to Overarching Recommendations ---------- Timeline ---------- Governance
ACCESS: MHS governance should standardize both access to care and customer service training across the direct care component.	Global Recommendation VI Campaign Plan Summit MHS Governance
QUALITY: DHA Education and Training Directorate should conduct an in-depth review and needs assessment of quality training to adequately assess the efficacy of training.	Global Recommendations V & VI Campaign Plan Summit DHA
QUALITY: MHS governance should determine the requirements to guide the development and implementation of a Quality expert career path.	Global Recommendation V Campaign Plan Summit MHS Governance
QUALITY: MHS governance should evaluate the utility of additional fellowship opportunities with TJC or other nationally recognized programs, and the Services should explore optimizing and standardizing Service fellow utilization with follow-on assignment after fellowship completion.	Global Recommendation V Campaign Plan Summit MHS Governance
SAFETY: Further define and standardize minimal patient safety training requirements as outlined in DoDM 6025.13 policy.	Global Recommendation V Campaign Plan Summit MHS Governance
SAFETY: Develop an executive leadership toolkit; this best practice guide will address integral areas of patient safety.	Global Recommendations II & IV Campaign Plan Summit MHS Governance
SAFETY: Clarify policy and educate healthcare staff on the Sentinel Event definition and event types to reduce the variation in interpretation.	Global Recommendation V Campaign Plan Summit MHS Governance

Appendix 6. Recommendations and Comments

Action Items for Campaign Plan Summit* **EDUCATION AND TRAINING**	Mapping to Overarching Recommendations ---------- Timeline ---------- Governance
SAFETY: Standardize leadership activities to drive a culture of safety (Executive toolkit).	Global Recommendations II & IV Campaign Plan Summit MHS Governance

Action Items for Campaign Plan Summit* **PARTNERSHIPS WITH EXTERNAL SYSTEMS**	Mapping to Overarching Recommendations ---------- Timeline ---------- Governance
QUALITY: DHA should develop a strategy to establish relationships with civilian Health Systems to foster collaboration and data sharing that leads to performance improvements within the MHS.	Global Recommendations II & III Campaign Plan Summit DHA
QUALITY: MHS governance should evaluate the feasibility of DoD and TRICARE regional contractor collaborations/MOUs with local purchased care organizations to support EHR accessibility.	Global Recommendations III & IV Campaign Plan Summit MHS Governance
QUALITY: MHS Governance should identify and implement leading healthcare industry methods for instilling and maintaining cultural changes throughout a large system.	Global Recommendation V Campaign Plan Summit MHS Governance
SAFETY: DoD develops formal partnership plan with external health care organizations, TRICARE contractors, and national governing bodies to improve as learning organization and be at forefront of national benchmark development and initiatives for patient safety	Global Recommendation IV Campaign Plan Summit MHS Governance

*The Campaign Plan Summit will take the form of a 2-3 week event that brings together leaders and subject matter experts to develop comprehensive, integrated plans for addressing MHS Review Proposed Action Items. The Summit will be scheduled after the 29 August 2014 release of the MHS Review Final Report to the Secretary of Defense.

Action Items for Further Review
ACCESS/QUALITY/SAFETY: DoD should review hiring processes, policies, and pay scales within the Civilian Human Resources Agency and DoD to decrease the difficulty in hiring and retaining qualified staff, which directly impacts access, quality and patient safety.
ACCESS: MHS governance should assess the discrepancy between the access to care data, which demonstrates timely appointments and satisfaction with access to care as reported on DHA surveys.
ACCESS: MHS governance should assess, by enrollment category and product, the extent to which patients are asked to call back for an appointment.
QUALITY: MHS governance should evaluate the use of the risk-adjusted standardized mortality ratio (SMR) model in direct care; facilities with higher than expected mortality should validate the risk-adjusted SMR model data and perform a root cause analysis as indicated.
QUALITY: MHS governance should assess the value of expanding the number of HEDIS® measures monitored to evaluate care provided to enrolled beneficiaries.
QUALITY: The Perinatal Advisory Group (PAG) should conduct a comprehensive review of clinical practices related to metrics where MHS is underperforming. Through a dashboard and standardized metric reporting requirements, intervention plans should be developed and actions prioritized.
QUALITY: MHS governance should investigate readmissions of mothers and infants. This clinical review of diagnostic codes at readmission will identify the medical conditions that drive these rates and help determine if lagging performance is a quality issue or related to military-unique issues and flexibility.
SAFETY: Further review by the Infection Prevention and Control Panel (IPCP) to determine the cause for the variance in performance in accordance with the Partnership for Patients Implementation Guide for CLABSI and VAP/VAE.
SAFETY: DHA should conduct a business case analysis that identifies the most effective method for staffing the Patient Safety Program.

Appendix 6.2
Comments of External Reviewers[12]

External Methodology Review: Report from Dr. Brent James

23 July 2104

Background and Qualifications

I am a licensed physician who serves as Chief Quality Officer at Intermountain Healthcare, based in Salt Lake City, Utah.

Intermountain Healthcare is an integrated delivery system with 22 hospitals, more than 185 community-based clinics, an integrated health insurance plan that provides funding for about 25 percent of all care delivered by the Intermountain system, a major home health business, a durable equipment group, and other associated care delivery support sub-businesses. Intermountain works with more than 4,000 Utah- and Idaho-based physicians. More than 1,000 of those physicians are employed through the Intermountain Medical Group (IMG), a wholly-owned subsidiary. Together with IMG physicians, a core group of about 1,800 affiliated (non-employed), community-based physicians supply over 90 percent of all patient care services delivered within the Intermountain system. Intermountain-associated care (using Intermountain funding or coming through Intermountain facilities) typically compromises more than 60 percent of all services delivered through those tightly-aligned affiliated practices. Nine of Intermountain's 22 hospitals, all located in highly urban parts of Utah, account for more than 95 percent of more than 160,000 inpatient admissions per year within the Intermountain system. Two of those hospitals are major teaching and research hospitals that deliver quaternary-level services (e.g., multi-organ in-bloc transplant). Three function as tertiary-level (e.g., high-risk pregnancy, open heart surgery) minor teaching hospitals, supporting Family Medicine residency training and nurse training programs. Four are community hospitals that provide general services. The remaining 13 Intermountain hospitals serve rural communities, often as the sole provider of care within a local geography. Intermountain clinics service more than 5 million outpatient encounters each year.

Intermountain is non-profit with a strong charitable mission. It is governed by an unpaid Board of Trustees consisting of high-profile community leaders, supplemented by local leaders from the healing professions as well as several national policy experts. Intermountain provides more than 50 percent of all health care delivery services across Utah, southeastern Idaho, and (at a tertiary level) 7 surrounding States. Intermountain is the source of the majority of all unpaid care delivery services within its service areas, including home health services.

Intermountain has a very long history successfully applying the principles of quality improvement to clinical care delivery in an inpatient and outpatient setting. In 1996, Intermountain's then-CEO, Mr. William Nelson, assigned me to create a strategic plan that

---

[12] For this review, external reviewers participated as individual experts in their personal capacities, and not as the employees or representatives of their affiliated institutions.

would make clinical quality of care and patient safety Intermountain's core business strategy. The resulting plan was based around Dr. W. Edwards Deming's quality theory, which showed that in most circumstances process management that produced better quality outcomes also eliminated process-based waste resulting in much lower operating costs. Called Clinical Integration, by 2006 the effort had produced a series clinical patient registries that tracked longitudinal clinical, cost, and patient satisfaction outcomes data for 58 key clinical processes, representing about 80 percent of care delivered in the Intermountain system. Clinical Integration also built a management structure of physicians and nurses. That combination – solid process-level data supporting effective front-line clinical management – had produced very significant improvements in clinical outcomes on a broad scale, accompanied by more than $400 million in structural operating cost reductions through process-based waste elimination.

In addition to leading Clinical Integration, I also conduct the Advanced Training Program in Clinical Process Improvement (the ATP). Since 1992 that course has trained more than 5,000 health care leaders in clinical quality improvement (42 percent physician executives, 25 percent nursing leaders, 17 percent support staff, 8 percent C-suite administrators). About 80 percent of ATP graduates come from outside Intermountain Healthcare and Utah. ATP graduates have started more than 50 "sister" clinical quality improvement training programs in their home institutions. Ten of those "sister" ATP programs exist outside the borders of the United States, with particularly strong instances operating in Canada, Sweden, France, Great Britain, Argentina, Australia, and Singapore. I regularly visit other health systems both inside and outside the United States, both to participate in "sister" ATP training programs and to consult with health system leaders on clinical quality and cost management. Further, I am familiar with and regularly contribute to an extensive research literature associated with clinical quality improvement and patient safety.

Finally, I am an elected member of the National Academy of Science's Institute of Medicine; and hold adjunct professorships at the University of Utah School of Medicine, the Harvard School of Public Health, and the University of Sydney, Australia, School of Public Health.

In order to provide this review, the DoD appointed me a temporary government worker (GS-15) for the 2 days I was in Falls Church, Virginia, working directly on the project. While I accepted reimbursement from the DoD for travel expenses associated with providing this review, I have declined any other compensation.

Scope of Review

Several months ago I was contacted to conduct an independent review of the methodology – data systems and organizational structure and function – that supports access to care, quality of care, and patient safety systems within the (DoD) health care delivery system. That care delivery system includes both care delivered in DoD Medical Treatment Facilities (MTFs) – various levels of hospitals and outpatient clinics operated directly by the DoD MHS – and services contracted from local non-military care delivery systems (contracted community services). In accordance with Dr. Guice's instructions I focused on the underlying content, structure and operations of the data systems and organizational structures that support high-quality care, reflected in timely access to care (access), excellent clinical patient outcomes (quality), and minimization of harms associated with care delivery (patient safety). I did not examine or assess final performance results in any area.

I evaluated the methodologies underlying DoD MHS access, quality, and patient safety systems on the basis on standard methods currently employed in competent care delivery systems across the United States. I have also included structure and process standards that I have observed in first-world nations outside the United States.

While my evaluation is based on current standards within the healing professions, those standards are in rapid evolution. I have labelled these evaluations "findings."

I have also included specific changes that the DoD MHS leadership might consider to move care delivery within the U.S. military to levels well beyond that currently seen in other civilian U.S. and non-U.S. care delivery systems. These often go well beyond the current generally-accepted standard of care. I have labelled these "recommendations."

Sources of Information

In support of my evaluation, MHS officers supplied a series of written documents. I reviewed these before traveling to Falls Church, Virginia to meet in person with DoD MHS representatives. These included

> Terms of Reference
> Memoranda defining the scope, timelines, and study questions of the overarching review process
> Documents describing the MHS's methods for metric selection, data collection, data analysis, and reporting methods
> An article published in the New York Times newspaper, dated 28 June 2014, authored by Sharon LaFraniere and Andrew W. Lehren, entitled "In Military Care, a Pattern of Errors but Not Scrutiny" – criticizing the DoD MHS for patient safety and clinical quality events.

I also was given full access to the internal web-based shared document store that all members of the MHS review group were using to conduct the review, including their summaries and source documents.

On Monday, 21 July 2014, I travelled to Falls Church, Virginia. There I was able to meet the internal MHS teams conducting the full review. These teams included:

> Dr. Michael Malanoski (Captain, US Navy, retired) – overview of project and deliverables
> Dr. Paul Rockswold (Captain, US Navy) – analytic methodologies used in producing access, quality, and patient safety reports

- John Savage (Colonel, US Air Force) – overview of MHS management structures across the Defense Health Agency (DHA), the National Capitol Region (NCR), and all 3 military services
- Julie Freeman, (LTC, US Army) – full review of methods employed in conducting in-depth site reviews at 7 MHS facilities
- Dr. Kenneth Iverson (Rear Admiral, US Navy) and support team – review of MHS access measures, with underlying data systems and reports examples
- Barbara Holcomb, BSN, MSN (Brigadier General, US Army) and support team – review of MHS patient safety measures and support system, with report examples
- Dr. Lee Payne (Colonel, US Air Force) and support team – review of MHS quality of care measures, including underlying data systems and report examples

In addition to reviewing the presentations and documentation that each team supplied, I was able to question each team in detail and at length. I addressed questions arising from the presentations, but also extended well beyond the presentations to other foundational elements of measuring and reporting access, quality, and patient safety data. All teams were completely open to my queries and, to the best of my judgment, responded honestly. Their responses, while not always complimentary to the MHS, were consistent and complete within each team and across the separate teams.

Finally, I was generally familiar with recently-reported problems associated with access to care in the Veterans Administration Hospital (VAH) system, through the general news media, professional journals, and from conversations with past and present clinical officers within the VAH system with whom I have personal acquaintance.

Findings and Recommendations

General underlying data systems

While some cause and effect relationships are readily apparent to the human eye, most are not. In those circumstances data systems provide a means for humans to accurately observe, establish causal relationships, and take effective action. Such data systems are essential when managing and improving the care delivery infrastructure associated with quality, patient safety, and access to care. Solid data systems provide an ability to see, which in turn is the foundation upon which all effective action rests.

To achieve maximum accuracy, efficiency, timeliness, and efficacy the best data systems form an integral part of front-line care delivery processes. They avoid data abstraction wherever possible. Data abstraction involves third parties making judgments of primary data and can be associated with very significant errors in interpretation and transcription. Even when founded on integrated data systems rooted in front-line care delivery, errors and misinterpretations can arise as the data move upward along a chain of command. Each level of upward movement usually involves consolidation of reported data, with purposeful loss of detail. This is essential. Otherwise, high-order management reports will contain so much detail as to be incomprehensible. A well-connected reporting system provides well-organized high-order summaries that can easily "drill down" through layers of increasing detail back to the front-line care that documented each individual case. Such reporting systems are nested layers of focused dashboard reports, where each lower layer adds detail to summary elements included within the next higher dashboard.

The site visits performed by the MHS review team are one way to link summary reporting systems, upon which senior leadership must routinely rely, to front line reality. The MHS review team created a sampling frame based on MTF type; military service group; performance levels (poor vs excellent, as reported in routine summary data); and geographic location. They used that frame to identify 7 site visit locations. They then created a structured set of questions that they applied at the level of local leadership and front-line operations. They reviewed relevant documentation systems within each unit visited, again based on a standardized approach. They very carefully insured that people at all levels – patients, front line caregivers, local leaders, and others – could speak freely without fear of criticism or reprisal at the time of the site visit or afterword. Attendance at Town Hall meetings was voluntary. Such voluntary reporting should automatically be regarded as biased. Usually, those who have had bad experiences or want to voice criticisms will have the energy to attend and speak out. Voluntary town hall meetings thus function mainly as a complaint tracking system – an important element of quality measurement – rather than providing any sort of objective measure of overall performance.

While the site visit team used reasonable and appropriate criteria, the units assessed in the site visits were not randomly selected; nor were the questions used in local assessments validated. These methodologic constraints limit full generalization of site visit findings to the entire MHS system. However,

> **Finding 1: Within the time constraints of the evaluation, the site visits conducted by the MHS review team were (a) appropriately selected; and (b) very competently structured and performed. Findings from the site visits generally aligned well with data reported in the MHS quality, safety, and access measurement systems. This produces a high, if not perfect, level of confidence that the current MHS measurement systems accurately represent actual front-line performance.**

While quality and patient safety measurement and analysis have shown dramatic improvement over the past 20 years, it still suffers from significant limitations. More specifically, there are problems with (references provided on request):

- The underlying medical science regarding sources of variation for specific conditions, that greatly attenuate appropriate risk-adjustment of outcome data even in ideal circumstances (Eddy).

- Data extraction and consolidation for inclusion, exclusion, stratification, and clinical assessment factors, including (i) whether critical factors identified in a related science review were measured during the process of clinical care delivery; (ii) whether clinical assessments were recorded in a medical record; (iii) whether the measurement process identified and extracted all such critical factors, across all institutionally and geographically dispersed medical records; (iv) variation in the formats in which critical factors were recorded, across medical records sources; and (v) whether all such data elements were accurately and consistently abstracted.

- Analytic techniques, particularly regarding (i) production of summary measures across multiple contributing subscales; and (ii) attribution within a complex care delivery system.

- Inherent mathematical problems with the precision of ranking systems (Swedish AMI; Royal Academy; others).

As a result of these limitations, with very rare exceptions, it is not possible to produce clinical quality or patient safety measures that can accurately rank care providers. While large sample sizes can produce results that appear to show statistical significance, they hide underlying problems with the data system. As a classic illustration of the fruits that such limitations, DeLoitte Consulting's Paul Keckly (formerly head of the Vanderbilt Health system, and since retired from DeLoitte) asked his DeLoitte summer interns to identify U.S. hospitals that had been ranked in a "Top 100" list among more than 130 governmental and independent commercial bodies that publish hospital rankings. Among about 5,500 U.S. acute care hospitals, 1,457 ranked in the "Top 100 Hospitals" on at least one list. That translates into about 26 percent of all U.S. hospitals falling into the top 2 percent of hospital performance – a statistic that far outperforms "all of the children being above average" in Keillor's Lake Woebegone.

Ranking systems suffer from other major malfunctions that often arise from unexamined assumptions among those who advocate their use. In specific contrast, strong evidence supports the following conclusions:

- Most patients do not use medical outcome performance rankings (statistical league tables) to choose hospitals or physicians. They rely on personal relationships and recommendations by trusted referring physicians instead. (Details: when asked, patients will consistently say that they value ranking data. They will report that they used such ranking data, when it was available to them, when making choices. However, that positive response disappears when one carefully measures actual choices. About 2 – 3 percent of patients will use statistical ranking data to select physicians or hospitals. This percentage may be much higher for a few selected conditions, such as bone marrow transplant) (IOM Performance Measures Committee report).

- Even if patients could "vote with their feet for quality," it is often transpires that there is no higher quality care delivery opportunity within reasonable geographic reach. Limitations in the capacity of the care delivery system constrain patients to local care providers, even when various rankings systems suggest that those systems perform poorly. People truly do prefer to be treated close to home. This response often overrides otherwise compelling quality data.

- In the face of public data showing poor performance, most healthcare delivery leadership teams will launch improvement efforts. However, most of these efforts do not change actual performance. Very common alternative management strategies are to (1) Concentrate resources in the area under the public spotlight until attention shifts away ("work harder"). Even though performance in the focus area may temporarily improve, that improvement typically doesn't sustain. Worse, it pulls resources from other areas where they were better deployed in terms of overall quality performance. (2) Many groups will "improve their documentation" (goal displacement: Improve the ranking, rather than addressing real patient outcomes). They closely manage quality tracking systems to report better results, while true underlying performance remains unchanged. Examples of this "gaming the data system" or "looking good, as opposed to being good," are almost endless across a wide range of human activities, to the level of criminal violations on a broad scale. It is a source of endless difficulties for senior management teams who make the mistake of being insensitive to its presence while provoking exactly this response through goal setting, incentives, and thoughtless accountability.

- Ranking data are only rarely useful for choosing targets for improvement. To illustrate, over the past 20 years Intermountain Healthcare has hosted more than 100 successful clinical improvement projects. Almost all of those projects came in areas where Intermountain already outperformed national standards and was top rank when compared to other care delivery groups.

  A far better method for choosing improvement targets uses estimates of the gap between current performance and theoretic "best possible" performance. Williamson called this ABNA – "achievable benefit not achieved" (Williamson 1979). It often leads to quite different conclusions than reliance on comparative performance rankings. Project prioritization should also consider the availability of strong clinical leadership and established measurement systems. Although these 2 factors can be created as part of a project, that additional effort will necessarily extend the amount of time and effort that the project requires. Finally, to legitimately improve outcomes a team must discover process-level changes that produce measurably better performance. Occasionally comparative performance data will identify a few "best in class" performers around a particular process. More rarely still, some of those top performers will have built an identifiable process (a defined road to performance success) that they are able and willing to share. Very often the overall care delivery field used to generate comparative outcomes will fall far short of theoretic best possible performance. Differences in comparative outcomes will be found to arise from differences in underlying science, data systems, and analytic methods rather than legitimate performance. As important, improvement teams have strong alternatives in the face of these limitations in comparative outcomes data as an improvement tool. Teams can and routinely do use process improvement methods (e.g., Rapid Cycle PDSA) to discover new processes that produce significantly better outcome performance. They simultaneously set new performance standards for the entire care delivery field.

Perhaps the most pernicious damage done when senior leaders focus on external comparative data has to do with resource allocation. Data systems designed to rank providers or otherwise produce comparative outcomes (selection systems) differ dramatically from data systems designed for process management and improvement (improvement systems). With good design, an improvement data system "contains" accurate, timely, and complete selection data. The quality of such process-based improvement data typically exceeds that of data systems specifically built to produce selection data. The opposite is not true. Data systems designed for comparative outcomes usually lack critical data elements, and use non-ideal data element definitions, necessary to improve performance. Investing in data systems designed primarily to track comparative outcomes, usually in response to regulators or other external overseers, consumes organizational resources. That leaves internal teams without the resources they need to measure at a process level, damaging the organization's ability to improve performance (Berwick, James, & Coye; 2003). Efforts launched by external overseers and senior management in the name of quality can thus actively damage front line quality, patient safety, and access performance (Casalino, 1999; and others).

Recommendation 1: MHS leadership should avoid internal or external attempts to rank MTF facilities; it should proceed with great caution when comparing overall MHS performance or individual MTF facility performance to external standards, systems, or groups.

Quality improvement provides very strong and demonstrably effective strategies to use in place of traditional ranking or external comparison methods. These center around building data systems that focus on care delivery processes as opposed to individual clinicians or facilities.

A subset of quality theory directly addresses the measurement systems upon which quality management rests. The engineers who first generated that body of knowledge called it "gauge theory." Within engineering, a "gauge" is a measurement tool. For example, it might be micrometer used to measure the diameter of a steel bar. Engineers quickly noted that their measurement tools were themselves "systems of causes," and so always contained some element of random variation in the measurement outputs they produced. A gauge functioned well when the amount of variation inherent in the measurement system itself was small compared to the amount of variation contained within the process that the gauge (measurement system) assessed. Any quality organization should pay as much attention to its gauges – its measurement and reporting systems – as it does to performance generated by its care delivery processes.

Recommendation 2: Where possible report MHS quality, safety, and access measures using statistical process control (SPC) charts.

SPC charts visually display current point levels as well as trend over time in process or outcome measures. They include associated p-values, displayed graphically as "control limits" bounding the data. These graphical displays make it possible to identify statistical outliers, either from single points that fall outside the control limits or from patterns of points in the trended data, using simple, well-established rules.

Technically a statistical outlier point or pattern on an SPC chart means, exactly, that if one tracks that point to its root causes, it is possible to accurately identify the source of variation.

By itself, outliers found SPC-charted outcomes data DO NOT identify source causes. This is critically important within gauge theory. With any unrefined data system, many of the initial outlier points will track back to the measurement system, not to the underlying clinical process. This provides a reliable mechanism for building robust measurement systems over time. It involves (a) tracking important process and outcome parameters using SPC; (b) identifying outlier points; (c) tracking those outlier points down to root causes; then (d) when the causes so discovered point back to the measurement system, refining the measurement system itself. Through this mechanism, over time it is possible to build very robust, reliable measurement systems with minimal internal variability, which are much more effective for monitoring and improving the underlying care delivery processes.

Recommendation 3: MHS leadership should employ SPC "data loopback" methods to routinely improve and validate underlying quality, safety, and access reporting systems.

Such an approach will give senior leaders the ability to verify that the underlying data upon which they rely when making decisions is reasonably accurate and complete. MHS data will become routinely trustworthy.

As a corollary, it is relatively easy to show that, in most circumstances, it is not possible to accurately rank care providers (physicians, treatment facilities, or even health systems) on the basis of carefully selected and risk-adjusted clinical process or outcomes data. However, it is possible to use SPC techniques to compare any unit to its appropriate peers. The method involves generating the frequency distribution used to calculate an SPC chart using peer data, then plotting the unit under analysis against the resulting SPC center line and control limits. The method lends itself nicely to stratification and risk adjustment. As before, many of those outlier points will track back to problems with underlying data systems. Over time, appropriate response to data system problems so discovered with greatly improve the data systems, allow a clearer view of the associated processes, and lead to significant improvements in documented best care.

Hospital Patient Safety

The MHS system tracks patient safety through an array of targeted measurement systems. Three of these measurement systems derive from widely-used national standard tracking systems. They collect consistent data across all MHS inpatient care delivery sites, and across all 3 services. They include:

1. Patient Safety Indicators (PSI-90) – a system that examines electronic discharge abstract data, used under Congressional mandate by the DHHS Agency for Healthcare Research and Quality (AHRQ) as the core of the annual National Patient Safety Report. The DHHS Centers for Medicare and Medicaid Services (CMS) uses PSI subscales for its Medicare Value-Based Purchasing initiative, and as contributory measures within it newly launched Hospital-Acquired Condition Medicare payment modification program.

A great many non-governmental hospital ranking agencies also use the PSI for assessing patient safety at a hospital level.

2. National Healthcare Safety Network (NHSN) – a system that tracks healthcare-associated infections, recently mandated for use in all U.S. hospitals by the CDC. NHSN uses robust standard definitions for infection identification and classification.

3. Sentinel event reporting, based on standards promulgated by the TJC.

Following standard practices for most high-quality U.S. hospitals, the MHS also supports a voluntary patient safety reporting system that extends across all MHS care delivery sites:

4. Patient Safety System – a web-based reporting tool through which care delivery professionals can report specific events or circumstances that they believe produce patient harm or hold the potential for patient harm. Those making reports have the option to choose complete anonymity. The reporting system asks a series of questions that, beyond reporting an event, begins to typify and classify it.

    This system was originally developed in Great Britain. It has served that country for more than 12 years, reporting more than 12,000 potential patient safety events each month. It is widely regarded as the "state of the art" sentinel event tracking system based on voluntary reporting.

MHS leadership also reported that they routinely perform Root Cause Analyses (RCA) on serious safety events detected by the Sentinel Event Reporting system or by the Patient Safety System. More important, they report that they seek patterns of similar failures using those systems, then do concentrated RCA to identify system-level issues, as recommended by Dr. James Bagian (founder of the VAH's original patient safety system some years ago, where he championed RCA methods).

Finally, Air Force leadership reports that they have conducted the AHRQ Patient Safety Culture Survey on a single occasion in both hospital and ambulatory settings.

For military system patients treated in community hospitals and clinics the MHS functions as a third party payor – that is, as an insurance plan. That greatly limits their ability to track detailed patient safety data. All event tracking and reporting happens within the contracted civilian facilities. By current contract, civilian facilities must report Serious Reportable Events (SREs) and Potential Quality Issues (PQIs). These are closely linked to TJC Sentinel events, but many hospitals extend their content in ways that are inconsistent across different settings. Upon questioning, the MHS leadership currently do not have effective ways to assess the quality of patient safety data reported by these external institutions. They instead are forced to rely on quality oversight functions (e.g., TJC, CMS) routinely used in civilian care delivery systems. They propose to tighten their oversight through as yet unidentified improvements in future contract requirements for civilian facilities.

Finding 2: The patient safety tracking systems employed across all military inpatient facilities by MHS leadership – PSIs, NHSN, and JCAHO Sentinel event reporting – represent typical "best practice" in high-performing hospitals across the United States. MHS leadership reports reasonable and appropriate use of the resulting data to oversee patient safety across all services and facilities in the MHS.

Finding 3: The data systems that the MHS uses to track performance in contracted civilian facilities meet current industry "best practices" for health care payers. Even with "better contracting," many of the contracted civilian care delivery facilities probably will lack the necessary leadership will and resources to create "state of the art" patient safety-based delivery systems. Such systems are very difficult for payers to impose, acting from outside a particular care delivery system.

While current MHS patient safety oversight methods legitimately represent current standard practice for U.S. health care delivery, the field of patient safety is evolving rapidly. This clearly does not represent the next generation of best practice, and provides real opportunities for patient safety leadership within the MHS. Some key points include:

- A recent "gold standard" evaluation found that the AHRQ PSI system found only 10 of 173 confirmed inpatient care-associated injuries. It did not find any patient injury event that was not detected by some other, more effective event detection system. Of 13 total events found by the AHRQ PSI system, 3 were judged false positives by 2 independent physician reviewers. In other words, the AHRQ PSI system had a 5.8 percent true positive rate and a 23.1 percent false positive rate for detecting true care-associated patient injuries (Classen et al., Health Affairs 2011 – unpublished subanalysis at Intermountain's LDS Hospital where independent case-level reviews were available).

    Civilian hospitals that treat Medicare patients are required to use PSI for the CMS Value-Based Purchasing system and, to a lesser degree, the CMS Hospital-Acquired Condition system. Both of those CMS approaches use specific PSI subindices that purport to track specific types of injury, rather than the summary score. The just-cited gold standard evaluation did not test the PSI system at a subindex level. The MHS does not use the PSI-90 index at a summary level, but does use it at a subindex level.

Recommendation 4: MHS leadership should seriously consider abandoning the PSI-90 as a measure of hospital-based patient safety. It adds little value to patient safety efforts, as it typically fails to detect any events found by more reliable methods. If political considerations – i.e., the fact that PSIs are broadly mandated in all other hospital care delivery settings – demand continued use of the PSI, study your own use of the PSI system in detail then train all MHS hospital chart abstractors with an aim to reduce the PSI-90's high false positive rate.

The same study that assessed the AHRQ PSI-90 system against "gold standard" detection demonstrated a common finding observed across many empiric evaluations of patient safety event systems: Voluntary reporting built around TJC Sentinel events and NQF Never Events (one commonly-used method to somewhat extend the TJC Sentinel event list) at best detect only about 1 in 10 actual patient injury events. More typically, they find only about 1 in 100 hospital care-associated patient injuries. This is true even when using a "state of the art" voluntary reporting system, like the British Patient Safety Reporting system currently used within the MHS. For example, in 3 leading patient-safety hospitals evaluated in the Classen et al. Health Affairs study cited above, voluntary reporting found only 4 of 352 confirmed patient injuries. Confirmed TJC Sentinel events detected by the IHI Global Trigger tool showed that LDS Hospital should have reported and estimated 132 such sentinel events during 2004. The hospital reported 9 such events to State of Utah regulators in a mandatory reporting system. All hospitals across the entire State reported a total of only 36 events for the entire year. Nebeker showed that for independently confirmed (using a prospective clinical review trigger system) adverse drug events (ADEs – the most common form of hospital care-associated injury, usually accounting for more than half of all such injuries) that care delivery teams failed to connect an injured patient's symptoms to the offending drug almost 80 percent of the time. If care delivery teams fail to make the mental connection, they obviously can't record an injury event in a voluntary reporting system. Evans showed that the vast majority of ADEs (about 96.5 percent) arise from physician failures in drug ordering – a heuristic task – not from pharmacist or nurse errors in preparing or delivering the medication.

At present, the "state of the art" system for finding hospital care-associated injuries is the IHI Global Trigger Tool. That tool is freely available from the Institute for Healthcare Improvement (IHI), along with training methods and management structures to correctly deploy the method. It is relatively inexpensive to operate at the levels recommended by IHI, and represents a very reasonable use of existing patient safety resources. It will dramatically increase the MHS's detected injury rates; provide far better information to plan and deploy safer systems of care; and, properly used, document significant improvements in patient safety over time. A related set of prospective clinical review trigger systems operate real time. Very often, they detect injury events early in their course while it is still possible to intervene and reduce patient harm associated with the event. AHRQ's website freely offers full implementation manuals for prospective clinical review trigger systems that address the 3 most common forms of patient injuries: adverse drug events (ADEs), hospital-acquired infections (HAIs), and hospital-acquired pressure injuries (bed sores).

A "culture of safety" is a key feature of high-reliability patient safety systems. Such a culture is based around widespread knowledge and commitment among all personnel working in a care delivery system to avoid care-associated patient injuries. While voluntary reporting is not effective for tracking true patient injury rates, it does form a critical part of a culture of safety. Its continued use, in the context of strong and regular leadership emphasis, helps reinforce an ethic of safety. If gives front-line care givers opportunities to identify unsafe conditions and actual events. It facilitates focused feedback, where system leaders report back on changes made in response to front-line caregivers' suggestions that make care safer – a primary tool in promoting local ownership and involvement. While prospective and retrospective (chart review) clinical trigger systems very ably detect known patterns of failure, voluntary reporting taps creative human minds that can recognize legitimate patient safety circumstances or events not yet built into trigger systems.

Voluntary reporting systems play another critical role. Most regulatory patient safety programs are built around Sentinel and other reportable events. Several health care systems have expanded their Sentinel event reporting systems to include other care-associated injuries, beyond those included in the TJC Sentinel event set and the NQF Never Event list. These extended lists are usually labelled Serious Safety Events (SSEs). They typically include any patient event that can place a hospital at risk for malpractice actions or negative news media exposure, including any significant patient complaint. SSE systems consistently rely on voluntary reporting. Three very competent implementations of SSE systems include Ascension Health System, where the effort is led by CQO Dr. David Pryor; University of Michigan Health System, whose Chief Safety Officer is Dr. James Bagian; and the Baylor Health System in Dallas, Texas, where the effort is led by Dr. Donald Kennerly. Each of those systems implemented organization-wide training that led to dramatic increases in the number of reported events. For example, across Ascension Health's 110+ hospitals SSE rates increased from 0.8 SSEs per 10,000 equivalent patient days to 1.6 SSEs per 10,000 equivalent patient days. On the foundation of better measurement all 3 programs then implemented the single method proven to significantly reduce SSE rates. Called Team Leadership training, it represents a large step up from the AHRQ TeamSTEPPS program currently used within MHS. Following deployment, while using a stable tracking system, SSE rates at Ascension fell to 0.56 SSEs per 10,000 equivalent patient days. Pryor further reports several million dollars in annual malpractice savings.

These two types of systems – SSE voluntary tracking and trigger-based event detection tools; team leadership training and system changes derived from far richer data associated with more sensitive detection methods – work hand in glove. One addresses serious safety events that draw public attention. The other addresses more profound but less publicly obvious sources of injury, that drive far more actual patient harm at great expense.

> **Recommendation 5:** Study "state of the art" SSE voluntary event tracking systems, associated management structures, and team leadership training approaches at Ascension Health, the University of Michigan Medical Center, and/or Baylor Dallas. Based on those learnings, upgrade the MHS's SSE voluntary reporting system and deploy better team leadership training methods, with an aim to significantly reduce patient injury events that reach the attention of external regulators and the public.

> **Recommendation 6:** In parallel with Recommendation 5, adopt and deploy the IHI Global Trigger Tool across all inpatient units in the MHS. Use the resulting data to design and deploy system fixes that make safe care much easier to achieve within the MHS, while producing significant reductions in total cost of care.

If MHS leadership fails to adopt methods beyond the current MHS voluntary reporting systems and PSI-90 to track patient safety events, MHS will likely continue to have frequent, significant events that surprise the system and its leadership as they find their way to external regulatory bodies and the press. Most hospitals in the U.S. have not yet deployed such systems. Leading hospitals are presently doing so. Over coming years they will probably become much more common.

Clinical Outcome Quality

As with Patient Safety, the MHS assesses clinical outcome quality across its entire internal and contracted care delivery networks. Internal clinical quality tracking measurement systems for patients treated in internal MHS hospitals include: TJC Oryx data; CMS Hospital Compare data; and a modified version of the AHRQ HCAPS patient satisfaction survey. Measures for contracted civilian hospitals center around CMS Hospital Compare data. The MHS assesses outpatient clinical quality performance primarily through standard NCQA HEDIS measures.

The data systems used by the MHS to assess inpatient and outpatient clinical quality and patient satisfaction use well-established measurement tools built, promulgated and overseen by national quality oversight groups (CMS, TJC, and NCQA). These tools form the routine core of clinical quality measurement across the entire U.S. care delivery industry. I know of no other "national standard" quality assessment tools that the MHS does not currently employ. Both HCAPS and NCQA HEDIS measures typically include built in data system validation; review and validation of JCAHO Oryx measures typically occurs in association with JCAHO review and accreditation visits.

Finding 4: Current MHS measurement systems for inpatient and outpatient clinical quality reflect standard good practice across the U.S. health care delivery industry, both in terms of measurement systems used and their operations.

Access to care

The MHS operates under a legal mandate to provide timely medical services the populations that it serves. It has established access goals that reflect those legal requirements, broken into categories of emergent, acute, and elective care in both inpatient and outpatient settings. The MHS provides the bulk of those services through its own care delivery operations (MTFs). It offloads patients to contracted civilian facilities for special care needs, or when MTF locations cannot deliver all needed care in a timely way. The MHS is also developing tools for electronic interactions, to further improve accessibility.

The MHS has established a broad set of measures that track closely to similar access measures used in civilian systems. The MHS measures are comprehensive. Compared to those used in high-quality care settings outside of the MHS, I could not identify any category or specific measure that was missing within the MHS data system.

MHS data systems that track timely delivery take 2 basic forms. The first is integrated into the MTF's appointment scheduling software. It automatically records critical times whenever an appointment for services is scheduled. The fully integrated nature of this monitoring system makes it very unlikely that those using the system could manipulate reported data to hide substandard access, as has occurred in some other government-associated institutions. During site visits and through other reports, MHS leadership has been able to identify a single circumstance where front-line personnel were maintaining any sort of manual scheduling tool (appointment waiting lists): That involved patients who wanted to schedule specialty follow up visits at long intervals, typically beyond 6 months in the future. The MHS scheduling software allows specification of a "maximum delay" when scheduling appointments. It is typically set at 6 weeks by many MTF sites. Therefore, some front-line care delivery teams maintain patient lists so that they can load distant appointments when the software will finally accept them.

The second major data system used to track access to care within military care delivery systems is a patient survey conducted independently from care delivery teams. This provides an important cross check of data received from the scheduling system itself. That system suffers from one significant limitation: As described to me by MHS leadership, it is a voluntary survey with a typical low response rate. By definition, its results are therefore systematically biased. Typically, though, such bias will attract those with complaints more heavily than it will attract those who have had a positive experience. It will over-report dissatisfaction within timely access to care, rather than under-report it.

> **Finding 5: The MHS systems for tracking timely access to care are well-constructed and effectively operated, compared to similar systems used by high-quality civilian systems. They are innately difficult to manipulate (game), and any inherent bias contained in resulting reports should err on the side of underestimating timely, high satisfaction access to care, rather than overestimating it.**

A final structural comment

Health care delivery leadership can view clinical quality measurement and management from 2 perspectives. The first takes the viewpoint of regulatory compliance. Care delivery administration focuses on those measures mandated by external reviewers, such as the TJC, the NCQA, and CMS. Leadership aims to meet external requirements and thus receive legal and societal license to deliver care. Most care system administrators therefore regard regulatory compliance as an uncompensated cost of doing business. They try to minimize resources consumed in their quality measurement and management activities, while still meeting all external regulatory requirements. They regard the external validation they receive through these approaches as confirmation that they are delivering adequately good patient care.

The second approach looks at quality as the natural product of process management. It derives from Dr. W. Edwards Deming's quality improvement theory. It rests on 2 of Deming's 3 axiomatic principles:

1. All productive work (including all clinical care delivery and ancillary support services) is accomplished through processes.

    The purpose of any organization is to serve the needs and wants of customers – patients, in the case of care delivery. Deming regarded the money that a company receives for its products or services primarily as a measure of customer satisfaction. If customers have a free and informed choice, and those customers persistently come to a particular company to get products or services that fill their needs, it means that that company is best satisfying those customers compared to alternatives.

The way that a company creates products or services that satisfy customers is through front-line work processes. Therefore, Deming argued, any successful company will necessarily organize literally everything – especially data systems and management structures – around value-added front-line work processes, where "value-added" is defined by the company's customers.

2. Every process produces 3 classes of parallel outcomes: a Physical outcome; a Cost outcome; and a Satisfaction outcome.

   The term "quality" refers to the features and attributes of a process's physical outcomes. For health care delivery processes, physical outcomes correspond to clinical outcomes.

   This means that quality outcomes and cost outcomes are inextricably linked. Processes changes made to produce better clinical quality results will necessarily modify the resource costs associated with the same process. Conversely, changes made to reduce operating costs will unavoidably change clinical quality outcomes. Those changes may be large or small, positive or negative, but they are always present.

   Deming' went on to explore specific mechanisms by which Physical (quality) outcomes interacted with Cost outcomes within a process management framework. He identified 3 high-order classes that contained all possible forms of interaction. He demonstrated that, for 2 of the 3 classes, improvements in Physical outcomes – better quality – caused operating costs to fall. He labelled these 2 classes "quality waste" and "inefficiency waste."

   These ideas transformed manufacturing. They fueled the Japanese quality revolution during the 1950s, 60s, and 70s before returning to their home shores in the United States during the 1980s and 1990s (Deming and his colleagues got their start with these methods supporting U.S. war materiel manufacturing during World War II; Deming introduced them to Japanese manufacturing while working as a census statistician for General Douglas MacArthur in Japan after the war ended). They produced higher quality products while simultaneously reducing production costs. Any company that couldn't "do Deming" simply died – it could not begin to compete with those companies that could.

   Best current estimates suggest that at least 35 percent, and probably over 50 percent, of all resources spent on health care delivery in the U.S. and other First World nations fall into Deming's 2 waste categories.

Under this second model, administrators don't see quality measurement and management as an unavoidable expense necessary for regulatory compliance, but as the core set of measurement systems, management methods, and tools that form the heart of care delivery operation.

In reviewing the materials that you sent and drawing upon the day of interviews that you presented, I perceive that MHS leadership may see clinical quality and patient safety primarily as compliance efforts.

Recommendation 7: MHS leadership should adopt clinical quality improvement as a core business strategy.

This involves 3 main elements (Baldrige model):

1. Set and maintain a strong shared vision to drive the necessary change. To help build and sustain that vision, start to teach clinical quality improvement principles broadly across the MHS.

2. Perform key process analysis to identify high-priority processes within MHS operations.

   To illustrate, when we implement this step within Intermountain we first conceptually divided our care delivery system into 4 complementary categories: (1) Clinical conditions – disease treatment processes that define care delivery, the way that patients experience care – this is the central definition of "patient centered care" that we identified on the IOM committee that first introduced the term, and that we published in Crossing the Quality Chasm. (2) Clinical Support Services – clinical processes that are not condition specific, such as pharmacy, imaging, lab, blood bank, a procedure room, or a nursing service. (3) Patient Perceptions of Care – patient satisfaction with their care experience. While patient satisfaction follows the same theory and uses the same tools as the other categories, it operates in manner that is largely independent of them. It primarily relies on positive personal relationships. (4) Administrative Support Processes.

   We identified more than 1440 clinical conditions, corresponding to disease treatment processes, that fell into category number 1. We prioritized them on the basis of (a) number of patients involved; (b) health risk to the patient, which correlated very highly to resource intensity and cost of care; and (c) internal variability within a case type, assessed through the risk / resource consumption metric developed in (b). On that basis, 104 clinical condition processes – 7 percent of the total – accounted for 95 percent of all Intermountain care delivery services. Rather than the traditional 80/20 rule, care delivery exhibited a 95/7 rule. It concentrated massively.

   We then pursued the following steps in size order, as quickly as we could address specific processes. Fifteen years later, we have almost 60 major clinical processes under active management, that account for roughly 80 percent of all Intermountain care delivery operations.

3. Evaluate data needs for each clinical process (in size order, process by process, as just described). Build process-aligned data systems that embed clinical (physical, technically), cost, and satisfaction intermediate (process step) and final (end outcome) data into front-line care delivery processes.

This is the heart of the Intermountain clinical analytics system, which has been independently evaluated and judged world class by 2 major IT groups (KLAS and Himformatics). We have a longitudinal clinical registry to each clinical process that we manage. They reside on the Intermountain enterprise data warehouse (EDW), and provide raw data for 17 statisticians (at the moment – this capability continues to grow) who support care delivery management and improvement efforts.

We adopted an evidence-based method for identifying data elements and reports for quality management, that was first published by the National Quality Forum's (NQF's) Strategic Framework Board. Despite having one of the richest automated clinical data environments in the world, when we applied this approach we discovered that we were missing between 20 and 50 percent of critical data elements, across different processes; and that large amounts of data that we were spending large sums to collect were not useful for effective operations (what Dr. Gerald O'Connor at Dartmouth University calls "recreational data collection"). We ended up with far more parsimonious and efficient data sets designed for clinical care delivery process management and improvement (which links tightly to clinical research embedded into routine care delivery, often called a Learning Health Care System).

4. Once the necessary clinical data are available, build a clinical management structure – hire and assign physician and nurse leaders to use those data for accountability and improvement.

It is this structure that underlies Intermountain's success in producing "the best medical result at the lowest necessary cost" – the short version of the Intermountain mission statement. It doesn't correspond precisely to regulatory oversight systems, which were not built for improvement, but it does form a foundational ability to manage and improve care delivery, that can be mapped into regulatory reporting systems.

Thank you for the opportunity to review your quality efforts. They reflect well on the noble mission, competence, and truly dedicated service of the people who make up America's military. I hope that this evaluation and my comments are useful as you strive to make what is already quite good even better.

Yours sincerely,

Brent C. James, M.D., M.Stat.
Chief Quality Officer and
Executive Director, Intermountain Institute for Health Care Delivery Research
Adjunct Professor, Departments of Family and Preventive Medicine and Biomedical Informatics,

University of Utah School of Medicine
Visiting Lecturer, Department of Health Policy & Management, Harvard School of Public Health
Member, Institute of Medicine, National Academy of Sciences

External Methodology Review: Report from Dr. Qi Zhou

Reviewed by Qi Zhou
July 10-11, 2014

Purpose: External expert is to evaluate and comment on the methodology used for the "Military Health System (MHS) 90-day review for meeting the goals and objectives outline in the approved Terms of Reference as below:

Goal: This MHS Quality Review assessed access to health care, quality of care and patient safety, across the Military Health System (MHS), as directed by the Secretary of Defense. Key questions answered by this review:
- Does the MHS performance meet established internal standards as defined by policy, with regard to access to care, quality of care and patient safety?
- Does the MHS meet or exceed relevant external civilian benchmarks, with regard to access to care, quality of care and patient safety?
- Are our patients satisfied with the care received, with regard to access to care, quality of care and patient safety?

Data Sources: My assessment and comments on the review methodology are based on reviewing documents provided by MHS 90-day Review team and meetings with the MHS Program Review Lead, Dr. Michael Malanoski; Action Officer Leads: BG Barbara Holcomb (Patient Safety), RDML Kenneth Iverson (Access), and Brig Gen (s) Lee Payne (Quality); CAPT Paul Rockswold (Analytics Lead); and CAPT Carter (Writing). Col. John Savage also provided a comprehensive overview binder containing the MHS 90-day Review's Terms of Reference, Memorandums defining scope, timeline, study questions, policy, review methodology, metrics selection, site visit methodology, review process, and example data analysis. The access to the Max system provided more detailed documents from work groups on Access, Quality, Safety of care, and Data Analytics.

Comments on the Overall Review Methodology

The MHS 90-day Review was conducted by a multi-service team with representatives from the Army, Navy and Air Force medical commands, as well as Defense Health Agency personnel including Health Affair. The structure of the review team was designed as work groups of Quality, Safety, Access, Analytics, and Central Cell for the site visit and final report. Each work group consisted of subject matter experts (SMEs) from the Army, Navy, and Air Force. I had a very positive impression of the team structure; it functions well. The work groups are well coordinated and work with each other smoothly. With a very tight timeline and a broad comprehensive review of Access, Quality and Safety of care, the review team defined the review methodology as a three-prong analysis: 1) system-wide data collection, 2) conducting on site observational assessment of 7 sites, and 3) benchmarking with 3 best practice civilian health care systems which has staff model closed system similar to MHS. This approach enhanced the validity of the review and strengthens the credibility of the review findings as well as reporting to the Secretary and to the public. A few comments on each prong of the analysis are summarized below:

A. <u>System-wide data collection and analysis:</u>
The criteria used for measure selection are appropriate: They are consistent with national definitions on quality measures (such as NQF, IOM, IHI); are comparable to national benchmarks and leading civilian health care systems; and the data sources are available and currently used by MHS. The sample analyses and graphics reporting to compare MHS performance with AHRQ average and statistical confidence interval for selected measures on quality, safety and access to care are very impressive. The historical performance data (3 years) at MTF level showing patterns of performance across all measure sets is the right approach – much better than using individual level measures for information and the quality story. For example, a summary table showing that a few MTFs had higher performance in all measure sets across all domains (access, safety, and quality) while a couple of MTFs had lower performance for most measure sets. This pattern may show the true organizational performance. Performance at individual measure level may not be able to tell the story of the organizational performance. I reviewed a summary table with color coded for the quality metrics. It is very impressive and story telling. Similar summary tables might also be available for safety and access measures.

Recommendation 1: As discussed, it may be beneficial to add one more factor to the 'selected measure set'. The criteria used to select measures for the review should also consider the importance of the diseases/conditions which may impact the specific population for access, safety, and quality of care as well as outcomes. For example, adding OB delivery care measures since OB care is high volume of services.

Some areas, such as care for beneficiaries with disability, mental health, end of life care, and health care disparity, were out of scope for this review due to either a past effort or are planned for future considerations. It might be a good approach to mention it in the final report to highlight these areas being taking care of and not a gap in the review.

The final measure set selection for MHS performance comparison with civilian systems may also depend on the data completeness, sample size, high volume services population, and ability to address the 6 domains of IOM quality definition.

Recommendation 2: In the analysis, some measures were found to be sensitive to data sources and coding variations. An example would be the hospital acquired condition (HAC) – for pressure ulcers basing this measure on claims data only could be an unreliable data source due to coding variation. Hospitals coding HAC aggressively will have higher HAC rates, but their actual quality and safety performance might be better compared to those hospitals not coding the HAC as aggressively. Consistent coding is very important for these measures (see more information in Recommendation 5.)

B. <u>Site Visit (MTF) and validation:</u>
The targeted on-site review was an efficient use of time given the short time frame. The goal of the site visit was to verify if the MTF's and Clinic's performance is consistent with the guidance and policy defined by higher headquarters and MTF leadership, especially as it related to culture

of safety, quality of care and patient satisfaction. The town hall meetings with staff and patients provided qualitative data for assessing access, safety, and quality of care.

Recommendation 3: This data source will provide rich information for future quality improvement program design and development. Caution should be exercised when analyzing this data due to potential bias from 'participant self selection'. If time permits, to supplement this data source, a review of patient grievance data collected through normal business process, employee engagement survey data, and Human Resources employee complains data, may shed some lights on culture of safety and leadership performance.

C. Benchmarking with civilian health care system:
Kaiser Permanente, Geisinger, and Intermountain Healthcare are well recognized high performing health care delivery systems in US. Their robust quality management systems have years of trending data available on access, safety, and quality of care for benchmarking.

Recommendation 4: If needed, other benchmark data such as Cleveland Treatment Outcomes books, are good resources for specialty care performance
comparison: http://my.clevelandclinic.org/about-cleveland-clinic/quality-patient-safety/treatment-outcomes.aspx;
For access, physician supply data could be used to assess if any specialty care may have a physician shortage: https://www.aamc.org/download/263512/data/statedata2011.pdf

Comments on Patient Safety Methodology

Patient safety measurement and improvement in health care have had some challenges over past 100 years since Dr. Codman first published his surgical mortality rate. Ernest Amory Codman, M.D., was one of the most important figures in the history of outcomes research in medicine. While his contemporaries scorned his efforts to create systematic procedures to evaluate the end results of medical care, his work foreshadowed many of today's most pressing issues in patient safety. Since then, The Joint Commissions (TJC) and other accreditation bodies and government regulations are requiring hospitals and health care organizations to report sentinel events, patient safety culture survey, root cause analysis, and safety training.

The Safety Workgroup selected 9 core measures for this review. Of the 9 measures, I personally liked the safety culture survey, sentinel events data, and root case analysis (RCA). These three measures would encourage MTFs leadership and staff to focus on creating a culture of safety and reporting of sentinel events. The site visit questions for the leadership team and town hall meetings are good resources not only for data collection for this review, but also for future training and safety culture building.

Recommendation 5: Due to concerns of the reliability of claims data based patient safety indicators (PSI), the best effort to improve the safety of care at this point is to focus on structure and process measures such as leadership, staff training, the universal protocols, etc. Claims data based measures could be used for tracking, monitoring and improvement purpose. When the data validity is improved through staff training and standard coding, these measures can be added for comparison and performance reporting.

To address this concern, AHRQ published a toolkit for provider system to improve coding consistency:
http://www.ahrq.gov/professionals/systems/hospital/qitoolkit/b4-documentationcoding.pdf

Comments on Quality Methodology

The quality of care measures were the most robust and available data for the review. The Work Group selected a 37 measure set, most of which are composite measures. Hospital measure sets covers most inpatient care quality including readmissions. Healthcare Effectiveness Data Information Set (HEDIS) and Patient Centered Medical Home (PCMH) measures cover most ambulatory care for prevention and chronic care for pediatric, women's health, disease management, and senior care. The most important domain of quality is patient centric care and services. The patient experience survey data is a key component to incorporate patient perspective in this review. All accreditations, certifications and program recognitions highlighted the strong quality program foundation and effective implementation of policies and procedures. On site review questions on Quality of care is good high level assessment from leadership, staff, and patient.

Recommendation 6: Since there are robust data sources for some key prevention and disease management measures, it might be valuable to add a health care disparity analysis section to identify potential disparity (or assurance of no disparity) by region, and demographics, such as race, income, education, language spoken, or other important factors.

Although mental health care is out of scope for this review, it might help to depict a picture of comprehensive care provided to beneficiaries if some measures are available such as antidepressant management.

If time does not allow for this additional analysis, I would recommend it as a future consideration.

Comments on Access Methodology

Access of care is the most important factor for assuring all military service men, women, and their family members get the highest level of quality of care. The Work Group identified a good set of measures for access to evaluate the access performance against the access standard (high bar comparing to civilian system), effectiveness of governance and leadership, and patient centered care. The Access Measure Set (23 measures) includes both actual time for appointment and relative to standards, as well as member satisfaction. I am delighted to see a couple of measures reflecting health care innovation and using technology to address access needs: encouraging members using "secure messaging" to facilitate communication and continuity of care and using 24/7 nursing line to answer questions of acute care issues. Research indicates that using high tech technology and "secure messaging" can improve access and quality of care, reduce medical cost, and improve patient satisfaction. This is very encouraging.

The only suggestion I have for future data collection is to include "no show" data. The reduction in "no shows" to appointment (mostly due to auto assigned) would further improve the appointment availability and system efficiency, as well as staff satisfaction (a few comments from town hall meetings mentioned the issue related to "no-show").

Conclusion

My overall impression of the methodology used for the MHS Quality Review is that it is valid and sound. The majority measures selected for Access, Safety and Quality of care have passed the scientific rigor test by national entities in measure development and the NQF endorsement process. The analytical approach for data collection and comparison is robust and meaningful.

The team composition for the Review is adequate and many of the subject matter experts (SMEs) are significantly involved in the study design and implementation. The Work Group members are coordinating their roles and responsibilities with smooth communication and trusted relationships. The process for moving the project along is huge task. I am amazed how fast and efficient the operation from commanding officers to the analysts in the work groups which completed more than 50% document review, data collection, and site visits in a short of time (2-3 weeks). This truly demonstrates effective and high performing team work.

The MHS 90 day Review is a fresh healthy starting point in assessing our MHS effectiveness to provider high quality care to our service men, women and their family members. The strength of the review is very comprehensive despite the short turn-around time. Lessons learned from the system wide data collection and on site review will provide insights to continue quality improvement for a safe, high quality, equitable, accessible, and high value care delivery system. It was my pleasure and honor to serve in the role as an external expert to support the MHS 90 day Review. I'd like to thank the Review team leaders and members for spending their precious time with me and a sharing the great work group documents. A special thanks to Col. John Savage for his leadership and support for my completion of this review.

Very Respectfully,

Qi Zhou
Executive Director
Performance Measurement Program Strategy
& Quality Programs Oversight
Blue Cross Blue Shield of Massachusetts

External Methodology Review: Report from Dr. Katherine Kahn

Purpose: This external expert evaluated the Military Health System (MHS) 90-day review methodology for meeting the goals and objectives outline in the approved Terms of Reference.

Data Sources: This external expert had access and reviewed the following information for the analysis: Terms of Reference, Memorandums defining scope, timeline, study questions, policy/document review methodology, metric selection, site visit methodology, review outline, process and outcome review methods, example analysis, and early drafts of some sections of the report. The reviewer also had meetings with the MHS Program Review Lead, Dr. Michael Malanoski, Action Officer Leads: BG Barbara Holcomb (Patient Safety), RDML Kenneth Iverson (Access), and Brig Gen (s) Lee Payne (Quality), CAPT Paul Rockswold (Analytics Lead) and LTC Julie Freeman (Site Visit Lead); and Karen Guice, M.D., M.P.P, Principal Deputy Assistant Secretary of Defense for Health Affairs.

Overview of the Methodology

Timeline

The 90-day timeline for the Report is sufficient for allowing the collection, consolidation, and systematic presentation of information about the MHS and access, quality, and safety. This ambitious timeline and Report has benefitted from a well-coordinated effort including the direct and purchased care components of MHS, inputs from Army, Air Force, and Navy branches, analyses using beneficiary, staff, provider, and administrative informants involving qualitative and quantitative data collection and analyses. In addition to analyses of MHS data, serious efforts were made to compare MHS data to national benchmarks and to civilian health systems.

Scope

The scope of report was defined to be inclusive of most aspects of access, quality, and safety with a small number of well-specified exclusions that are readily justifiable on the basis of the limited timeline for this review and/or because of concurrent separate reviews and/or reports.

Processes of the Review

The thoroughness of the approach to the Report was apparent in its inclusion of multiple data sources, stakeholders, and analysis methods. The process for generating the Report appeared extremely well coordinated with the goal of providing a transparent look at access, quality, and safety records that characterizes the MHS through the summer of 2014.

Commentary on the Overall Methodology for Assessing Patient Access, Quality and Safety

The overall methodology for assessing patient access, quality, and safety is, by design, similar across the domains of access, quality, and safety. The strengths of the approach include an aggressive effort to consolidate a wide variety of qualitative and quantitative data across the three domains characterizing both direct and purchased MHS care, to organize the data according to review goals and study questions, to provide data about successes and failures, and to comment on the effectiveness of governance and leadership.

Stated review goals[13] include determining if the MHS as defined by standards in the Office of the Secretary of Defense (OSD) for Health Affairs (HA), service specific Military Department policies and guidance, and TRICARE contract specifications
- Provides ready access to medical care;
- Meets or exceeds the benchmarks for health care quality; and
- Has created a culture of safety with effective processes for safe and reliable care for beneficiaries?

For each of the three domains of access, quality, and safety, the stated study questions[14] are:
- Does the MHS performance meet established internal standards as defined by policy, with regard to access to care, quality of care and patient safety?
- Does the MHS meet or exceed relevant external civilian benchmarks, with regard to access to care, quality of care and patient safety?
- Are our patients satisfied with the care received, with regard to access to care, quality of care and patient safety?

There is substantial merit to this selection of these three study questions. The first study question addresses performance within MHS across three domains of access, quality and safety and prompts reporting of internal comparisons recognized as important to MHS. These include multiple well-conceived internal comparisons.

The second question motivates comparisons between MHS data and national benchmarks, as well as between MHS data and three comparable civilian benchmarks across three domains. The third question requires reporting of data of patient satisfaction across three domains.

For each of the three domains of access, quality, and safety, a revised and more explicit set of study questions address the following constructs:
- **Performance** which asks about the current state of indicators within MHS, whether the indicators meet or exceed internal standards, national benchmarks or civilian health systems.
- **Effectiveness of Governance & Leadership** which asks if policies systematically support access, quality, and safety throughout the MHS, and how well military health facilities (MTFs) comply with access, quality, and safety policies.
- **Patient-Centeredness** which asks about reported perceptions of MHS's patients regarding access, quality, and safety, as well asking how patient satisfaction regarding access, quality and safety compared with external benchmarks.

With this framework the Report is designed to systematically provide both performance data using standard definitions of access, quality, and safety and also patient centeredness data through reports of beneficiary satisfaction across the same three domains. Where possible, each

---

[13] Original Guidance Goals from the Terms of Reference
[14] Original Guidance Study Questions

of these reports is presented in terms of current MHS performance, variability in MHS performance across specified comparators internal to MHS, and in relation to national and civilian benchmarks. All of these features of the Report are well-presented. However, some areas could benefit from improvement.

The Report could be improved with a systematic discussion of data quality pertinent to performance and patient-centeredness. The reader of the report is provided an occasional glimpse into the completeness of data across strata examined. However, the presentation of data quality is not systematic which is necessary in order for the reader to gauge the completeness and the validity of the data presented. This Report is designed for a broad readership and these readers will want some basis for understanding potential biases associated with the data. This problem could be readily remedied with text or a table providing a basic characterization of all data sources presented. In a report such as this, it is not possible for all aspects of all of the data to be characterized. However, some simple characteristics of the analyzed data sets should be systematically included to help the reader understand potential biases associated with the data, and also to help the reader begin to understand the effectiveness of leadership and governance in designing a system for successful monitoring of access, quality, and safety. Example variables that could be included are: the year of data collection, the sample size, the number of sites included and the number not included, the response or participation rate, evidence for the generalizability of the data, and a listing of variables that have major problems with missing values.

Data quality is a critical component of any quality monitoring system. The absence of systematic reporting about data quality inhibits the readers' confidence in data validity and in transparency which is cited as a key feature of this report. Additionally, providing the reader with a framework for understanding data quality will allow the reader to contextualize results. When positive and negative performance data are reported, they are most likely to be interpreted correctly when associated with meaningful information about the quality of the data.

Adding a brief, but systematic data-set-specific section on data quality will substantially enhance the reporting of answers to the data presented pertinent to **performance** and **patient-centeredness**. The third category of study question pertains to **Effectiveness of Governance & Leadership**. The methods presented for answering this question are predominantly confined to a description of leadership, and documentation of the number of policies and reports that have been reviewed. Follow-up to prior recommendations for responding to deficits in quality noted in prior reports are occasionally presented. This information is helpful. However, in order to answer this very broad and important set of questions about the effectiveness of governance and leadership, additional documentation is required. First, the Report should help the reader understand the ways in which governance and leadership support the data systems and other infrastructure required to systematically examine access, quality, and safety. While some reports suggest excellent performance, many of the reports of performance and patient satisfaction suggest less than ideal access, quality, and safety. What role is governance and leadership playing in assuring that data systems for capturing problems with access, quality, and safety are identified in a timely manner? Is the combination of the electronic health record and the billing records adequate for supporting a robust monitoring system? The reader should be informed about how data systems have recently improved, what problems have been identified, and what solutions governance and leadership are playing to assure that data quality is adequate to support a system for timely monitoring of access, quality, and safety across both the direct and purchased care components.

There are many challenges to all health care systems in developing and sustaining an adequate monitoring system. Additionally, the MHS faces unique challenges including high volumes of patients and providers, high turnover rates, challenges with training, challenges with settings of various size and rurality. The efforts that governance and leadership are making to build and sustain a rigorous data monitoring system in light of these challenges should be presented. Challenges that remain to achieving an adequate monitoring system should be noted including expectations for when challenges are likely to be addressed and/or overcome if they cannot be addressed now. Additionally, patient cohorts that could be vulnerable to problems with access, quality, or safety as a consequence of inadequate data systems should be mentioned. This section of the Report would allow MHS to highlight important advances that are emerging with the new Defense Health Agency (DHA) and its newly coordinated approach to spanning military services. This section of the Report would also allow MHS to showcase the many external measures of access, quality, and safety in which it participates. When MHS participation is less than that of others, reasons for this should be noted and strategies for developing comparable monitoring systems should be noted.

The results of the Performance and Patient-Centeredness sections of the Report will show findings that are better than hoped and also show finding that are less good than hoped. These findings should be presented in a very objective manner. One approach that should be considered is to divide each summary section into a segment that focuses on results to be emulated and another segment that focuses on results that should be improved. A health care delivery system with a serious approach to quality monitoring and improvement will highlight every opportunity to improve care as one an opportunity. This approach would than set the stage for showing how governance and leadership have helped or need to help address the construct that the data are showing.

For example, if satisfaction data are improving, it would be useful to show what structural changes have been implemented that are likely responsible for these improvements. Furthermore, any systematic efforts by governance and leadership to disseminate the structures and processes associated with good outcomes should be highlighted. If this is not known, then MHS should indicate what they are doing to learn how to evaluate the relationships between their governance and leadership decisions and performance and patient-centeredness metrics.

A similar approach should be taken to results that need improvement (even if the suboptimal results are improved compared with last year or in relation to a comparator). All suboptimal findings can be improved but limited resources typically mandate that they cannot all be improved now. Strategies taken by leadership to prioritize resources including personnel, data and monitoring systems, fiscal resources should be made clear in relation to the large number of domains of care that can be improved. Without addressing the approach leadership is taking to recognize high and low performance, it is difficult to believe the report is meaningfully addressing the question of the effectiveness of governance and leadership.

There are major changes in health systems throughout the nation that involve the integration of electronic health records, a systematic commitment to quality monitoring, and the exploration of how population health should be monitored and explored. It is not expected that the MHS singularly will have mastered all of these issues. This Report should highlight the approach governance and leadership is taking to guide data monitoring so that analyses of access, quality, and safety can lead to ongoing improvements in care and outcomes.

Overall, the specific measures selected for reporting, the benchmarks, and comparisons are meaningful. The measures are valuable only when their analysis is used to identify problems and to improve them. The importance of these measures will be enhanced when basic features of data quality are shown, and when the approach of governance and leadership to data quality and the performance indicators is made more explicit.
Submitted by:

Katherine L. Kahn MD
Senior Scientist RAND
Professor of Medicine, David Geffen School of Medicine at UCLA

External Review of Findings and Recommendations: Report from Dr. Janet Corrigan

Date: July 30, 2014
External Expert Review Conducted By:
Janet M. Corrigan, PhD.
Distinguished Fellow
The Dartmouth Institute for Health Policy and Clinical Practice

Purpose: The purpose of this external expert review is to evaluate the Military Health System (MHS) 90-day review findings and recommendations with reference to the goals and objectives outline in the approved Terms of Reference.

Data Sources: This review was informed by the following information: Terms of Reference; memoranda defining scope, timeline, and study questions; policy/document review methodology; metric analysis methodology; site visit methodology; process and outcome review methods; site visit histograms and analysis; and draft final report. I participated in a 1-day meeting on July 14, 2014, that included briefing sessions by MHS Program Review Lead, Dr. Michael Malanoski, and Action Officer Leads: BG Barbara Holcomb (Patient Safety), RDML Kenneth Iverson (Access), Brig Gen (s) Lee Payne (Quality), CAPT Paul Rockswold (Analytics Lead) and LTC Julie Freeman (Site Visit Lead).

Summary Comments

Considering the time constraints imposed on this MHS review, leadership should be commended for having conducted a thorough and balanced review of access to health care and the quality and safety of services provided in both the direct and purchased care components. Performance information was gathered from both the enterprise-wide data and measurement system and the conduct of site visits and town hall meetings; and, whenever possible, MHS results were compared with external benchmarks and those of leading systems.

Overall, the results are mixed. MHS meets or exceeds many internal and external standards and benchmarks in the areas of access, quality, and safety, but there is variability within MHS and some performance gaps.

Following are comments on the overarching goals and recommendations, followed by comments on the specific findings and recommendations pertaining to system-wide improvements, access to care, and quality and safety.

Overarching Goals and System-wide Improvements

I strongly support MHS's overarching goal of becoming a high reliability organization. In its pursuit of excellence, MHS should take full advantage of opportunities to enter into partnerships and to learn from others, for example, the Malcolm Baldrige National Quality Program and the Institute for Healthcare Improvement have substantial track records in helping health care organizations achieve high reliability.

I also encourage MHS to consider whether more fundamental changes in the health care delivery and financing systems might be necessary to achieve the goal of high reliability, specifically:

- Planned and coordinated approach to direct and purchased care. DHS provides beneficiaries with ready access to network providers, which has certain benefits (e.g., serves as a safety valve when the direct care component lacks capacity; provides access to specialized services that may not be a priority for MHS to develop itself due to low demand). However, MHS makes *extensive* use of purchased services and this raises concerns about care coordination and continuity, which are key to beneficiary satisfaction and outcomes. MHS also has less influence over the quality and safety of purchased services than it does over direct services. MHS would benefit from being more explicit about the beneficiary needs it intends to satisfy directly and the circumstances under which it is best to purchase services (these will undoubtedly vary across services and service areas); and carefully designing and operating a delivery system with the proper capacity and resources to meet identified beneficiary needs.

- Flexible and timely human resource policies and practices. Human resources are critical to producing high quality health care. The 90-day review surfaced numerous concerns about staffing including: impact of furloughs on all levels of the system; restrictions on creating and filling positions that impede hiring key personnel (e.g., safety officers); frequent rotations of staff; and the glacial pace of the hiring process. These issues will need to be addressed to create a high-performing health system.

- Enhanced beneficiary-engagement. There are opportunities for DOD to benefit from greater engagement of beneficiaries. Beneficiaries have direct experience with the DOD system and can provide immediate feedback on performance. Beneficiary input is critical to the redesign of care processes to be more patient-centered. Beneficiary engagement in all aspects of patient safety (e.g., reporting errors, root cause analyses, design of safe systems) is an integral part of a culture of safety and transparency. DOD should identify ways to enhance beneficiary involvement in governance, planning and system redesign, operations, monitoring and reporting.

- Comprehensive approach to managing health care costs. It was noted that health care accounts for a sizable proportion of the DOD budget, and there will continue to be upward pressures on cost as the covered population grows and ages and with the introduction of new medical advances and technology. The Institute of Medicine has estimated that 30% or more of health care expenditures constitute waste. To contain health care costs without reducing access and quality, the DOD, like private sector health care systems, must redesign care processes to remove waste. This will require systems that can measure and manage the total cost of care for various types of patients, whether services are provided by MTFs or purchased (budgeting systems for direct and purchased care are currently separate). Enhancements may also be needed in DOD's information system and budgeting processes to support making wise health investment decisions. For example, it was noted that budgeting constraints may have slowed down hiring of patient safety experts at various MTFs, yet investing in safety expertise yields a very positive return in terms of better outcomes *and lower total costs.*[15]

Recommendation 1: MHS should develop a performance management system adopting a core set of metrics regarding access, quality, and patient safety; further develop MHS dashboards with system-wide performance measures; conduct regular, formal performance reviews of the entire MHS, with the DHA monitoring performance and supporting MHS governance bodies in those reviews.

DOD will benefit greatly from alignment of measures between the purchased and direct care components. I also urge alignment with national standardized measurement and reporting systems, such as those sponsored by CMS, AHRQ, NCQA and others. Lastly, MHS might consider real-time monitoring systems for front-line teams that include run charts and other timely and actionable displays of data.

Recommendation 2: The MHS should develop an enterprise-wide quality and patient safety data analytics infrastructure, to include health information technology systems, data management tools, and appropriately trained personnel. There should be clear linkage between the Defense Health Agency's analytic capabilities, which monitors the MHS overall, and the Service level analytic assets.

This is an extremely important recommendation. A sophisticated and adequately funded analytics infrastructure is a necessary prerequisite to becoming a high reliability organization.

Adequate investment in patient safety analytics is also particularly important at this point in time when DOD is transitioning to a new electronic health record system. EHRs offer great promise for improving safety (by providing clinicians with access to more complete patient information along with clinical decision-supports), but the introduction of a new EHR system, like any new technology, can result in new types of errors and safety issues, especially during the early phases of adoption.

Recommendation 3: The MHS should emphasize transparency of information, including both the direct and purchased care components, with visibility internally, externally, and to DOD beneficiaries. Greater alignment of the measures of the purchased care component with those of the direct care component should be incorporated in TRICARE regional contracts.

I encourage DOD to make extensive use of a public and beneficiary portals to display performance information along with descriptions of improvement efforts; and to provide opportunities for beneficiaries to comment and make suggestions and to participate in improvement efforts.

---

[15] For example, estimated additional health care costs associated with health care -acquired infections include $20,000 for a surgical site infection, $40,000 for ventilator-associated pneumonia, and $46,000 for a central line-associated blood stream infection. Zimlichman, JAMA Internal Medicine, 2013.

Recommendation 4: Through MHS governance, policy guidance can be developed to provide the Services with common executable goals. While respecting the Services individual cultures, this effort would advance an understanding of the culture of safety and patient-centered care across the MHS.

As a part of developing an enterprise-wide strategy, MHS leadership might consider paring back the total number of performance goals that services and MTFs are currently expected to meet. It was noted during interviews that there are currently service-specific goals, enterprise-wide goals, and externally set goals. Focusing on a limited number of very high priority goals will allow leadership and front-line staff to devote the necessary attention and resources to rapidly achieve measureable improvements, thus boosting morale.

Recommendation 5: The MHS should continue, where it makes sense either fiscally or from a quality perspective, to standardize processes and outcomes across the enterprise in the areas of patient safety, quality, and access.

It is also important to empower front-line care teams to fix quality and safety problems in a timely manner.

Access Findings and Recommendations:

Overall, the MHS direct care component performs well compared with both DOD and external standards and with other leading private sector health systems across a wide variety of indicators. A deeper dive into the results indicates that overall system performance may be masking some important performance gaps:
- Across service and MTF variability. There is a good deal of variability in performance across services (e.g., Air Force meets the MHS standard for Average Number of Days to Acute Appointment, but other services do not), and MTFs (e.g., Average Days to Third Next Acute Appointment).
- Signs of pent-up demand. MHS should be commended for establishing the Nurse Advice Line in March 2014; high use of this service (over 1000 calls per day) clearly points to need for access to health care professionals for a variety of situations (e.g., emergency care, appointment scheduling, referrals to the private sector, and advice). Some beneficiaries participating in Town Hall meetings also expressed a good deal of frustration gaining access with some choosing to bypass the central appointment system and go directly to the clinic, and others being advised to call back at a later time for an appointment.
- Weak beneficiary survey results. Results for key access questions on beneficiary surveys are either below or barely meeting external benchmarks.

Moving forward, MHS will want to obtain a more complete picture of access by measuring and monitoring at the level of individual facilities and care sites (hospitals, ambulatory surgery centers, medical homes); and procedures (an area that lacks established standards is time to procedure).

Unlike the MHS direct care component, far less is known about access in the purchased care component. As recommended in the report, this is an area for improvement.

I concur with the specific access-related recommendations in the report. Removing barriers to use of the Secure Messaging System (currently not used by many clinicians) and the online appointment scheduling system (experiencing technical problems and lack of beneficiary support) should be high priorities. I also encourage use of nationally standardized beneficiary survey instruments, such as CAHPS, accompanied by routine benchmarking with other systems in the public and private sector.

Lastly, continued development and enhancement of PCMHs would be wise. Utilization data indicate that beneficiaries are responding very positively to the medical home concept (the proportion of primary care delivered in the direct care component has increased steadily since the inception of PCMHs), and a core competency of PCMHs is establishment of an ongoing relationship between the primary care clinician and the patient. All beneficiaries should have a designated medical home (if they so choose to have one) and the medical home should be responsible for assuring that patients have appropriate access and know how to navigate the health care system.

Quality Findings and Recommendations:

MHS has conducted a thorough review of quality using national standardized measure sets developed and used by leading accrediting organizations, professional and specialty societies, government agencies, and others. The measures cover prevention, acute care and specialty care; and medical care processes, patient outcomes and patient satisfaction.

Overall, MHS performance mirrors what we see in the private sector, a good deal of mediocrity, pockets of excellence, and some serious gaps. For example,

- On the National Committee for Quality Assurance's HEDIS Measures (a tool used by 90% of health plans in the US), MHS direct services falls below the 50 percentile for most of the 18 selected measures and below the 25 percentile for three measures (cholesterol management for patients with cardiovascular conditions, and Hemoglobin A1c and LDL cholesterol screening for diabetics). For purchased care, 7 of the 12 measures monitored fell below the NCQA 25th percentile in 2012.
- When compared to the three selected health plans on HEDIS measures, MHS performs at or above the benchmark for about half of the measures and below the benchmark for the remaining half.
- On The Joint Commission's ORYX measures, MHS direct care performs below the benchmark on 9 of 13 composite measure sets. For the purchased care component, comparative data was available for only 5 measures, but performance compared well to national benchmarks. Compared to the three external health systems, MHS had the lowest rates on 17 of 20 measures.
- MHS performed better on AHRQ's Prevention Quality Indicators that measure the occurrence of conditions that are potentially preventable with good outpatient care. MHS direct care performance met or exceeded national benchmarks on 89% of these measures.

- Results for the most recent reporting period of the National Surgical Quality Improvement Program (sponsored by the American College of Surgeons) found that three MTFs are performing at the top tier nationally, but surgical morbidity is significantly higher than expected at eight MTFs. Urinary tract infections, surgical site infections, return to the OR, and pneumonia were major contributors to poor performance.
- MHS performed well on some measures of perinatal care, but poorly on others (e.g., shoulder dystocia, postpartum hemorrhage, postpartum and infant readmissions).

The 90-day Review has provided MHS with a wealth of information on clinical performance, and MHS leadership have formulated strong sets of recommendations pertaining to each of the areas reviewed. I applaud the emphasis on: development of a strong data platform; use of standardized measures; ongoing collaboration and benchmarking with civilian health services; development of MHS dashboards at the MTF and provider levels; education and training for staff in quality improvement, rapid cycle improvement, Six Sigma and other proven approaches to process improvement; strong analytic support for implementation of targeted interventions and tools (e.g., surgical checklists, hand washing protocols and practices); transparency and scaling of successful results.

Although the site visits and town hall meetings provided useful input and suggestions from staff, MHS may want to consider conducting regular surveys of staff to obtain input on quality and safety issues; and also to elicit suggestions for maximizing the impact of the many quality improvement efforts that will likely be implemented over the coming months and years. It will also be important to "free up" staff time to engage in improvement activities, especially in light of the concerns voiced at town hall meetings about current workload and volume of patient visits.

DHS is well on the road to having a robust and comprehensive measurement system. Additional enhancements might include:
- Nursing sensitive indicators (which are being used in some locations but not enterprise-wide). Nursing sensitive indicators provide important information on quality and safety and adequacy of nurse staffing.
- Patient-reported outcome measures (e.g., ability to return to work, pain, functioning (e.g., SF-12), depression (e.g., PSQ-9)). Sometimes collected through web portals or on tablets at the time of a visit, patient-reported outcome measures provide useful information in support of patient and clinician decision-making and important feedback on whether a patient's goals for treatment are being achieved.
- Measures of care coordination, continuity and transitions (e.g., Care Transitions Measure). Given the rotation of staff and the use of direct and purchased care components, MHS has real challenges in providing seamless care to beneficiaries.

MHS may also want to explore whether there are additional opportunities for MTFs to participate in condition/procedure-specific registries. Registries, such as the one maintained by the Society for Thoracic Surgeons, provide useful benchmarking information and targeted educational programs.

Safety Findings and Recommendations

There are only a limited number of national patient safety benchmarks available, but overall, MHS direct care compares favorably. Gaps that should be addressed include:
- Surveys on Patient Safety Culture. The hospital culture survey identified several areas for improvement: including response rates, supervisor/manager expectations, organizational learning, non-punitive response, teamwork, and staffing. As noted above, human resource issues (e.g., staffing, turnover) appear to be a systemic and pervasive problem that needs to be addressed. MHS should also consider fielding the AHRQ Medical Office Survey of Patient Safety Culture in the PCMHs or expanding use of the current ambulatory survey being used in some settings.
- Healthcare Acquired Infections. Attention should be focused on CLABSI and VAP, as well as, measuring and reducing infection rates that occur outside ICUs.

The MHS direct care has many of the building blocks of a comprehensive patient safety system already in place and a great deal has been accomplished over the last decade. Investments have been made in safety metrics and measurement systems; policies and processes for reporting near misses and adverse events; teamwork collaboration and communication strategies; and a central mechanism to capture patient safety information. The 90-day review has identified many very promising opportunities to strengthen and enhance this infrastructure including: clarity of definitions and policies pertaining to sentinel events and what constitutes a root cause analysis; greater reliance on global trigger tools for manual or automated extraction of data from medical records along with "attainable" goals for reporting of near misses; development of a system-wide closed loop mechanism to ensure documentation and disposition of alerts and advisories; education and supports to enhance executive leadership engagement and safety training at all levels; and expanded system-wide transparency of patient safety information. Successful implementation of these recommendations will require strong leadership at the highest levels, sustained commitment, adequate resources, and accountability mechanisms.

As noted above, patient and family engagement is key to building a safe health system. Additional steps that might be taken to enhance safety through patient and family engagement include:
- Establish strong policies that demonstrate leadership commitment (e.g., open access to medical records).
- Invite patients and family members to participate in safety oversight committees, root cause analyses and subsequent improvement efforts.
- Provide training to staff on how best to foster patient engagement including: overcoming health literacy challenges, inviting patient input, being attentive to input received, and acknowledging and thanking patients for their input.
- Establish formal processes (surveys, error reporting) to obtain patient input.

- Provide adequate information and supports to patients to manage their health conditions and medications including 24/7 advice lines and written care plans and instructions (at appropriate literacy levels).

A culture of safety is also one that protects, respects, and attends to the needs of the members of the care team. MHS should measure and design care processes to minimize injuries to staff (e.g., falls, needle pricks, back strain, violence, and stress). Many health systems, especially those with hierarchical structures, have found that leadership, staff training and disciplinary systems are needed to make sure that all members of the care team are treated respectfully and are comfortable speaking up on behalf of the patient. Lastly, the vast majority of errors stem from "systems issues," not incompetence or willful misconduct; staff that make errors should be treated with compassion and provided with emotional supports to overcome the guilt and shame that often accompanies such situations.

Military Health System Review – Final Report
August 29, 2014

External Review of Findings and Recommendations: Report from Dr. Pamela Cipriano

Purpose: The external expert will evaluate the Military Health System (MHS) 90-day review findings and recommendations with reference to the goals and objectives outline in the approved Terms of Reference.

Data Sources: The external expert had access and reviewed the following information for her analysis: Terms of Reference, Memoranda defining scope, timeline, study questions, policy/document review methodology, metric analysis methodology, site visit methodology, process and outcome review methods, site visit histograms, analysis, and draft final report. The reviewer also had access to speak with the MHS Program Review Lead, Dr. Michael Malanoski, Action Officer Leads: BG Barbara Holcomb (Patient Safety), RDML Kenneth Iverson (Access), Brig Gen (s) Lee Payne (Quality), CAPT Paul Rockswold (Analytics Lead and LTC Julie Freeman (Site Visit Lead).

Results

Reviewers were asked to characterize current performance, identify any urgent areas for attention, and recommend actions to achieve top tier performance. As such, I offer the following observations:

Access: Current performance exceeds Department standards for primary care and is commendable. Areas for improvement relate primarily to consistency of provider and overall perception/satisfaction.

Quality: Quality measures at a composite level show average performance. MHS results are below the selected top performing civilian systems in most areas. Specific areas that are underperforming are noted throughout the findings and should be addressed with focused improvement plans. These include but are not limited to measures within HEDIS, NSQIP, NHSN, and Perinatal measures. Current performance is, for the most part, at average levels, but not in keeping with the MHS expectations of top tier outcomes. As noted, cross Service policies and methods will be needed to formulate and implement a coordinated improvement effort that uses best practices (within MHS and externally validated). The MHS is its own reference group and does not enjoy some of the external group/registry comparisons where civilian hospitals report data or are reviewed by rating or 'watchdog' type groups. For example, the University Hospital System Consortium provides comparison of quality performance of like institutions. Similarly, hospital systems produce internal comparisons of their institutions.

Safety: Most important and urgent is the need to be aggressive in establishing a culture of safety. Despite prior efforts, the culture does not seem to have permeated below leadership ranks. Until rank and file internalize their roles in promoting safety and preventing harm, performance will be mediocre. Leadership must declare and then demonstrate their commitment to a culture that encourages reporting, is not punitive, and is dedicated to improvement.

The foundation for achieving top performance is already in place and is being enhanced with new approaches that will provide for system wide goals, measures, and review of performance.

Further coordination and use of dashboards, consistent review, use of appropriate external comparisons may require additional training, IT infrastructure, and collaborations as noted in the findings and recommendations. It may not be clear who the "champions" are for quality improvement in each MTF. This is also an essential ingredient for staff to understand, beyond normal chain of command, who else is the leader for quality improvement.

In the sections that follow, I have addressed the recommendations for each area: Access to Care, Quality, and Safety. Comments follow each recommendation or are summarized in sections. General comments follow as well.

Access Findings and Recommendations

The Department's clearly articulated guidance and standards for access to health care (based on urgency of patient need) has resulted in clear expectations and ability to measure performance in direct care with some challenges for measurement in purchased care. Contemporary technologies in use such as secure messaging, TRICARE On-Line, and the Nurse Advice Line, are enhancing beneficiary access which is consistent with civilian systems as well.

Performance for Direct Care acute and specialty care appointments are excellent and outperform MHS and CA standards. Given this high level of performance it may not be necessary to continue to measure "days to third available appointment in primary care" as it is no longer applicable; some civilian systems have abandoned this measure in favor or same day or 'open' access (whenever the patient wants to come) for primary as well as some specialty care. There should be reconsideration of the standard for specialty care visits of 28 days. This far exceeds patient expectations and civilian systems in most specialties. With the average number of days being 12.4 days (median 11.6) a revised standard of 14 calendar days (10 business days) would be an achievable goal.

Overall, data sources were adequate, as were benchmark and external system comparisons. The lack of data from purchased service facilities (as pointed out in the recommendations) is an area for improvement.

Recommendations to Improve Access to Care

Please note, recommendation numbering and language listed here were taken from a previous draft of the Final Report. A table that maps the recommendation numbers used here with the recommendations listed in Appendix 6.1 of this report is provided at the conclusion of Dr. Cipriano's comments.

1. The DHA should, through governance, commission an external study to evaluate purchased care access for TRICARE Prime enrollees as it relates to 32 C.F.R. § 199.17. This study should include a review of all data available and a recommendation for data that should be incorporated into the current and future TRICARE contracts. (Mapped to Finding 2)
   Reviewer comment: Agree—it is important to be able to assess these other services and hold them to the same standards as MTFs.

2. MHS governance should increase the focus on the standardization of specialty care, including creation of the Tri-Service Specialty Care Advisory Board, funding requirements to standardize specialty product lines, business rules for access, and performance review metrics for specialty care product lines. (Mapped to Finding 3)
   Reviewer comment: Agree with continued implementation of the Specialty Care Advisory Board, etc. This will improve the ability to have a more comprehensive measurement of care that is either a complex episode or requires chronic management beyond primary care.
3. The Services should, through governance, standardize MHS access to care business practices by replacing the MHS Guide to Access Success with a MHS policy memorandum and subsequent DoD Instruction. (Mapped to Finding 4)
   Reviewer comment: no comment
4. The Services and DHA should, through governance, continue implementation of the Joint Service survey tool. (Mapped to Finding 5)
   Reviewer comment: Agree
5. DHA should, through governance, standardize reporting from the TROs to Services. (Mapped to Finding 6)
   Reviewer comment: Agree
6. The Services should, through governance, establish a measure to assess patient satisfaction with office waiting times through the new Joint Service satisfaction survey tool. (Mapped to Finding 7)
   Reviewer comment: In addition to measuring office waiting times, setting a goal to improve the rating of "getting care when needed" to closer approximate the CAHPS benchmark of 85%.
7. The Services and DHA should, through governance, promote SM and TOL through direct care component-wide standardized business processes and a strategic marketing approach. (Mapped to Finding 8)
   Reviewer comment: Greater use of these technologies can enhance access perception/response, and satisfaction. As soon as the electronic record system is upgraded, TOL capabilities should be expanded to mirror patient portals with greater self-service capabilities (some of this may be available now but was not apparent in the review materials).
8. The Services and DHA should, through governance, standardize both ATC and customer service training across the direct care component. (Mapped to Finding 9)
   Reviewer comment: This should be a priority and should include cross training for scheduling functions to address staffing shortages. A system should be developed that eliminates the need for the patient to call back, i.e. service their call until an appointment has been made or another appropriate disposition. The beneficiary town hall responses reinforced the dissatisfaction and barriers this has presented in the past.

Quality Findings and Recommendations

The Quality and Safety dimensions of any health system are inextricably linked, thus recommendations in the following Safety section will overlap with Quality. Some recommendations of this sections also address improved access and the dimension of patient satisfaction. Similar to recommendations in Access, there is a need for data from the purchased services component of care particularly as it relates to coordination of services and specialty care outcomes. This has been raised in prior external surveys as well.

Policy guidance across the Services and the NCR is insufficient to establish a system wide view of quality even though the MTF Directors ensure that hospitals maintain comprehensive Clinical Quality Management and Patient Safety Programs. Efforts to standardize and provide central guidance from the Clinical Quality Forum (CQF) which is relatively new with the formation of the DHA should continue. The CQF can be a driving force to effect improvement in clinical quality across the MHS. Each service develops its own quality improvement efforts which is appropriate but could benefit from an overarching framework that combines joint quality goals and metrics.

Upon hearing presentations in advance of reviewing the draft report, the Quality Improvement efforts appeared nascent in comparison to the depth of work in progress to address access and in some cases safety. Thus the number of recommendations is voluminous although not unrealistic given the size and complexity of the MHS. The detailed results presented in the report suggest areas for clinical improvement (HEDIS, NSQIP, and IPI) and should be addressed at the MTF level. A contemporary look at using mortality as an indicator should be considered.

Oral presentation referenced construction of a data warehouse which will be useful for generating reports for both (Alat and Ecentris data) that will allow comparative data, custom analyses, and presentation of dashboards.

It is important to continue to focus on skill development through education, and establishing a culture that values quality improvement. There must be infusion of this value from executive leadership to front line staff. Ensuring data transparency and creating a "just culture" will create the right mindset for embracing the need to improve.

Recommendations to Improve Quality of Care

Please note, recommendation numbering and language listed here were taken from a previous draft of the Final Report. A table that maps the recommendation numbers used here with the recommendations listed in Appendix 6.1 of this report is provided at the conclusion of Dr. Cipriano's comments.

1. MHS Governance should identify and implement leading healthcare industry methods for instilling and maintaining cultural changes throughout a large system.
   Reviewer comment: As evidenced by site visit reports, executives and quality management staff have a more significant level of awareness of quality initiatives and organizational performance than do staff and patients. This is only addressed through education and establishment of a culture that embraces quality and safety (similar finding with AHRQ Culture of Safety Survey); early report findings speak to a "standardized and intentional approach" to improving quality and safety will be beneficial. It will be essential to involve front line staff in performance improvement

activities and to achieve staff empowerment and commitment that will not only improve but sustain quality improvements.
2. DHA should establish relationships with civilian Health Systems to participate in collaboration and data sharing to facilitate more complete comparisons.
Reviewer comment: agree but probably not top priority; publicly available data may be sufficient for established benchmarks for initial comparisons.
3. MHS governance should develop and implement an enterprise performance management system that links to MHS and Service strategy with dashboards and common performance measures to support visibility of those measures across the enterprise.
Reviewer comment: Absolutely essential. This will also allow sharing and spread of best practices. Evidence suggests posting (can be just internal to staff or to your public) of data enhances quality improvement efforts.
4. MHS governance should create and task an MHS data analytics cell to provide actionable information to the Services and DHA at the enterprise level.
Reviewer comment: While it is possible that there is actionable data at both Service and DHA levels, it may be more appropriate to define desired outcomes and metrics at the DHA level, then implement and measure at the Service and MTF level. (similar to what is currently done)
5. ASD (HA) and DHA should develop policy guidance in support of DoDI and DoDM 6025.13 with specific direction on quality measurement, performance improvement, and requirements for education and training.
Reviewer comment: Policy guidance will help standardize education and training which is not only disparate but difficult to ascertain/measure at this time. It would be wise to exercise caution in expanding training in Lean and Six Sigma, but rather focus on training the larger number of staff who must understand principles and approaches to performance improvement and not necessarily the leadership skills to analyze processes and provide statistical support. What appears to be lacking is the more general wide spread understanding of process improvement, simple data interpretation, and use of control charts to create a common understanding of performance.
6. ASD (HA) should develop and implement a process to manage and track compliance of Services and DHA with applicable DoD policies and directives.
Reviewer comment: Agree
7. DHA Education and Training Directorate should conduct an in-depth review and needs assessment of quality training to adequately assess the efficacy of training. (#11, #49)
Reviewer Comment: Agree, consistent with #5 above
8. DHA should integrate requirements for Purchased Care clinical quality data on TRICARE beneficiaries into the TRICARE Operations Manual and future TRICARE regional contracts.
Reviewer comment: Agree—this is a consistent recommendation of prior reviews and this review.
9. MHS governance should commission a study to assess development of a Quality expert career path.
Reviewer comment: There are a number of available courses that prepare individuals for leadership roles in quality management and leadership. I do not believe a study is necessary. The emphasis should be on cultivating a knowledge base in the broad range of

leaders and front line staff with only a few experts needed to lead the execution of quality plans which include the measurement and reporting of quality outcomes.

10. MHS governance should establish a mechanism to aggregate and communicate accreditation findings across the MHS.
    Reviewer comment: Agreed. This should be relatively simple aggregation perhaps through the MOG.
11. MHS governance should consider expanding fellowship opportunities to include other national quality and accreditation organizations (e.g. Institute for Healthcare Improvement, AAAHC, etc.). Optimize utilization of fellows after completion of training.
    Reviewer comment: Agree, and consistent with responses to broader training; these individuals could easily rise to leadership roles.
12. DHA Health Plans should give purchased care contractors the authority to utilize supplemental databases to improve the capture of clinical information for purchased care enrollees.
    Reviewer comment: Agree

See comments under #18 for recommendations 13-18

13. DHA Health plans should explore alternative methods of incentivizing contractors and/or providers to improve the provision of clinical preventive services and HEDIS® performance. This may require statutory or regulatory changes, since new, innovative payment mechanisms may have to be developed to encourage compliance.
    Reviewer comment:
14. MHS governance should commission a study to assess the value of expanding the number of HEDIS® measures monitored to evaluate care provided to enrolled beneficiaries.
    Reviewer comment:
15. MTFs should capture and verify clinical data regarding preventive services that are obtained outside of the direct care component and enter that information into AHLTA.
    Reviewer comment:
16. DHA should develop plans to improve Other Health Insurance documentation in DEERS for all beneficiaries to ensure those with Other Health Insurance are not included in HEDIS® calculations.
    Reviewer comment:
17. MHS governance should increase efforts to understand the determinants of PQI performance and evaluate whether age adjustment of PQI data would enhance its accuracy.
    Reviewer comment:
18. MHS governance should implement a monitoring program for PQI measures and require plans for improvement if a facility is a statistical outlier for performance for two consecutive quarters.
    Reviewer comment: **Items 13-18 Agree with the recommendations.** *The performance on HEDIS® and PQI measures is disappointing. It would be beneficial to have dashboards by Service and NCR for comparisons and ultimately sharing of best practices to gain improvements. Better data collection methods are needed to be more inclusive. The*

detailed analysis in the report can guide the locus of improvement efforts including the expansion of HEDIS® measures, action lists, and documentation in DEERS, etc.

19. MHS governance should establish an implementation plan for MHS Population Health Portal readmissions site to ensure maximum utilization to reduce avoidable readmissions.
    Reviewer comment: Performance in reducing readmissions is admirable and is much stronger than in the civilian world. The benefit is in improving patient experience and improving coordination of care which has positive benefits for the patient and care team/system.
20. DHA Healthcare Ops Directorate should complete transition to the HEDIS® All-Cause Readmission standardized measure which is risk-adjusted and has national benchmarks.
    Reviewer comment: Agree but should follow any further developments in changes approved by National Quality Forum regarding all cause readmission measure(s).
21. DHA HIT should prioritize electronic medical record upgrades by aligning needed data elements into Essentris®. Move to remote access for all inpatient MTFs by utilizing the recently available Application Virtualization Hosting Environment (AVHE), allowing earlier collection of data.
    Reviewer comment: Agree would be beneficial
22. MHS governance should establish goals for increasing the number of Top Performers each year.
    Reviewer comment: Agree and couple with appropriate recognition and rewards as powerful incentives.

See comments under #26 for Recommendations 23-26

23. MHS governance should explore expanding NSQIP® participation to all remaining Direct Care inpatient facilities performing surgery. In addition, ensure our ambulatory surgery platforms all participate in a similar surgical quality improvement program.
    Reviewer comment:
24. DHA Healthcare Operations Directorate should partner with the American College of Surgeons to build a more effective collaboration between our facilities using their experience in building collaborative partnerships to capitalize on our top performing facilities best practices.
    Reviewer comment:
25. DHA Healthcare Operations Directorate should partner with the American College of Surgeons to evaluate MHS morbidity data in assisting the MHS and its facilities in developing plans for improvement.
    Reviewer comment:
26. MHS governance should task the NSQIP® working group to assess surgical morbidity shortfalls to the Medical Operations Group (MOG) for Tri-Service/DHA engagement, collaborative support, and facility action.
    Reviewer comment: Agree further conversation with NSQIP® and ACS officials would be beneficial before changing approach dramatically. Of great concern is the higher morbidity. Exploration with civilian high performing institutions may be instructive. If not already developed, the MHS might offer to initiate the ambulatory program. CMS reports the following on their website regarding the ASCQR: "The Ambulatory Surgical Center Quality Reporting (ASCQR) Program is a pay-for-reporting, quality data program finalized by the Centers for Medicare & Medicaid Services (CMS). Under this

program, ASCs report quality of care data for standardized measures to receive the full annual update to their ASC annual payment rate, beginning with Calendar Year (CY) 2014 payments."

27. The Perinatal Advisory Group (PAG) should lead efforts to increase the number of comparative measures in which MHS outperforms the NPIC average, utilizing a dashboard and reporting requirements for the Services.
Reviewer comment: Dashboards are an effective improvement tool. The perinatal review was very thorough and identified key areas for improvement such as shoulder dystocia, PPhemorrhage, readmissions of mothers and newborns.

28. HA policy is needed to support the collaborative standardized targets for perinatal metrics and to standardize annual and interval training requirements.
Reviewer comment: Agree

29. MHS governance should task the Perinatal Advisory Group to conduct a comprehensive review of clinical practices related to metrics where MHS is underperforming; develop intervention plans and prioritize actions.
Reviewer comment: Agree, consistent with #27 above

30. MHS governance should require a review of provider documentation and coding practices at MTFs to validate data integrity. Standardization of accurate coding practices should be implemented across Direct Care.
Reviewer comment: This recommendation should be edited to reflect its relationship to the perinatal measures. If there are other areas where documentation and coding lag then standard procedures could be applied there as well.

31. MHS governance should further investigate readmissions of mothers and infants. Require a clinical review of diagnostic codes at readmission to identify the medical conditions that drive these rates and help determine if lagging performance is a quality issue or related to military-unique issues and flexibility.
Reviewer comment: Agree; consistent with #27 and #30

32. MHS governance should integrate measures of mortality into their quality monitoring and performance improvement programs.
Reviewer comment: Agree. Health systems today are struggling between mortality indices, absolute numbers, and risk adjustment strategies. However, it is important to measure and look for areas where unexpected mortality can be reduced through implementation of sepsis protocols, assessment of rapid response teams, adherence to infection prevention bundles, etc.

33. MHS governance should commission a study to assess the validity of the results of the IQI measures.
Reviewer comment: Before commissioning a study, refer to the Value Based Purchasing section of the CMS website to see if there is updated information from Mathematica or others on the reliability of IQI measures.

34. MHS governance should require Service facilities with higher-than-expected mortality on an IQI measure for more than one quarter should perform an investigation using the tool referenced in recommendation above and implement improvement activities as indicated.
Reviewer comment: Agree

35. MHS governance should commission a study to assess the validity of the results of the risk-adjusted mortality measures. All risk-adjusted SMR model data should be validated

and a root cause sought in all those with validated, statistically significantly increased mortality.
Reviewer comment: Before undertaking a study, it might be appropriate to consult on existing risk adjustment methodologies that are reliable for age, gender, etc. There is also much work going on to establish a risk adjustment for sociodemographic factors by CMS that is under review and consideration by NQF.

36. MHS Governance should set MHS goals to meet or exceed civilian benchmarks in satisfaction with primary care for every MTF.
Reviewer comment: Agree; reasonable target.

37. Add to MTF leader and staff mandatory annual training requirements; PCMH concepts and operations, Relay Health, Nurse Advice Line (NAL) utilization, and customer service.
Reviewer comment: Agree. Strengthening PCMH operations should yield higher customer satisfaction. Rating of personal doctor fell below civilian systems and CAHPS.

38. Specialty Care Advisory Board should gather and distribute "best practices" from highest rated facilities.
Reviewer comment: Agree; approaches will likely build on customer serviced training and efficiency.

39. MHS governance should expand MHS Perinatal Advisory Group work on improving beneficiary perception of OB quality of care.
Reviewer comment: Agree

40. Services and DHA should continue PCMH concept development in all MTFs to increase probability of achieving primary care satisfaction to levels equivalent to the civilian benchmark. (#44-45)
Reviewer comment: Agree; concept has proven successful.

41. PCMH Advisory Board should assess processes that affect PCM continuity at high performing PCMH sites and promulgate across the MHS to support improvement initiatives.
Reviewer comment: Agree; may want to look at a model of care that accommodates provider reassignments. Is it possible to introduce patient to team that may cover one another? Even in teaching medical centers, 'continuity clinics' allow for handoffs to another provider.

42. DHA should establish clear and consistent guidelines for the CONUS TRICARE Regions and the OCONUS Area Offices on reporting and processing quality and patient safety issues identified from the purchased care.
Reviewer comment: Agree. The ability to secure performance from purchased service providers is a pervasive theme and calls for inclusion of contract language that will direct these activities.

43. MHS governance should identify a strategy to market and utilize Clinical Practice Guidelines.
Reviewer comment: When possible, include guidelines in the build of health record order sets; adherence is challenged in many medical centers. Auditing of adherence to order sets and/or guidelines included in decision support systems is gaining traction in civilian systems but can be difficult to accomplish.

44. Establish DoD and TRICARE regional contractor collaborations/MOUs with local purchased care organizations to support EHR accessibility.
   Reviewer comment: Agree; may need to work with state entities involved in HIE.
45. MHS governance should develop processes to ensure standardized notification requirements for laboratory and radiology.
   Reviewer comment: Agree and this is consistent with Joint Commission expectations.

Patient Safety Findings and Recommendations

The Patient Safety Program of the DoD is twelve years old however various portions took years to implement, thus performance overall is at an average level. Underlying the MHS performance and similar to many civilian organizations is the slow journey to evolving a culture of safety and establishing a high reliability organization. Results of the AHRQ survey on a culture of safety showed little to no change in repeated administrations over the past decade. This was surprising given the emphasis on safety in civilian organizations as well as the emphasis by the IOM.

A prior study (Lumetra) shed light on some of the same recommendations being made in this review, namely the need to improve reporting of events both real and near misses, and improving the follow up to these reports. The prior report also brought into question the appropriate resources need to staff the patient safety program.

The review focused on both processes and outcomes. Training and education, root cause analyses conducted for sentinel events, and safety tools were identified as areas that could be improved. Overall findings using the PSI#90 (Patient Safety Indicators) showed comparable performance of MTFs to the reference population of AHRQ. Evaluation of its use for improvement should be considered at this time.

Performance on measures used in other pay for performance systems is consistent with other organizations although some are outliers. Major measures of preventable events and hospital acquired conditions varied when compared to civilian systems.

Recommendations to Improve Patient Safety

Please note, recommendation numbering and language listed here were taken from a previous draft of the Final Report. A table that maps the recommendation numbers used here with the recommendations listed in Appendix 6.1 of this report is provided at the conclusion of Dr. Cipriano's comments.

1. Refine DoDM 6025.13 policy to establish more than one mechanism for capturing harm events. (mapped to Finding #1)
   Reviewer comment: Agree. Aggressive reporting is key to improving.
2. Clarify the definition of "sentinel event" in the DoDM 6025.13. (mapped to Finding #2)
   Reviewer comment: Agree.
3. Incorporate and define appropriate policy for patient/family engagement. (mapped to Finding #3)
   Reviewer comment: Agree

4. Establish clear expectations in DoDM 6025.13 for the RCA process. (mapped to Finding #4)
   Reviewer comment: Agree
5. Establish a system-wide closed loop mechanism. (mapped to Finding #5)
   Reviewer comment: Agree. This may be easier with new EHR as it relies on recording the reporting event and then documenting who takes action and result.
6. Ensure that the policy establishes attainable goals for "near miss" reporting. (mapped to Finding #6)
   Reviewer comment: Low reporting of near misses was identified as a problem including perception of staff that they did not need to report; suggest this be heightened awareness in training and the importance of counting and understanding near misses as a prevention strategy.
7. Establish a system-wide structure to fully expand internal transparency of patient safety information in compliance with 10 US Code 1102. (mapped to Finding #7)
   Reviewer comment: Agree; an important aspect of a culture of safety.
8. DHA conducts a business case analysis that identifies the most effective method for staffing the Patient Safety Program. (mapped to Finding #8)
   Reviewer comment: Agree, this is consistent with prior external studies. Given slow progress over time, dedicated personnel might be a strategy that is needed in some areas.
9. Authorize the Service-level and DHA patient safety officers direct access to senior executives for pre-defined critical events and messages. (mapped to Finding #9)
   Reviewer comment: Agree; necessary role for leadership to be available.
10. Define and standardize minimal patient safety training requirements in DoDM 6025.13 policy. (mapped to Finding #10)
    Reviewer comment: Agree; essential for transparency, understanding, and commitment to safety culture.
11. Develop an executive leadership toolkit; this best practice guide will address integral areas of patient safety. (mapped to Finding #11)
    Reviewer comment: Agree; also identified in prior reviews; executive leaders need to role model knowledge and use skills to help address safety issues.
12. MHS Governance must determine safety culture expectations, set targets based on opportunities. (mapped to Finding #12)
    Reviewer comment: Agree; fundamental to improved safety.
13. Consider PSI #90 composite utilization as a component of a comprehensive safety measure set and develop an educational plan to support implementation. (mapped to Finding #15)
    Reviewer comment: Agree
14. This finding requires further review by the Infection Prevention and Control Panel (IPCP) to determine the cause for the variance in performance in accordance with the Partnership for Patients Implementation Guide for CLABSI. (mapped to Finding #17)
    Reviewer comment: Agree further investigation is indicated.
15. This finding requires further review by the IPCP to determine the cause for the variance in performance in accordance with the Partnership for Patients Implementation Guide for VAP/VAE. (mapped to Finding #18)

Reviewer comment: Agree since these rates are higher than desired and many hospitals are making significant improvement to zero.

16. The IPCP will develop a comprehensive plan to standardize requirements for monitoring device-related infections. (mapped to Finding #18)
    Reviewer comment: Agree
17. Clarify policy and educate healthcare staff on the Sentinel Event definition and event types to reduce the variation in interpretation. (mapped to Finding #20)
    Reviewer comment: Agree
18. MHS Governance should pursue an enterprise-wide improvement process addressing top five reported SEs and improve distinction between SEs occurring within ambulatory versus hospital settings, and monitor SE occurrence by rates using appropriate denominator estimates. (mapped to Finding #21)
    Reviewer comment: Agree but must be part of comprehensive reporting process that encourages reporting and then stratifies all events and determines those for RCA.
19. Establish clear expectations for the RCA process and the follow up that will occur. (mapped to Finding #22)
    Reviewer comment: Agree; should be part of PSP.
20. Standardize PI RCA process with focus on event type classification, centralized repository and dissemination of lessons learned. (mapped to Finding #24)
    Reviewer comment: Agree; consistent with recommendations above.
21. Standardize event type components of the event reporting process. (mapped to Finding #25)
    Reviewer comment: Agree; consistent with recommendations above.
22. Standardize leadership activities to drive a culture of safety (Executive toolkit). (mapped to Finding #26)
    Reviewer comment: Agree; consistent with other recommendations.
23. Adopt a chart audit based methodology such as the IHI Global Trigger Tool (GTT) to determine harm rate. (mapped to Finding #27)
    Reviewer comment: A chart based methodology has its limitations and is not timely. Education and setting expectations for more robust real time reporting is the more contemporary approach to understanding safety events.
24. Incorporate best practices from all three contractors to develop a more standardized process that enhances transparency, minimizes variation, and incentivizes reporting for process improvement. (mapped to Finding #29)
    Reviewer comment: Agree; aggregate best practices for use across all Services.
25. DoD direct care systems should pursue tracking infection rates at the unit level beyond ICUs. (mapped to Finding #31 and 32)
    Reviewer comment: Agree; will need to have accurate tracking given patient movement and the transit of devices inserted in different locations.
26. Establish rate-based SE reporting for DoD or other recognized frequency tracking. (mapped to Finding #34)
    Reviewer comment: This can be accomplished and should be accompanied by an overall push to increase reporting that adjusts for an increase in events over at least a year until new rates plateau.

General Findings

The data sources analyzed for this review were numerous and thorough as was the identification of external benchmarks. Given the aggressive time frames for both the internal and external views, the data were more than adequate. The data were analyzed appropriately to produce meaningful information; presentation was clear and relevant. Appendices were provided to augment the highlights in the report. A few additional recommendations at the strategy level are offered in some of the recommendations.

The review addressed key relevant issues and challenges. Accurate reporting and interpretation of information allowed for identification of high and low performance areas.

Conclusions

Strengths of the findings and recommendations:

The report represents, without bias, both areas were the MHS excels and where improvement is needed. One of the interesting report findings was the presence of prior external reviews that had, in some cases, reached similar conclusions and posed consistent recommendations. In a few areas, improvements have been made but are still in need of attention.

Overall performance in providing timely access to care meets or exceeds standards. Quality measures are more often average when compared to benchmarks; there is a serious attempt to use most available measures, and be inclusive of all areas of care including behavioral health, care of children, and obstetrics along with standard acute and primary care of adults. The journey to achieve a culture of safety is ongoing. There are opportunities to accelerate these activities which address the Patient Safety Program and its measures, along with additional quality measurement.

Reviews were fairly comprehensive and demonstrate leading edge practices such as well-developed PCMH, use of technology for patient engagement, and an emerging desire for internal collaboration and sharing with the new DHA and its structures. Leadership should be commended for its vision in not only recognizing the synergy and common purpose of unifying guidance and policies around health delivery, but also the desire to provide the tools and support the local leadership efforts of the MTFs and NCR facilities.

Whenever possible, external benchmarks were used for comparison. In some cases, benchmarks are not well developed or it is difficult to access the data.

Weaknesses of the findings and recommendations:

The report recognizes the need for a more robust commitment to a Culture of Safety. Most important is that this culture penetrate to front line staff and not rest with leadership. Reframing expectations for access, quality, and safety within a culture of safety can be a powerful means to improving many different types of results it also reinforces a patient and family centric approach to care.

One of the consistent findings is the lack of data from the purchased service component of care. This has been noted in previous reviews and cannot be ignored going forward. It is not unreasonable to include an expectation for quality measurement and performance in this sector as it is now standard operating procedure and expectation within accrediting bodies and for CMS reimbursement.

Bidirectional flow of data is an area for improvement not only from a technical perspective but also from an interpretation and planning perspective. The growing interest and demand for cross service comparisons via dashboards can help with the spread of best practices and evoking a healthy competitive spirit to improve outcomes.

Given the sophistication of quality measurement systems and techniques, it was surprising that the MHS is not leading the way in terms of quality measurement and outcomes. Again the roadmap of areas ripe for improvement is embedded in the reported findings. There is a sincere interest in making these improvements. Participation in external measurement systems should continue in order to mark progress and have a consistent compare group. Training from established organizations (IHI, Intermountain, etc.) can produce resident experts and offer methodologies for increasing effectiveness in PI efforts.

Comparison to the Pay For Performance measures and methods employed by CMS can be a useful comparison. Similarly, continuing to use high performing organizations as an informal comparison can provide a high bar for those measures where MHS lags behind.

Timelines for Addressing Recommendations

There are several considerations for determining timelines for implementation of the recommendations. First, there is some urgency to address improvement strategies where performance is in the lowest quartile of quality outcomes at the facility level within a Service. Action plans may already be in place, but otherwise should be instituted within 90 days. Ongoing measurement and monitoring should occur monthly with quarterly review of progress.

Second, the imperative to merge cultures and systems requires a one to two year time frame. Laying the foundation by establishing expectations and providing training will likely take a year to complete. Establishing sufficient culture change to actualize a culture of safety that is embraced at all levels of the enterprise will require a second year to measure and see results, achieve expected performance, and reinforce positive gains. Some areas will respond more quickly than others. Because of the long trajectory, it is essential to begin this work as quickly as possible.

Third, the need to implement enterprise policies, practices, data collection methods, and reporting will require a more robust analytic infrastructure.

The following rough timeline is offered as an example for parsing activities for some of the major areas of recommendations. It is only a guide based on experience, and is intended to reflect a dynamic processes.

Time Frame	Activity to address recommendations
0 – 3 months	<ul><li>Address quality measures at <25th percentile (HEDIS, Core measures, NPIC, NSQIP)</li><li>Outline steps for setting expectations of a Culture of Safety and communicate leadership's commitment and expectations</li><li>Establish training requirements for all levels of personnel for Culture of Safety</li><li>Evaluate requirements for improving analytic infrastructure of MHS data systems</li></ul>
3-6 months	<ul><li>Harmonize governance policies for management of quality programs (establish system-wide measures, time frames for reporting, benchmarking, etc.)</li><li>Communicate expectations to Purchased Care Network</li><li>Begin Culture of Safety training and address associated programmatic improvements</li></ul>
6-12 months	<ul><li>Complete Culture of Safety training—this will address many of the Patient Safety Recommendations</li><li>Add expectations to TRICARE contracts</li><li>Determine mortality measurement methodology</li><li>Continue to build out tools for increasing Access</li><li>Develop recognition program to highlight improvement and better performers across the enterprise</li><li>Implement actions to close horizontal quality gaps and create consistent approaches to care (e.g. Pain Management)</li><li>Status check initial/urgent improvement goals</li></ul>
12-18 months	<ul><li>Provide enterprise information such as aggregate accreditation findings</li><li>Integrate more PQI measures into quality plan</li><li>Do complete review of status for addressing recommendations</li></ul>
18-24 months	<ul><li>Establish appropriate external review collaborations for comparisons and exchange data</li><li>Repeat site visits and hold focus groups to assess changes</li><li>Repeat Culture of Safety survey</li></ul>

Thank you for the opportunity to participate in this review.

Pamela F. Cipriano

Pamela F. Cipriano, PhD, RN, NEA-BC, FAAN
President, American Nurses Association

The following table maps the recommendation numbers used in Dr. Cipriano's comments with the recommendation numbers listed in Appendix 6.1 of this report.

Recommendation # in Dr. Cipriano's Review	Recommendation # in Appendix 6.1
ACCESS	
1	3
2	1
3	2
4	4
5	5
6	Wrapped into #4
7	6
8	7
QUALITY	
1	8
2	9
3	10
4	10
5	11, 14
6	13, 15
7	12, 16
8	17
9	18
10	19
11	20
12	21
13	22
14	23
15	24
16	25
17	27
18	27
19	28
20	29
21	30
22	31
23	32
24	33
25	33
26	34
27	35
28	36
29	35
30	37, 38
31	39
32	40
33	Does not appear in list of recommendations included in Appendix 6.1

Recommendation # in Dr. Cipriano's Review	Recommendation # in Appendix 6.1
34	41
35	42
36	43
37	44
38	43, 45
39	43
40	45
41	46
42	47
43	48
44	49
45	50
SAFETY	
1	54
2	55
3	56
4	57
5	58
6	59
7	60
8	61
9	62
10	63
11	64
12	65
13	66
14	67
15	67
16	68
17	69
18	70
19	71
20	72
21	73
22	74
23	75
24	76
25	77
26	Does not appear in list of recommendations included in Appendix 6.1

External Review of Findings and Recommendations: Report from Dr. Peter Pronovost

Purpose: The external expert will evaluate the Military Health System (MHS) 90-day review findings and recommendations with reference to the goals and objectives outline in the approved Terms of Reference.

Data Sources: The external expert had access and reviewed the following information for their analysis: Terms of Reference, Memoranda defining scope, timeline, study questions, policy/document review methodology, metric analysis methodology, site visit methodology, process and outcome review methods, site visit histograms, analysis, and draft final report. The reviewer also had access to speak with the MHS Program Review Lead, Dr. Michael Malanoski, Action Officer Leads: BG Barbara Holcomb (Patient Safety), RDML Kenneth Iverson (Access), Brig Gen (s) Lee Payne (Quality), CAPT Paul Rockswold (Analytics Lead) and LTC Julie Freeman (Site Visit Lead).

Results

DOD leadership should be commended for embarking on this 90 day review, conducting a detailed self-study to evaluate the safety, quality and access in the MHS. The methods and discipline and transparency are impressive, even more impressive given the 90 day review period. The leadership of the MHS and the engagement of the MTFs speaks strongly to a culture committed to patients, devoted to decreasing preventable harm, committed to continuously improving patient outcomes, experience, and access.

The study provides answers to two key questions: one addressing accountability, the other addressing learning. The accountability question is whether the review identified signals to suggest that the safety, quality or access in the MHS has significant and substantive deficiencies such that patients receiving care in the MHS suffer lower safety, quality and access than patient receiving care in non-MHS facilities; does MHS have dark spots in its care delivery? The report provided no evidence of substantive deficiencies in the safety, quality, and access to care at MHS that would warrant broad and urgent changes. Though care in MHS and civilian facilities can improve, there was no evidence that care in MHS facilities is worse overall than civilian healthcare.

The learning question is whether the report identified opportunities to learn and to improve. Here the report provides many bright spots. The report provides opportunities for improvement in culture and leadership, in structures, in processes, and in the science of quality and safety. Though it is difficult to ascertain the culture of the MHS through this report, the culture around safety, quality and access seems to be one of mediocrity rather than one of national leadership. The tone of the report was largely seeking to confirm that the MHS provides average care and is not inferior to civilian care. This is understandable given the purpose of this report. Yet this type of leadership message is not inspirational and not likely to lead to excellent care. The MHS should declare and commit to be national leaders in safety, quality and access. Also, several signals suggested that the culture of one of fear, or judging rather than learning. This might warrant further investigation.

The structure also can also be improved to provide an opportunity for peer learning and accountability. The MHS might consider implementing a fractal model of performance improvement in which they define roles, skills and accountability at each level of the organization and each level, is tasked with creating a structure to accommodate safety and quality leaders from the lower level. For example, a MTF quality and safety leader might ensure that each department has a quality and safety leader and meet regularly with them. This type of structure seems similar to the structure the MHS has for creating accountability for reducing mortality in trauma patients. In this system, there is a clear chain of command from front-line medic to care at a quaternary medical facility.

One significant opportunity to improve MHS, and have MHS lead the US healthcare systems is in the governance for access, quality and safety. The report comments how the business analytics in MHS (and civilian healthcare) are more developed than safety and quality analytics. As a goal, the DOD can work so that the oversight and accountability for access, quality and safety functions with the same discipline and rigor as the oversight of financial performance. This would include clearly defined goals and targets, enabling support systems to collect and report data, local engagement in meeting targets and transparency and accountability for meeting performance goals. Healthcare can learn much from finance and efforts to support this learning within MHS might prove beneficial.

The report identified a number of process improvements; from improving contracting, to reducing ICU infections and they are all appropriate. It might be helpful for DOD leaders to clearly define the accountable leaders to achieve these goals. The different services have a large number of structures responsible for safety, quality and access. It is not clear how all of them interact or overlap. On the one hand, this is important since they all look at different components of access, safety and quality. On the other hand, some of the work overlaps and could potentially be made synergistic. It might be helpful to explore ways to link them, perhaps under an umbrella quality and safety and access group, carefully balancing the independence and interdependence of each group.

Patient Safety Findings and Recommendations

Overall, the DOD did an amazing job looking at a large amount of data to evaluate their quality and safety. Quality and safety data are much less standardized and mature than financial data and the DOD did a remarkable and valid job of making the most of the data. Appropriately, the data was largely used to answer the accountability question. After this review is complete, there is opportunity to use these data to learn. This would include evaluating variation in performance at the MTF level and units within the MTF, identifying units or areas in which there is a cluster of concerns about safety, and using these data to create a regular safety dashboard, modeling the reporting of financial performance. There are also opportunities to follow up this study with more qualitative work to better understand the culture. Some of the signals suggested that there were pockets of staff who perceived a culture of retaliation and fear, who were not comfortable speaking up or speaking out. The lack of voice behaviors can pose risks to patients and the MHS. While civilian healthcare also has these concerns, it would serve patients and the MHS to better understand these cultural concerns and work to improve them.

The MHS work in patient safety is exemplar. In particular, its Patient Safety Reporting Systems and its focus on teamwork training are models for civilian hospitals. In addition, the MHS has been extremely responsive to the finding of prior reviews, especially the 2008 Lumetra study, demonstrating strong leadership commitment to safety.

The recommendations to improve safety and quality are wise, responsive to the study, and will improve care within the MHS. As such, I support all of the recommendations and did not comment on each individual recommendation. However, below I offer some reflections on the report and opportunities to further improve care in the MHS.

MHS leaders may want to further define what work is in safety and what is the appropriate level of the MHS for mitigating risks. Safety overlaps with quality and defining what functions are housed in quality and which in safety could allow synergy. Though there is a lot of data in safety, most of it is not rate based. Rather the data identifies risks. MHS might think of how it could aggregate the large amount of safety data to help prioritize risks (and improvement efforts) at the Unit, MTF, Service and MHS levels. For example, risks might be grouped into risky providers, risky units, and risky systems. MHS might look at these risks at the Service, MTF and unit levels and describe accountability for mitigating these risks. One novel method, used more in Europe than in the US, is the safety case, in which a care area takes the risk data, conducts their own risk assessment, prioritizes these risks and then reports how they will defend against the major risks. This type of approach engages local leaders, is sensitive to local context yet still allows accountability. In addition, the MHS might seek to learn more from efforts to identify and mitigate risks from submarines, aircraft carriers and other areas of the military. These programs are well regarded as models for risk reduction and the MHS likely can learn from them and in doing so, lead all of healthcare. This learning also applies to more disciplined contracting. The DOD has skilled contractors who helped to create intraoperability in aviation and other military areas; the MHS can learn from this DOD experience.

Given the immaturity of the science of safety, it seems there would be opportunities for the services to learn from each other, and from other parts of the DOD, balancing independence, yet supporting interdependence. For example, they may have an annual meeting about how they are organizing safety work and what they are learning.

The MHS might consider more clearly describing what they do with the safety culture data. It is great that they measure culture. The next step might be to standardize how they present culture data to each MTF and what they require of each MTF in presenting their culture data to each unit within the MTF. They might clarify who would be responsible for such a debriefing, consider if they have the proper skills and create an accountability system to monitor improvement plans at the unit and MTF levels. Ideally every unit and every MTF would have plans to improve culture. The MHS might also prioritize these efforts on units with the lowest culture scores.

Given the complex organizational structure of the MHS, they might consider organizing their quality and safety efforts using a "fractal" conceptual model. For example, the MHS could clearly define the knowledge, skills, resources and accountability for safety (and quality) at every level of the MHS and create structures in which each higher level meets regularly with each lower level group (ie at MTF safety leaders meet with department safety leaders who in turn meet with unit level safety leaders). Such a fractal system creates a structure to link horizontal teams in peer learning communities, which have the largest impact on improving quality and safety. Such a fractal system also creates a structure for vertical accountability and organizational learning.

It seems the MHS includes patient experience under safety. Given the importance of this area and the skills required to improve it, the MHS might consider separating the patient experience work into its own domain. The patient experience work could be combined with patient relations work (ie complaint management) and access to ensure the MHS has a more complete picture of patient experience, and has goals, enabling systems, performance measures and accountability for patient experience.

In defining goals, the DOD should seek to ensure that goals are linked to measures that are collected in units as close to the patient as possible (ie individual provider or unit or clinic) and then aggregated to higher levels. Similar to the chain of command for the transport of a trauma patient, MHS leaders need to ensure a chain of accountability for safety and quality from unit, to department, to MHF to service to DOD.

DOD should ensure that it supports a culture in which goals, measures and enabling systems are centralized, yet local MTF and units have some flexibility to implement practices based on their local context and resources and are accountable for meeting goals. While healthcare is generally under-standardized, too much standardization may reduce safety and worsen productivity; leaders need the flexibility to find the balance. For example, in our work using checklists to reduce infections, there were 5 evidence-based practices to reduce infections. Each unit and each hospital made their own checklist, all included the 5 items. While the checklists were 90% similar, the flexibility to make the checklist their own lead to its use and to reduced infections. Each hospital thought their checklist was the best; and it was for their culture and resources. Had we required that all hospitals use the exact same checklist, the checklist would likely not have been used and infections would remain high. MHS should standardize goals, measures and principles of practice, and encourage local variation in how those principles are applied, ensuring the application aligns with the principles.

Quality Findings and Recommendations

The evaluation of the quality program was impressive. They collected a large number of measures, most of which are used in public reporting and pay for quality in the civilian sector. The analysis was robust and they made use of the large amount of data. Like safety, the report provides confidence that there is no significant accountability problem with quality within the MHS. The focus could be on learning and improving. The recommendations are all valid and sound and will help improve the MHS. Many of the general comments I made about safety and the need for a fractal infrastructure and peer learning apply to quality.

The report identified gaps in understanding of goals for quality between unit, MTF and service leaders. This suggests that a more robust structure, such as the fractal structure, may provide a mechanism to narrow those gaps and allow for peer learning.

The MHS appears to have robust analytics for quality and it would be helpful (if not already done) to produce standardized and integrated quality reports, modeled after financial reports for each MTF, Service and overall MHS. The reporting of financial performance could serve as a model. This type of approach should come with clearly defined roles and accountabilities.

Though the MHS was doing significant and laudable work in quality, it was hard to find clearly declared and communicated goals; such as zero ICU blood stream infections or 96% performance on all core measures. Without clear goals it is difficult for the MHS to lead in quality. The MHS can consider declaring some goals. It might be helpful for accountability to monitor achievement of goals as dichotomous: either the goal is met or not. The MHS should also ensure that it has sufficient enabling systems to help the MTF meet those goals. Accountability absent engaging systems leads to gaming and potentially false reports. Yet with goals, and enabling systems, MHS leaders should hold MTF leaders accountable for realizing the goals.

Given the size of the MHS and the importance of quality, safety and access, the MHS might consider creating more formal career paths for clinician and administrative leaders in quality and safety. This could include a defined set of skills and an explicit career ladder with elevated levels of responsibility. Importantly, leaders in quality and safety require skills in evaluation, in process and system redesign, and in leadership, especially in influencing. The MHS training programs can ensure quality and safety leaders obtain all of these skill sets.

The report talks about the use of overall MTF mortality as a measure of quality; this measure should be used cautiously. Though overall hospital mortality has face validity, there is substantial evidence that it might not be valid and may lead to inaccurate inferences. For example, a study in the New England Journal of Medicine by Dave Shehan demonstrated that among Massachusetts hospitals 42% of hospitals classified as having above average mortality were classified as having below average mortality when they changed the methods of risk adjustment. If overall hospital mortality is used, it should be used as a screen to obtain future data. On the other hand, disease or procedure specific mortality can be more accurate, (because they have more accurate risk adjustment) and more useful.

Areas that the report did not evaluate, understandable given the charge, are care coordination, population health, and value (ie eliminating waste in healthcare while maintaining quality). These are important areas for patients, policy makers and the MHS. Future work on quality should explore these areas and measures of these should be included in future quality reports.

Access Findings and Recommendations

The study did an exemplary job evaluating access. The amount of data and the rigor with which they analyzed it is impressive. A notable strength of the MHS is having explicit standards for performance regarding access. All of the recommendations regarding access are wise and robust and will help make the MHS leaders in access. Below are some reflections regarding access.

The report recommended the MHS build specifications regarding access, quality and safety into its contracts. This seems to be a key and high impact intervention. The MHS should define goals, accountabilities and milestones for achieving this.

While the analysis of access is important, the MHS could stratify measures of access by product lines important to its members. For example, the MHS could identify areas of concerns and interest, such as mental health, and monitor access for specific product lines. Just as with all the other analyses, the average access, while informative, likely misses variation in performance among individual product lines. MHS should define these important services and stratify access by these product lines

The MHS should consider making performance on access part of routine quality and safety reports that go to management.

The MHS might consider linking access, patient experience, patient relations, and perhaps patient education into a common function. For example, the report notes that some patients reported difficulties with access. These comments report a rich opportunity to learn and improve. Yet is was unclear what would be done with these comments and who is responsible to understand them and improve. By looking at access by product line and by linking access to data regarding patient satisfaction, and patient complaints, the MHS might have a more comprehensive picture of access.

Conclusions

MHS should be commended for its dedication to improve access, quality and safety, for the rigor with which it conducted this review, and for the commitment to improve the MHS. MHS leaders, its employees and patients should take comfort that access, quality and safety in the MHS is comparable to civilian health systems. The MHS staff should be commended for its dedication to patients and to improving safety and quality. Though there are opportunities to improve care, the report did not identify significant accountability issues that would require urgent and immediate action on behalf of the MHS.

The report identified significant opportunities to learn and improve. The recommendations contained within the report are thorough and comprehensive and will likely improve access, quality and safety. I support the recommendations and made additional comments and recommendations.

Thank you for inviting me to serve on the review panel to help improve care in the MHS. All Americans who live in freedom are indebted to those who serve to maintain it. It is an honor to serve the men and women who protect our great country.

Name/Title
Peter Pronovost, MD, PhD, FCCM
Johns Hopkins Medicine Senior Vice President for Patient Safety and Quality
Director of the Armstrong Institute for Patient Safety and Quality
The C. Michael and S. Ann Armstrong Professor of Patient Safety, The Johns Hopkins University School of Medicine.

APPENDIX 7. ACRONYMS

Appendix 7.1
List of Acronyms

AAAHC	Accreditation Association for Ambulatory Health Care
AAFP	American Academy of Family Physicians
AAR	After Action Report
ABO	ABO Blood Group System
ACE	Angiotensin-Converting Enzyme
ACOG	American Congress of Obstetricians and Gynecologists
ACP	Army Campaign Plan
ADE	Adverse Drug Event
ADFM	Active Duty Family Member
ADLS	Advanced Distributive Learning System
ADSM	Active Duty Service Member
AE	Adverse Event
AES	Aeromedical Evacuation
AETC	Air Education Training Command
AF	Air Force
AFI	Air Force Instruction
AFMOA	Air Force Medical Operations Agency
AFMOA/SGHQ	AFMOA Surgeon General Headquarters
AFMS	Air Force Medical Service
AF/SG	Air Force Surgeon General
AFSO21	Air Force Smart Operations for the 21st Century
AHLTA	Armed Forces Health Longitudinal Technology Application
AHRQ	Agency for Healthcare Research and Quality
AIWG	Access Improvement Work Group
AM2020CP	Army Medicine 2020 Campaign Plan
AMDOC	Advanced Medical Department Officer Course
AMEDD	Army Medical Department
AMEDD CS	Army Medical Department Center and School
AMI	Acute Myocardial Infarction
AMI-8a	Primary Percutaneous Coronary Intervention
ANOVA	Analysis of Variance
APIC	Association for Professionals in Infection Control and Epidemiology
APLSS	Provider Level Satisfaction Survey
AQD	Additional Qualification Designator
AR	Army Regulation
ARC	Air Reserve Component
ASCQR	Ambulatory Surgical Center Quality Reporting

ASD(HA)	Assistant Secretary of Defense for Health Affairs or Assistant Secretary of Defense (Health Affairs)
ATC	Access to Care
AWHONN	Association of Women's Health, Obstetrics and Neonatal Nursing
BB	Black Belts
BCA	Business Case Analysis
BHOP	Behavioral Health Optimization Program
BP	Blood Pressure
BPR	Business Process Reengineering
BPSM	Basic Patient Safety Manager
BRAC	Base Closure and Realignment
BUMED	U.S. Navy Bureau of Medicine and Surgery
CA	California State Department of Managed Health Care
CAC	Children's Asthma Care
CAHPS	Consumer Assessment of Healthcare Providers and Systems
CAP (1)	College of American Pathologists
CAP (2)	Community-Acquired Pneumonia
CAPER	Comprehensive Ambulatory/Professional Encounter Record
CAUTI	Catheter-Associated Urinary Tract Infections
CBPCC	Community Based Primary Care Clinics
CBT	Computer-Based Training
CDC	Center for Disease Control and Prevention
CDRL	Contract Data Requirements List
CE	Continuing Education
CFR	Code of Federal Regulations
CHAMPUS	Civilian Health and Medical Program of the Uniformed Services
CHCS	Composite Health Care System
CHF	Congestive Heart Failure
CIN	Cervical Intraepithelial Neoplasia
CJCS	Chairman of the Joint Chiefs of Staff
CLABSI	Central Line-Associated Bloodstream Infection
CLIP	Clinical Laboratory Improvement Program
CM	Case Management
CMAC	CHAMPUS Maximum Allowable Charge
CMC	Commandant of the Marine Corps
CMS (1)	Centers for Medicare & Medicaid Services
CMS (2)	Command Management system
CNO	Chief of Naval Operations
CONUS	Contiguous United States
CoP	Community of Practice
CPAD	Clinical Performance Assurance Directorate
CPG	Clinical Practice Guidelines
CPI/LSS	Continuous Process Improvement/Lean Six Sigma

CPIMS	Continuous Process Improvement Management System
CPI-MT	Continuous Process Improvement Management Tool
CQF	Clinical Quality Forum
CQM	Clinical Quality Management
CQMP	Clinical Quality Management Program
CSA (1)	Chief of Staff, Army
CSA (2)	Clinical Support Agreement
CSAF	Chief of Staff, Air Force
CTLDTS	Command Team Leader Development Training Session
CY	Calendar Year
DASD	Deputy Assistant Secretary of Defense
DA SG-ZB	Deputy Surgeon General/Deputy Commanding General (Operations)
DC	Direct Care
D/C	Discharge
DEERS	Defense Enrollment Eligibility Reporting System
DEXCOM	Deputy's Executive Committee
DHA	Defense Health Agency
DHHQ	Defense Health Headquarters
DIACAP	Department of Defense Information Assurance Certification and Accreditation Process
DMAG	Deputy's Management Action Group
DMIS	Defense Medical Information System
DoD	Department of Defense
DoDD	Department of Defense Directive
DoDI	Department of Defense Instruction
DoDM	Department of Defense Manual
DON	Department of the Navy
DP	Designated Providers
DPPO	Designated Provider Program Office
DSI	Directorate of strategy and Innovation
DTMS	Digital Training Management system
DVT	Deep Vein Thrombosis
E	Enlisted
EAR	Enhanced Ambulatory Record
EBP	Evidence Based Practice
ECRI	Emergency Care Research Institute
ED	Emergency Department
EHR	Electronic Health Record
EMS	Emergency Medical System
eMSM	Enhanced Multi-service Markets
EOD	End-of-Day
ER	Emergency Room
ERSA	External Resource Sharing Agreements

EST	Established
EXSUM	Executive Summary
FARM	Fiscal Accountability and Recovery Mission
FBCH	Fort Belvoir Community Hospital
FFRDC	Federally Funded Research and Development Centers
FMEA	Failure Mode Effects Analysis
FY	Fiscal Year
GAO	Government Accountability Office
GB	Green Belts
GBS	Group B Streptococcal
GPM	Group Practice Manager
GS	General Schedule
GTT	Global Trigger Tool
HA	Health Affairs
HAC	Hospital Acquired Conditions
HAF/SG3	Headquarters Air Force Directorate of Healthcare Operations
HAI	Healthcare-associated Infections
HAIMS	Healthcare Artifact and Image Management Solution
HAS	Hospital Specialty Care and Ambulatory [Procedure]
HbA1c	Glycosylated Hemoglobin
HBIPS	Hospital Based Inpatient Psychiatric Services
HCAHPS	Hospital Consumer Assessment of Healthcare Providers and Systems
HCSDB	Health Care Survey of DoD Beneficiaries
HCUP	Healthcare Cost Utilization Project
HEDIS®	Healthcare Effectiveness Data and Information Set
HF	Heart Failure
HFC	Heart Failure Clinical
HF1	Discharge Instructions
HMO	Health Maintenance Organization
HMPC	Home Management Plan of Care
HPV	Human Papilloma Virus
HQDA	Headquarters, Department of the Army
HR	House Report
HREC	Health Record
HRO	High Reliability Organization
HS	External Hospital System
HS1	Health System 1
HS2	Health System 2
HS3	Health System 3
HS-A	Health System A
HS-B	Health System B
HSOPS	Hospital Survey on Patient Safety Culture
IAW	In Accordance With

ICU	Intensive Care Unit
IDIQ	Indefinite Delivery, Indefinite Quantity
IE	Industrial Engineering
IG	Inspector General
IHI	Institute for Healthcare Improvement
IMIT	Information Management Information Technology
IMM	Immunization
IMM 1a	Pneumococcal Immunization
IMM 2	Influenza Immunization
IOM	Institute of Medicine
IQI	Inpatient Quality Indicator
IQR	interquartile range
IPCP	Infection Prevention and Control Panel
IRIS	Integrated Resource and Incentive System
IRMAC	Integrated Referral Management Appointing Center
ISMP	Institute for Safe Medication Practice
JCAHO	Joint Commission on Accreditation of Healthcare Organizations
JPC	Joint Pathology Center
JSS	Joint Staff Surgeon
JTF CAPMED	Joint Task Force for the National Capital Region Medical Directorate
JTF-CQM	Joint Task Force Clinical Quality Manual
KePRO	Keystone Peer Review Organization Inc.
LAN	Learning Action Network
LBP	Low Back Pain
LCL	Lower Control Limit
LDL	Low-Density Lipoprotein
LDL-C	Low-Density Lipoprotein Cholesterol
LIP	Licensed Independent Practitioners
LSS	Lean Six Sigma
LVS	Left Ventricular Systolic
M3	(BUMED) Clinical Operations
MAE	Market Analysis and Evaluation
MAJCOM	Major Command, Air Force
MBB	Master Black Belts
MBOG	Medical Business Operations Group
MCSC	Managed Care Support Contractors
MDG	Medical Group
MDAG	Medical Deputies Action Group
MDRO	Multidrug-Resistant Organism
MEC	Medical Executive Committee
MEDCEN	Medical Centers
MEDCOM	United States Army Medical Command
MERIT	Medical Enterprise Resource Information Tool

MEPRS	Medical Expense and Performance Reporting System
MHP	Medical Home Ports
MHS	Military Health System
MHSER	Military Health System Executive Review
MHSPSP	Military Health System Patient Safety Program
MHSSI	Military Health System Support Initiatives
MOES	Mobile Obstetric Emergencies Simulator
MOG	Medical Operations Group
MPOG	Manpower and Personnel Operations
MQA	Medical Quality Assurance
MQIP	Medical Quality Improvement Program
MSC	Major Subordinate Commands
MTF (1)	Medical Treatment Facility
MTF (2)	Military Treatment Facility
NAL	Nurse Advice Line
NCQA	National Committee for Quality Assurance
NCR	National Capital Region
NCR MD	National Capital Region Medical Directorate
ND	No data
NEC	Navy Enlisted Classification
NME	Navy Medicine East
NHSN	National Healthcare Safety Network
NMW	Navy Medicine West
NPIC	National Perinatal Information Center
NPSF	National Patient Safety Foundation
NPSG	National Patient Safety Goals
NQF	National Quality Forum
NSQIP®	National Surgical Quality Improvement Center
O	Officer
OASD (HA)	Office of the Assistant Secretary of Defense for Health Affairs
OB	Obstetrics
OCONUS	Outside of the Contiguous United States
OHI	Other Health Insurance
OIP	Organizational Inspection Program
OLS	Ordinary Least Squares
OP	Hospital Outpatient
OR	Operating Room
ORYX®	No acronym - unofficially: Outcome Research Yields Excellence
OSD	Office of the Secretary of Defense
OTJ	On-the-job
OTAD	Other Than Active Duty
OTR	Outpatient Treatment Record
OTSG	Office of the Surgeon General

PA	Privacy Act
PAC	Policy Advisory Council
PAG	Perinatal Advisory Group
PAP	Papanicolaou Test
PAS	Patient Appointing System
PBAM	Performance Based Budget Model
PC (1)	Perinatal Care
PC (2)	Purchased Care
PC01	Elective Delivery
PC02	Cesarean Section
PCDB	Perinatal Center Data Base
PCM	Primary Care Manager
PCMH (1)	Patient Centered Medical Home
PCMH (2)	Primary Care Medical Home
PCS	Permanent Change of Station
PCS	Permanent Change of Station
PCTS	Patient CaringTouch System
PDASD	Principal Deputy Assistant Secretary of Defense
PDCA	Plan-Do-Check-Act
PDSA	Plan-Do-Study-Act
PE	Pulmonary Embolism
PfP	Partnership for Patients
PI	Performance Improvement
PII	Personally Identifiable Information
PMR	Performance Management Review
PMRM	Practice Management Revenue Model
PN	Pneumonia
PN3b	Blood Cultures Performed in the ED Prior to Initial Antibiotic in Hospital
POA	Present on Admission
POD 1	Postoperative Day 1
POD 2	Postoperative Day 2
PPD	Postpartum Depression
PPH	Postpartum Hemorrhage
PPO	Preferred Provider Organization
PPV23	Pneumococcal Immunization
PQI	Prevention Quality Indicators
PRO	Peer Review Organization
PS	PowerSteering
PSA	Prime Service Area
PSAC	Patient Safety Analysis Center
PSI	Patient Safety Indicator
PSI #90	Patient Safety for Selected Procedures Composite
PSIC	Patient Safety Improvement Collaborative

PSM	Patient Safety Manager
PSP	Patient Safety Program
PSS	Patient Satisfaction Survey
PPSPCC	Patient Safety Planning and Coordinating Committee
PSQAC	Patient Safety and Quality Academic Collaborative
PSR	Patient Safety Reporting
PT	Physical Therapy
Q	Quartile
QA	Quality Assurance
QAS	Quality Analytic Services
QC	Quality Committee
QI	Quality Issues
QPSEA	Quality and Patient Safety Educators Academy
QPSRMTF	Quality Patient Safety Risk Management Task Force
QSPAR	Quality Systems Program Assessment Review
R&A	Review and Analysis
RCA	Root Cause Analysis
Rh	Rhesus Blood Group System
RMC (1)	Referral Management Center
RMC (2)	Regional Medical Command
RMO	Referral Management Operations
RN	Registered Nurse
ROFR	Right of First Refusal
ROI	Return on Investment
ROUT	Routine
ROR	Return to Operating Room
RVU	Relative Value Unit
R_x	Prescription
SAC	Senior Action Council
SAP	Scientific Advisory Panel
SBAR	Situation, Background, Assessment, and Recommendation
SCIP	Surgical Care Improvement Project
SCIP2a	Prophylactic Antibiotic Selection for Surgical Patients
SCIP Card-2	Surgery Patients on Beta-Blocker Therapy Prior to Arrival Who Received A Beta-Blocker During the Perioperative Period
SCIP VTE-2	Surgery Patients Who Received Appropriate Venous Thromboembolism Prophylaxis within 24 Hours Prior to Surgery to 24 Hours after Surgery
SCMH	Soldier-Centered Medical Home
SDA	Service Delivery Assessment
SE	Sentinel Event
SEIPS	Systems Engineering Initiative for Patient Safety
SERC	Senior Executive Review Committee
SF	Standard Form

SG	Surgeon General	
SHIP	Strategic Health Incentivization Program	
SIC	Super Integration Council	
SID	State Inpatient Database	
SIDR	Standard Inpatient Data Record	
SM	Secure Messaging	
SME	Subject Matter Expert	
SMMAC	Senior Military Medical Action Council	
SMR	Standardized Mortality Ratio	
SMS	Strategic Management System	
SRE	Serious Reportable Events	
SSI	Surgical Site Infection	
SSP	Support Staff Protocol	
STK	Stroke	
SUB	Substance Use	
T-3	TRICARE Third Generation of Contracts	
TAO	TRICARE Area Office	
TCQF	TRICARE Clinical Quality Forum	
TJC	The Joint Commission	
T-Nex	Tricare Next Generation of Contracts	
TMA	TRICARE Management Authority	
TOB	Tobacco Treatment	
TOC	TRICARE Operations Center	
TOL	TRICARE Online	
TOM	TRICARE Operations Manual	
TOP	TRICARE Overseas Program	
TRISS	TRICARE Inpatient Satisfaction Survey	
TRO	TRICARE Regional Office	
TROSS	TRICARE Outpatient Satisfaction Surveys	
TSG	The Surgeon General	
TUC	Tobacco Use Cessation	
UC	Urgent Care	
UCC	Urgent Care Clinic	
UCL	Upper Control Limit	
UEI	Unit Effectiveness Inspection	
UP	Universal Protocol	
USAF	United States Air Force	
USAFSAM	USAF School of Aerospace Medicine	
USC	United States Code	
USD(P&R)	Under Secretary of Defense for Personnel and Readiness	
USPSTF	U.S. Preventive Services Task Force	
USU	Uniformed Services University	
USUHS	Uniformed Services University of the Health Sciences	

UT	University of Tennessee
UTI	Urinary Tract Infection
VA	Department of Veterans Affairs
VAE	Ventilator Associated Events
VAP	Ventilator Associated Pneumonia
VHA	Veterans Health Administration
VTC	Video Teleconference
VTE	Venous Thromboembolism
WEA	Web-enabled Appointments
WG	Work Group
WRNMMC	Walter Reed National Military Medical Center
WSS	Wrong Site Surgeries

www.ingramcontent.com/pod-product-compliance
Lightning Source LLC
Chambersburg PA
CBHW081138180526
45170CB00006B/1846